Essentials of
NURSING
Research and Biostatistics

Essentials of
NURSING
Research and Biostatistics

As per the Revised INC Syllabus for BSc Nursing, 2021
(Also Covering the Old Syllabus)

Second Edition

Bijayalaskhmi Dash MSc (N)
Assistant Professor-cum-Principal in-charge
SCB Government College of Nursing
SCB Medical College Campus
Cuttack, Odisha, India

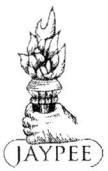

JAYPEE BROTHERS MEDICAL PUBLISHERS
The Health Sciences Publisher
New Delhi | London

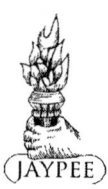
Jaypee Brothers Medical Publishers (P) Ltd

Headquarters

Jaypee Brothers Medical Publishers (P) Ltd
EMCA House, 23/23-B
Ansari Road, Daryaganj
New Delhi 110 002, India
Landline: +91-11-23272143, +91-11-23272703
+91-11-23282021, +91-11-23245672
Email: jaypee@jaypeebrothers.com

Corporate Office

Jaypee Brothers Medical Publishers (P) Ltd
4838/24, Ansari Road, Daryaganj
New Delhi 110 002, India
Phone: +91-11-43574357
Fax: +91-11-43574314
Email: jaypee@jaypeebrothers.com

Overseas Office

J.P. Medical Ltd
83 Victoria Street, London
SW1H 0HW (UK)
Phone: +44 20 3170 8910
Fax: +44 (0)20 3008 6180
Email: info@jpmedpub.com

Website: www.jaypeebrothers.com
Website: www.jaypeedigital.com

© 2022, Jaypee Brothers Medical Publishers

The views and opinions expressed in this book are solely those of the original contributor(s)/author(s) and do not necessarily represent those of editor(s) of the book.

All rights reserved. No part of this publication may be reproduced, stored or transmitted in any form or by any means, electronic, mechanical, photocopying, recording or otherwise, without the prior permission in writing of the publishers.

All brand names and product names used in this book are trade names, service marks, trademarks or registered trademarks of their respective owners. The publisher is not associated with any product or vendor mentioned in this book.

Medical knowledge and practice change constantly. This book is designed to provide accurate, authoritative information about the subject matter in question. However, readers are advised to check the most current information available on procedures included and check information from the manufacturer of each product to be administered, to verify the recommended dose, formula, method and duration of administration, adverse effects and contraindications. It is the responsibility of the practitioner to take all appropriate safety precautions. Neither the publisher nor the author(s)/editor(s) assume any liability for any injury and/or damage to persons or property arising from or related to use of material in this book.

This book is sold on the understanding that the publisher is not engaged in providing professional medical services. If such advice or services are required, the services of a competent medical professional should be sought.

Every effort has been made where necessary to contact holders of copyright to obtain permission to reproduce copyright material. If any have been inadvertently overlooked, the publisher will be pleased to make the necessary arrangements at the first opportunity.

Inquiries for bulk sales may be solicited at: jaypee@jaypeebrothers.com

Essentials of Nursing Research and Biostatistics

First Edition   : 2017
Second Edition : **2022**
ISBN 978-93-90595-35-8

Printed at

Dedicated to

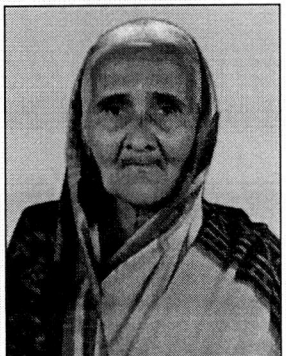

My mother-in-law Mrs Sakuntala Dash for her continuous support and encouragement

Preface to the Second Edition

It's said, **"There is only one thing that can replace a book, a new book".** With constantly changing environment, evolution of latest technology and accuracy in data, the research process and outcomes change continuously. The second edition of *Essentials of Nursing Research and Biostatistics* comes bearing all the necessary alterations and changes. Nursing research has tremendous influence on current and future professional nursing practice. It is also a vital component to healthcare field which helps in implementing new changes in the lifelong care of individuals. National Institute of Nursing Research (NINR) defines the aim of nursing research as the development of knowledge to build scientific foundation for clinical practice, prevent disease and disability, manage and eliminate symptoms caused by illness and enhance end-of-life and palliative care. Indian Nursing Council (INC) being a statutory body encourages nursing research and evidence-based practice in different set-up.

The second edition has been formulated with many modifications. Each and every chapter starts with learning objectives and ends with summary. Readers can also test their knowledge, by solving subjective and objective type questions, provided at the end of each chapter. It is way more comprehensive and includes a lot of diagrammatic representation of facts and is designed to provide in-depth coverage of all the aspects of nursing research, with suitable examples. Topics that are rarely dealt with in different nursing research books, like use of Microsoft Excel and **SPSS** (statistical package for social science) in data analysis, application of theories in nursing research, newer methods and tools for data collection and detail application of biostatistics in nursing research are also covered in this edition.

For nursing students, this textbook can form a basis of identifying research problem, planning and implementing a research plan, enabling the students to evaluate research studies and utilize research findings to improve quality of nursing practices. It is expected that the information provided in this textbook will be interesting and useful for the readers. They are more than welcome to give their valuable and constructive feedback.

Growth of nursing research is the key to the development of nursing profession. This textbook has been enhanced to reflect continuous improvements in the field of nursing research, and act as the primary source of information for nursing students.

Bijayalaskhmi Dash

Preface to the First Edition

Nursing research has tremendous influence on current and future professional nursing practice. It is also a vital component to the health care field which helps in implementing new changes in the lifelong care of individuals. Indian Nursing Council being a statutory body encourages nursing research and evidence-based practice in different set-up. Nursing students of different courses like GNM, BSc and MSc are expected to gain knowledge and skills in nursing research which may help them to input their knowledge in different settings. This book has been developed to supplement knowledge on research, make the students clear about research concepts and provide a solid understanding on research methodology. The first edition of this book includes all aspects of nursing research and has been written in simple language with suitable examples. This textbook is designed to provide in-depth coverage of all aspects of nursing research with avoidance of unnecessary vague thing which confuses the students. Several topics that rarely dealt with existing nursing research books like different types of qualitative researches, application of theories in nursing research, application of biostatistics in nursing research in detail and newer methods and tools for data collection are also covered in this book. This book has also a separate chapter on research critique which helps the researcher to evaluate quantitative and qualitative research studies.

For nursing students, this book can form a basis for identifying research problem, planning and implementing a research plan, enabling the students to evaluate research studies and utilize research findings to improve quality of nursing practice. It is expected that the information presented in this textbook will be interesting and useful for the readers. Readers are welcome to give valuable and constructive suggestions in the content which will help to enrich the future editions and will be appreciated.

The growth of nursing profession is possible by the growth of nursing research. This book has been evolved to reflect the continuous advancements in the field of nursing research, and to meet the growing information source required for nursing students.

Bijayalaskhmi Dash

Acknowledgments

This book *Essentials of Nursing Research and Biostatistics* is not only the result of my own wisdom and experience, but also a collective effort of so many around me. I have tried to made a considerable effort to make it authentic and quality possible but I owe a deep sense of gratitude to those who contributed for the successful completion of the endeavor.

First of all, I especially acknowledge the contributions of all the editors and scholars who have applied their editorial expertize with valuable comments which helped me to move forward.

I wish to express my deepest gratitude and sincere thanks to my teachers especially Dr Laxmi Rana, PhD (Nursing) for her support, encouragement and blessings which was an input to write this book.

I convey my sincere thanks to Jaypee Brothers Medical Publishers (P) Ltd, New Delhi, India for their efforts and suggestions, especially, Shri Jitendar P Vij (Group Chairman), Mr Ankit Vij (Managing Director), Mr MS Mani (Group President), Dr Madhu Choudhary (Publishing Head–Education), Ms Pooja Bhandari (Production Head), Ms Sunita Katla (Executive Assistant to Group Chairman and Publishing Manager), Mr Sabyasachi Hazra (Commissioning Editor, Kolkata branch), Ms Seema Dogra (Cover Visualizer), Mr Rajesh Sharma (Production Coordinator), Ms Anjali (Development Editor), Mr Kulwant Singh (Typesetter), Ms Geeta Rani (Proofreader), Mr Sanjeev (Graphic Designer) and the whole team members for helping me throughout the period. I also express my gratitude to them, for accepting my proposal and encouraging me to complete this book by providing me timely corrections.

Finally, I am thankful to all my family members, friends, and colleagues for their support and encouragement.

Contents

Chapter 1: Introduction to Nursing Research   1
- Methods of Acquiring Knowledge in Nursing   4
- Problem-solving   7
- Scientific Method/Research   9
- Nursing Research   14
- Nursing Research and Evidence-based Practice   27

Chapter 2: Research Process   39
- Major Phases in the Quantitative Research Process   39
- Qualitative Research Process Steps   49
- Terminology   53

Chapter 3: Research Problems, Objectives, Variables Hypothesis, Delimitation, and Assumptions   81
- Definitions of Research Problem   82
- Meaning of Research Problem   82
- Sources of Research Problems   82
- Research Problems to be Avoided   85
- Characteristics of a Good Research Problem   86
- Qualities of a Good Research Questions   89
- Steps in Developing a Research Problem   89
- Criteria for Developing Problem Statement   91
- Research Objectives   91
- Variables Concept   96
- Hypothesis Concept   100
- Delimitations   104
- Limitations   106
- Assumptions   107

Chapter 4: Review of Literature   112
- Meaning of Literature Review   113
- Definitions   113
- Purposes of Literature Review   114

- ❖ Importance of Literature Review *114*
- ❖ Sources of Literature Review *115*
- ❖ Steps Followed for Good Literature Review *118*
- ❖ Tips to Remember When Doing Literature Review *121*

Chapter 5: Theoretical and Conceptual Frameworks 124

- ❖ Some Common Terms *124*
- ❖ Concepts of Theories and Nursing Theories *125*
- ❖ Definitions *125*
- ❖ Purpose of a Theory *126*
- ❖ Characteristics of a Theory *126*
- ❖ Nursing Theory *126*
- ❖ Types of Theory *127*
- ❖ Characteristics of a Theory *131*
- ❖ Uses of Theories *131*
- ❖ Research Framework *132*

Chapter 6: Ethics in Research 146

- ❖ Definitions *146*
- ❖ Importance of Ethics in Nursing Research *147*
- ❖ Historical Background *147*
- ❖ Codes of Ethics in Nursing Research *147*
- ❖ Ethical Principles in Nursing Research *148*
- ❖ Inform Consent *152*
- ❖ Ethical Responsibilities of a Nurse Researcher *154*
- ❖ Dilemma in Nursing Research *155*
- ❖ Ethical Committee in Research *156*

Chapter 7: Concept of Research Design 161

- ❖ Definitions *161*
- ❖ Meaning of Research Design *162*
- ❖ Elements *162*
- ❖ Factors Affecting Selection of Research Design *162*
- ❖ Classification of Research Design *164*
- ❖ Experimental Research Design *168*
- ❖ Nonexperimental Research Design *178*
- ❖ Qualitative Research Design *184*

Chapter 8: Sampling and its Design 197

- ❖ Concept of Population *197*
- ❖ Definition of Population *198*
- ❖ Eligibility Criteria of Population During Selection *198*
- ❖ Process of Selection of Sample *199*
- ❖ Concept of Sample *200*
- ❖ Sampling *200*
- ❖ Sampling Process *204*
- ❖ Sampling Errors *206*

- Nonsampling Errors *207*
- Sampling Bias *207*
- Sampling Technique *207*

Chapter 9: Methods of Data Collection   221

- Data *221*
- Types of Research Data *222*
- Data Collection Plan *223*
- Dimensions of Data Collection Approaches *224*
- Developing Data Collection Plan *225*
- Steps of Developing Data Collection Plan *227*
- Methods and Tools of Data Collection *229*
- Interview *229*
- Questionnaire *238*
- Observation *245*
- Biophysiological Methods *252*
- Projective Techniques *254*
- Vignette Method *256*
- Visual Analogue Scale or Visual Analog Scale *257*
- Development of Tools *259*
- Construction of Schedules and Questionnaires *265*
- Ordinal Scale *267*
- Interval Scale *267*
- Ratio Scale *267*

Chapter 10: Analysis of Data and Application of Biostatistics in Nursing Research   279

- Definitions *280*
- Analysis of Quantitative Data *280*
- Application of Statistics *283*
- Descriptive Statistics *284*
- Inferential Statistics *331*
- Use of Computer in Quantitative Data Analysis *333*
- Probability *355*
- Analysis of Qualitative Data *364*

Chapter 11: Research Critique   376

- Introduction to the Concept of Research Critique *376*
- Definitions *377*
- Importance of Research Critique *377*
- Purposes of Critique *377*
- Principles of Research Critique *377*
- Four Key Aspects of Critique *378*
- Critique Skills *378*
- Critique Process for Quantitative Studies *380*
- Steps for Critiquing Quantitative Research Studies *380*
- Qualitative Research Critique *387*
- What to be Avoid During Critique? *392*

Chapter 12: Communication and Utilization of Research — 395

- Steps for Communicating the Research *396*
- Writing a Research Report *397*
- Types of Report *398*
- Guidelines for Writing Research Report *399*
- Steps in Writing Report *400*
- Format of a Thesis or Dissertation *401*
- Writing the References/Bibliography *405*
- Style of Writing Reference/Bibliography *406*
- Vancouver Referencing Style *409*
- Publication of Article in Journal *411*
- Utilization of Research Findings *417*
- Development and Presenting a Research Proposal *422*
- Importance of a Proposal Before Conducting a Research *426*
- Format of Research Proposal *426*
- Sample of a Research Proposal *430*
- Computer in Nursing Research *435*

Index — *443*

Nursing Research and Biostatistics

(Revised INC BSc Nursing Syllabus, 2021)

PLACEMENT: VII SEMESTER

THEORY: 2 Credits (40 hours)

PRACTICUM: Lab/Skill Lab: 1 Credit (40 hours), Clinical Project: 40 hours

DESCRIPTION: The course is designed to enable students to develop an understanding of basic concepts of research, research process and statistics. It is further, structured to conduct/participate in need-based research studies in various settings and utilize the research findings to provide quality nursing care. The hours for practical will be utilized for conducting individual/group research project.

COMPETENCIES: On completion of the course, students will be competent to:
- Identify research priority areas
- Formulate research questions/problem statement/hypotheses
- Review related literature on selected research problem and prepare annotated bibliography
- Prepare sample data collection tool
- Analyze and interpret the given data
- Practice computing, descriptive statistics and correlation
- Draw figures and types of graphs on given select data
- Develop a research proposal
- Plan and conduct a group/individual research project

COURSE OUTLINE

T – Theory, P – Practicum

Unit	Time (hours) T	Time (hours) P	Learning outcomes	Content	Teaching/ learning activities	Assessment methods
I	6		• Describe the concept of research, terms, need and areas of research in nursing • Explain the steps of research process • State the purposes and steps of evidence-based practice	**Research and research process** • Introduction and need for nursing research • Definition of research and nursing research • Steps of scientific method • Characteristics of good research • Steps of research process—overview • Evidence based practice: concept, meaning, purposes, steps of EBP process and barriers	• Lecture cum-discussion • Narrate steps of research process followed from examples of published studies • Identify research priorities on a given area/ specialty • List examples of evidence based practice	• Short answer • Objective type

Contd...

Contd...

Unit	Time (hours) T	Time (hours) P	Learning outcomes	Content	Teaching/ learning activities	Assessment methods
II	2	8	Identify and state the research problem and objectives	**Research problem/question** • Identification of problem area • Problem statement • Criteria of a good research problem • Writing objectives and hypotheses	• Lecture-cum-discussion • Exercise on writing statement of problem and objectives	• Short answer • Objective type • Formulation of research questions/ objectives/ hypothesis
III	2	6	Review the related literature	**Review of literature** • Location • Sources • On line search; CINHAL, COCHRANE etc. • Purposes • Method of review	• Lecture-cum-discussion • Exercise on reviewing one research report/ article for a selected research problem • Prepare annotated bibliography	• Short answer • Objective type • Assessment of review of literature on given topic presented
IV	4	1	Describe the research approaches and designs	**Research approaches and designs** • Historical, survey and experimental • Qualitative and quantitative designs	• Lecture-cum-discussion • Identify types of research approaches used from examples of published and unpublished research • Studies with rationale	• Short answer • Objective type
V	6	6	Explain the sampling process Describe the methods of data collection	**Sampling and data collection** • Definition of population, sample • Sampling criteria, factors influencing sampling process, types of sampling techniques • Data—why, what, from whom, when and where to collect • Data collection methods and instruments • Methods of data collection • Questioning, interviewing • Observations, record analysis and measurement • Types of instruments, validity & reliability of the instrument Research ethics Pilot study Data collection procedure	• Lecture-cum-discussion • Reading assignment on examples of data collection tools • Preparation of sample data collection tool • Conduct group research project	• Short answer • Objective type • Developing questionnaire/ interview schedule/ checklist
VI	4	6	Analyze, interpret and summarize the research data	**Analysis of data** Compilation, tabulation, classification, summarization, presentation, interpretation of data	Lecture-cum-discussion Preparation of sample tables	Short answer Objective type Analyze and interpret given data

Contd...

Contd...

Unit	Time (hours) T	Time (hours) P	Learning outcomes	Content	Teaching/ learning activities	Assessment methods
VII	12	8	Explain the use of statistics, scales of measurement and graphical presentation of data Describe the measures of central tendency and variability and methods of correlation	**Introduction to statistics** • Definition, use of statistics, scales of measurement • Frequency distribution and graphical presentation of data Mean, median, mode, standard deviation • Normal probability and tests of significance • Co-efficient of correlation • Statistical packages and its application	• Lecture-cum-discussion • Practice on Graphical presentations • Practice on computation of measures of central tendency, variability and correlation	Short answer Objective type Computation of descriptive statistics
VIII	4	5 40 Hrs (clinical project)	Communicate and utilize the research findings	**Communication and utilization of research** • Communication of research findings • Verbal report • Writing research report • Writing scientific article/paper • Critical review of published research including publication ethics • Utilization of research findings • Conducting group research project	• Lecture-cum-discussion • Read/ presentations of a sample published/ unpublished research report • Plan, conduct and write individual/group research project	• Short answer • Objective type • Oral presentation Development of research proposal • Assessment of research project

Nursing Research and Biostatistics

(As per INC BSc Nursing Syllabus)

Fourth Year
Internship

Time - Theory – 45 Hours
Practical - 45 Hours

COURSE DESCRIPTION: The course is designed to enable students to develop and understanding of basic concepts of research, research process and statistics. It is further, structured to conduct/participate in need based research studies in various settings and utilize the research findings to provide quality nursing care. The hours for Practical will be utilized for conducting Individual/group research project.

Unit	Time (hours)	Learning outcomes	Content	Teaching/ learning activities	Assessment methods
I	4	• Describe the concept of research, terms, need and areas of research in Nursing • Explain the steps of research process	**Research and research process** • Introduction and need for nursing research • Definition of research & nursing research • Steps of scientific method • Characteristics of good research • Steps of Research process- overview	• Lecture discussion • Narrate steps of research process followed from examples of published studies	• Short answer • Objective type
II	3	Identify and state the research problem and objectives	**Research problem/question** • Identification of problem area • Problem statement • Criteria of a good research problem • Writing objectives	• Lecture discussion • Exercise on writing statement of problem and objectives	• Short answer • Objective type
III	3	Review the related literature	**Review of literature** • Location • Sources • On line search; CINHAL, COCHRANE etc. • Purposes • Method of review	• Lecture discussion • Exercise on reviewing one research report/ article for a selected research problem • Prepare annotated bibliography	• Short answer • Objective type
IV	4	Describe the research approaches and designs	**Research approaches and designs** • Historical, survey and experimental • Qualitative and quantitative designs	• Lecture discussion • Explain types of research approaches used from examples of published and unpublished research studies with rationale	• Short answer • Objective type

Unit	Time (hours)	Learning outcomes	Content	Teaching/ learning activities	Assessment methods

V	8	Explain the sampling process
		
		Describe the methods of data collection
			Sampling and data collection
			• Definition of population, sampling criteria, factors influencing sampling process, types of sampling techniques
			• Data—why, what, from whom, when and where to collect
			• Data collection methods and instruments
			  ◊ Methods of data collection
			  ◊ Questioning, interviewing
			  ◊ Observations, record analysis and measurement
			  ◊ Types of instruments, validity & reliability of the instrument
			  ◊ Research ethics
			  ◊ Pilot study
			  ◊ Data collection procedure
				• Lecture discussion
				• Reading assignment on examples of data collection tools
				• Preparation of sample data collection tool
				• Conduct group research project
					• Short answer
					• Objective type

VI	4	Analyze, interpret and summarize the research data	**Analysis of data** Compilation, tabulation, classification, summarization, presentation, interpretation of data	• Lecture discussion • Preparation of sample tables	• Short answer • Objective type
VII	15	Explain the use of statistics, scales of measurement and graphical presentation of data Describe the measures of central tendency and variability and methods of correlation	**Introduction to statistics** • Definition, use of statistics, scales of measurement • Frequency distribution and graphical presentation of data • Mean, median, mode, standard deviation • Normal probability and tests of significance • Co-efficient of correlation • Statistical packages and its application	• Lecture discussion • Practice on graphical presentations • Practice on computation of measures of central tendency, variability and correlation	• Short answer • Objective type

VIII	4	Communicate and utilize the research findings	**Communication and utilization of research**
			• Communication of research findings
			  ◊ Verbal report
			  ◊ Writing research report
			  ◊ Writing scientific article/paper
			    » Critical review of published research
			    » Utilization of research findings
				• Lecture discussion
				• Read/presentations of a sample published/unpublished research report
				• Writing group research project
					• Short answer
					• Objective type

Chapter 1

Introduction to Nursing Research

Learning Objectives

After completion of this chapter, the students will be able to:
- Explain the concept of research and nursing research.
- Enumerate the aims of research and nursing research.
- Identify the characteristics of nursing research.
- Describe problem-solving process and scientific method.
- Explain about different types of research.
- Identify the methods of acquiring knowledge in nursing.
- Enumerate importance and scope of nursing research.
- Recall historical evaluation of nursing research.
- Explain the use of nursing research in various practice field.
- Recognize the problems in nursing and other field of sciences.
- Explain the concept of evidence-based practice in nursing.

INTRODUCTION TO RESEARCH

Meaning of Research

Research in common parlance refers to a search for knowledge. Once can also define research as a scientific and systematic search for pertinent information on a specific topic. Research is diligent, systematic inquiry or investigation to validate and refine existing knowledge and generate new knowledge with some specific goals. It is a systematic process which focused on uncovering new knowledge to help understand phenomena, answer questions, or address problems. The main goal of research is the gathering and interpreting of information to answer questions. Research is an academic activity and as such the term should be used in a technical sense. According to Clifford Woody, research comprises defining and redefining problems, formulating hypothesis or suggested solutions; collecting, organizing and evaluating data; making deductions and reaching conclusions; and at last carefully testing the conclusions to determine whether they fit the formulating hypothesis. D Slesinger and M Stephenson in the Encyclopaedia of Social Sciences define research as "the manipulation of things, concepts or symbols for the purpose of generalizing to extend, correct or verify knowledge, whether that knowledge aids in construction of theory or in the practice of an art". A number of different definitions for research exist however common to all of them is an agreement that research is systematic, disciplined and focused on gathering information to understand a phenomena, answer questions or solve research problems. The systematic nature of the research process means that research is undertaken in a methodological fashion using a rigorous approach to collect information (data) about a phenomena or research problem and to analyze and interpret that information in order to begin to answer questions or solve problems since research is directed at ultimately helping us to answer a question or address a problem. In general research means, the research process which deals with the ways and strategies used by researchers to understand the world around us. In the broadest sense of the word, the definition of research includes any gathering of data, information and facts for the advancement of knowledge.

The strict definition of scientific research is performing a methodical study in order to prove a hypothesis or answer a specific question. Finding a definitive answer is the central goal of any experimental process.

Definitions of Research

'A careful enquiry or examination in seeking facts or principles, a diligent investigation to ascertain something.'
—*Clifferd Woody*

'A honest, exhaustive, intelligent searching for facts and their meaning or implications with inference to a given problem. It is a process of arriving at dependable solutions and systematic collection and analysis and interpretation of data'.
—*PM Cook*

'Systematic search for answers to questions about facts and the relationship between and among the facts.'

- Research is a systematic attempt to provide answers to questions   —*Tuckman*, 1999.
- Research may be defined as the systematic and objective analysis and recording of controlled observations that may lead to the development of generalizations, principles, or theories, resulting in prediction and possible control of events   —*Best and Kahn*, 1998.
- Research is a systematic way of asking questions, a systematic method of inquiry
—*Drew, Hardman and Hart*, 1996.

Characteristics of Research

- Research must be systematic and follow a series of steps and a rigid standard protocol.
- The rules for research are broadly similar but may vary slightly between the different fields of science.
- Scientific research must be organized and undergo planning, including performing literature reviews of past research and evaluating what questions need to be answered.
- The scientific definition of research generally states that a variable must be manipulated, although case studies and purely observational science do not always comply with this norm.
- Research must be directed towards solution of problem.
- They requires clear articulation of a goal.
- Researches should be logical and systematic in nature.
- Should be relevant to what is required.
- Should be empirical and replicable in nature.
- Procedure should be reproducible in nature.
- Controlled movement of the research procedure.
- Often divides main problem into sub problems.
- Guided by specific problem, question, or hypothesis.
- Accepts certain critical assumptions.
- Requires collection and interpretation of data.
- Cyclical (helical) in nature.
- It is carried out to find out cause and effect relationship.
- Researches emphasizes on development of generalizations, principles of theories and help in predicting future occurrences.
- Applying all possible tests to validate the procedure and tries to eliminate bias.

- ❖ Should be carried out by based upon observable experiences or empirical evidences to establish knowledge and concepts through verifications.
- ❖ It demands accurate observation and description.
- ❖ Helps in answering various pertinent questions.
- ❖ Involves gathering information from primary or firsthand information sources using existing data for a new purpose.

General Aims of Research (Fig. 1.1)
Observe and Describe

This aim is especially applicable for descriptive research where the researcher observe and describe the gather information that illuminates relationships, patterns and links between variables. An example would be an investigation of the link between students' study skills and course drop-out rates.

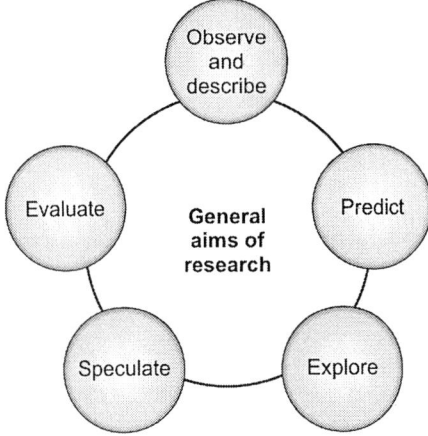

Fig. 1.1: General aims of research.

Predict

Prediction in research fulfils one of the basic desires of humanity, to discern the future and know what fate holds. Such foresight used to involve studying the stars or looking at the entrails of animals. To a certain extent, most scientists regularly use prediction in research as a fundamental of the scientific method, when they generate a hypothesis and predict what will happen. For example, some environments were unhealthier than others, especially in a hot climate where gangrene was a problem. The purpose of this type of research is to develop a model that predicts the likely course of events given particular intervening variables or circumstances.

Explore

The main aim of research is to explain the phenomena. Exploratory type of research investigates an area or issue on which little previous work has been carried out. In an organizational setting it may be used to discover whether or not a problem exists. Explanatory type of research also aims to show why relationships, patterns and links occur. For example, how could study skills support improve student retention? And does this depend on other factors, such as different types of support available. Like descriptive research, exploratory research begins with a phenomenon of interest; but rather than simply observing and describing it, exploratory research investigates the full nature of the phenomenon, the manner in which it is manifested, and the other factors to which it is related.

Speculate

Sometimes research is implemented strategically, where researchers take account of current situations and speculate as to their future implications. For example, the introduction of a specific government policy might raise implications for practitioners involved in its implementation. Research of this nature might speculate as to what these implications might be and develop a program of inquiry that can inform future responses to these issues.

Evaluate

Evaluation is also one of the general aim of research. Through evaluation we can evaluate the impact of something, e.g., a new policy, event, law, treatment regime or the introduction of a new system. The process of gathering information and analyzing to give feedback is called evaluation which is also done by research.

METHODS OF ACQUIRING KNOWLEDGE IN NURSING

A well-developed and reliable body of knowledge is a foundation for any profession. This most sought-after knowledge can be acquired from highly structured as well as loosely arranged processes or methods. Traditionally unstructured or loosely arrange structure method, such as trial and error, tradition, experience, authority and intuitions, are followed to gain knowledge. However with complexity of development the researcher developed more structured methods, such as logical reasoning, problem-solving and scientific methods to gain knowledge. Nursing knowledge is drawn from a multifaceted base and includes evidence that comes from science (research and evaluation), experience and personally derived understanding. Scientific knowledge is developed through enquiry and can use the research approaches. It is, however, not the only form of evidence used by nurses in their practice. Nurses also use experience gained from practice itself and their own personal learning. Problem-solving is a primitive way of gaining knowledge in comparison to scientific methods. The method of acquiring the nursing knowledge **(Fig. 1.2)** may be classified under two broad categories, i.e:
1. Unstructured methods of acquiring the knowledge
2. Structured methods of acquiring the knowledge

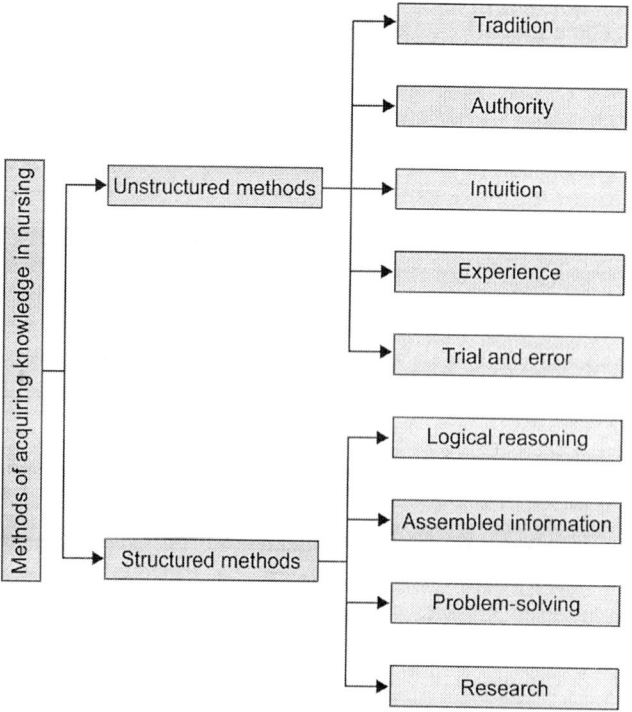

Fig. 1.2: Methods of acquiring knowledge in nursing.

Unstructured Methods

Tradition

Tradition means the transmission of customs or beliefs from generation to generation. Here the knowledge passed down through generations of nurses form the basis of traditional understanding. Traditional practices can be conveyed through observed practice, role modeling, written documents, books, journal articles, and often from 'experienced' practitioners. These practices can be imposed by our seniors and elders that "This is the way it should be done because this is the way it has always been done". Such an approach can lead to the development of a nursing culture that accepts practices as being right, without questioning their foundation and evidence base. Examples from current practice can include the daily washing or bathing of patients before mid-morning, recording observations of temperature, respirations, blood pressure and pulse on a regular basis. Some traditional practices can have a useful place in today's nursing. Team handovers serve a useful purpose in ensuring the transfer of patient and other ward-related information from the out-going to the in-coming nursing team. The practice can also facilitate learning for student nurses and new staff members and offers an opportunity for socialization of the team. But every time the science and technology was changing and it is not right to follow the traditional methods.

Authority

Perhaps one of the most common unstructured methods of acquiring knowledge is authority. This method involves accepting new ideas because some authority figure states that they are true. These authorities in nursing include our seniors, doctors, head nurses, etc. Sometime the expert persons in particular fields also show their authority. Nevertheless, much of the information we acquire is through authority because we do not have time to question and independently research every piece of knowledge we learn through authority. This is the unstructured method to gain knowledge.

Intuition

It is known as information obtained through sixth sense without conscious thinking but in this the rationalizing the information may not be obtained. When we use our intuition, we are relying on our guts, our emotions, and/or our instincts to guide us. Rather than examining facts or using rational thought, intuition involves believing what feels true. The problem with relying on intuition is that our intuitions can be wrong because they are driven by cognitive and motivational biases rather than logical reasoning or scientific evidence. It is suggested that a lack of objectivity and ability to identify a rationale behind decisions taken using intuitive and tacit knowledge prevents it being viewed as a phenomenon for scientific study and adversely affects its recognition and standing as a knowledge base for practice.

Experience

Experience is best unstructured source/method of gaining knowledge. What we as a nurses or midwives gain knowledge by our own experience by our practice, we never get such type of knowledge from others. Nursing is a practical subject which skill and expertise is essential. We will get a greater extent on the experience of our own rather than a lesser extent on the experience of others. Often experience is developed through observing role models in practice, and as such can be developed to include traditional and tacit knowledge.

Trial and Error

In this approach, alternatives are tried successively until a solution to a problem is found. In day-to-day life, everybody uses this techniques to solve much type of problem, including professional ones. There are probably examples of drawing on trial and error to develop personal knowledge that we can identify considered an aspect of practice.

Structured Methods

Logical Reasoning

Logical reasoning is one of the fundamental skills of effective thinking. Logical reasoning is mental processing to solve the problem, when we try to thinks what is the logic behind it means how it proved through logic. Using this method premises are stated and logical rules are followed to arrive at sound conclusions. There are two types of logical reasoning methods inductive reasoning and deductive reasoning.

1. **Inductive reasoning:** Induction is a form of logical reasoning in which a generalization is induced from a number of specific, observed instances. For example, when a nurse always observe that that always the children are getting stress when they entered into immunization room. So the nurses can predict that the children get stressed when they entered into immunization room.
2. **Deductive reasoning:** It is the process of developing specific prediction from general principles. Deduction is the form in which specific conclusions are inferred from more general premises or assertions. For example, if we assume that separation of children from the parents is stressful for all children then we can assume it for individual child.

Assembled Information

In making clinical decision healthcare professional also rely on various information that has been assembled for variety of purposes. Here reasoning proceeds from general assertions to specific conclusions. The information assembled from various sources, such as national, international and local data on different issues to solve the problems.

Problem-solving

Problem-solving is a method to obtain the solution of a problem by following a series of steps. Nurses use problem-solving process to solve a particular problem and find a particular intervention effective which may also be effective for similar other situations. Thus, problem-solving for one situation contributes to the nurse's knowledge for problem-solving in other similar situations.

Scientific Method/Research

It is the most structured way of gaining knowledge. Research conducted within a disciplined format is the most sophisticated method of acquiring knowledge. Findings from rigorous research investigations are considered to be at pinnacle of the evidence hierarchy for establishing evidence-based nursing (EBN) practices. Scientific knowledge is positioned at the highest levels the hierarchy of evidence and makes a significant contribution to the development and application of nursing practice. Scientific evidence also informs nursing education, policy and management.

PROBLEM-SOLVING

A human child has to meet and solve his problems. The problems which present themselves in his physical surroundings, his intellectual association and in his social contacts can grow in number and complexity as the child grows older an older. His success in life is in large measure determined by individual's capacity and competence to solve them. Problem exists for him at every step; his growth, development and living lie in their solution. In school, the child is to be trained in the art and craft of problem-solution.

The problem-solving method aims at presenting the knowledge to be learned in the form of a problem. It beings with a problematic solution and consists of continues, meaningful, well-integrated activity. The problems are set to the students in a natural way and it is ensure that the students are genuinely interested to solve them. Problem-solving approach is considered to be specific to a situation and individuals involved in a particular problem at a particular time. Decision-making and problem-solving processes are interdependent. There are also intangible its effect only can be felt. So, analytical and critical thinking and decision-making is a thinking process that requires skills in rational and logical thinking.

Definitions of Problem-solving Method

According to Yoakum and Simpson: 'A problem occurs in a situation in which a felt-difficulty to act is realized. It is a difficulty that is clearly present and recognized by the thinker. It may be purely mental difficulty or it may be physical and involve the manipulation of data. The distinguishing thinks about a problem however is that it impresses the individual who meets it as needing a solution. He recognizes it as a challenge.'

LA Averill has said, 'the only worthwhile life is a life which contains its problem; to live without any longings and ambitions is to live only half-way.'

Purposes of Problem-solving

- Train students in the act of reasoning
- Give practical knowledge
- Discover new knowledge
- Solve a puzzling problem
- Improve knowledge of the students
- Overcome inferences in the attainment of objective

Problem-solving Process

The problem-solving process consists of a series of steps that are followed depending on the type of problem to be solved. These are **(Fig. 1.3)**:
- Problem definition or identification of problem
- Problem analysis
- Generating possible solution
- Analyzing the solution
- Selecting the best solution
- Implementing the solution
- Evaluation and revision

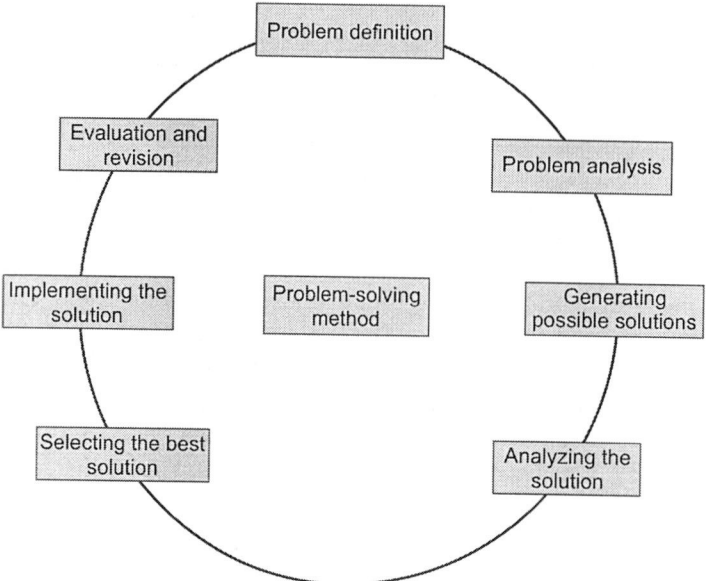

Fig, 1.3: Steps of problem-solving process.

Problem Definition

The normal process for solving a problem initiating involves defining the problem which is to be solved. In this first stage, there is a need to write down what exactly the problem entails, which helps to identify the real problem that is under study and needs an immediate solution. This is considered as the most essential steps of the problem-solving, because by defining the problem it helps in proper perceiving which helps in analyzing the problems. Without this next steps cannot be executed. Eminent author of the subject are of this opinion that a problem well-defined is half solved. Sufficient time should be spent on defining the problem as it is not always easy to define the problem and to see the fundamental thing that is causing difficulty and that needs correction. Right answer to the right question can be possible by having only clear definition.

Problem Analysis

After perceiving the problem the next step is to analyze how the problem affects the researcher and his or her current situation and the other people involved in this situation. In addition, the gravity of the problem and all the factors which are contributing to the problem are determined. Furthermore, the analysis helps in understanding the source of the problem and how it affects the current development and researcher's environment.

Generating Possible Solution

When the real problem is discovered, its contributing factors should be investigated. At this stage, focus must be on identifying and generating all possible solutions for a problem. Each potential idea for solution of a problem must be considered without discarding it through value judgment, however, each idea should be treated as a new idea in its own right and worthy of consideration.

Analysis the Solution

In this section of the problem-solving process, various factors about each of the potential solutions are investigated where in the entire positive and negative aspects of each solution against the problem are analyzed. The feasibility of each solution are also analyzed.

Selecting the Best Solution

At this stage, an attempt is made to compare the available solutions. The available solutions cannot only compared in terms solving the problem but also in terms of feasibility, resources needed and time taken. The eventually the best solution is selected based on careful judgment, which is supposed to solve the problem swiftly and smoothly. The alternatives also evaluated on three matters those are:
1. *Suitability:* Will it solve the problem partially, permanently or temporarily?
2. *Feasibility:* Will it work and how much will it cost/can we afford it?
3. *Acceptability:* It is acceptance to know involved and responsible.
    The decision maker should list benefits, cost and risks associated with each alternatives. Each alternative and improvement, its benefits any cost of action be weighed then the best solution should be chosen.

Implementing the Solution

Implementing the solution is the step of the problem-solving process which is putting plan into action. Here we practically solve the problem by implementing the selected solution.

Evaluation and Revision

This is the final stage of the problem-solving process where after implementation of the most potential solution and evaluation is made to judge the effectiveness of the solution in resolving the problem. This stage also helps to redefine the problem and revise the problem-solving process in case the initial solution fails to manage the problem effectively.

Advantages of Problem-solving

- Improves problem-solving abilities
- Student centered rather than teacher centered
- Collaboration among learners
- Constructivism of learners with guidance of teachers
- Allows for multiple intelligence
- Extended time frames
- Deeper understanding of knowledge
- Multidisciplinary

SCIENTIFIC METHOD/RESEARCH

The scientific method is a logical and rational order of steps by which scientists come to conclusions about the world around them. The scientific method helps to organize thoughts and procedures so that scientists can be confident in the answers they find. Scientists use observations, hypotheses, and deductions to make these conclusions, various possibilities using the scientific method is to eventually come to an answer to the original question.

The scientific method, as defined by various scientists and philosophers, has a fairly rigorous structure that should be followed.

Characteristics of Scientific Method

- *Empirical:* Science is based purely around observation and measurement, and the vast majority of research involves some type of practical experimentation.
- *The scientific method relies upon data:* The scientific method uses some type of measurement to analyze results, feeding these findings back into theories of what we know about the world. There are two major ways of obtaining data, through measurement and observation. These are generally referred to as quantitative and qualitative measurements.
- *The scientific method is intellectual and visionary:* Science requires vision, and the ability to observe the implications of results. Collecting data is part of the process, and it also needs to be analyzed and interpreted.
   However, the visionary part of science lies in relating the findings back into the real world. Even pure sciences, which are studied for their own sake rather than any practical application, are visionary and have wider goals.
- *Science uses experiments to test predictions:* This process of induction and generalization allows scientists to make predictions about how they think that something should behave, and design an experiment to test it.
   This experiment does not always mean setting up rows of test tubes in the laboratory or designing surveys. It can also mean taking measurements and observing the natural world.
- *Systematic and methodical:* Scientists are very conservative in how they approach results and they are naturally very sceptical. It takes more than one experiment to change the way that they think, however loud the headlines, and any results must be retested and repeated until a solid body of evidence is built up. This process ensures that researchers do not make mistakes or purposefully manipulate evidence. Scientific method always follows order and it is a systematic processes.
- *Scientists' attempt to control external factors that are not under direct investigation:* The scientist in the laboratory or in the field should control external factors influencing investigation. For example, when the scientist prepare some analgesic medicine and observe their effectiveness she has to control other pain relief method like avoidance of yoga.
- *Findings of scientific methods can be generalized:* The conclusion drawn from any scientific method can be generalized for general population which means that they can be used in situation other than the one under study. Theory can drawn from it. Sometimes based on the findings we can suggest recommendations what can be done further.
- *Scientific methods are based on assumptions or hypothesis:* Before starting any investigation the researcher adopt some assumption for his/her research which forms the basis for the research and devolve some hypothesis which indicate the tentative result for the study. The two things are very essential without which study cannot be started.

Table 1.1 shows difference between problem-solving and research.

Types of Research

Basic versus Applied

Research can be functionally divided into basic (or pure) research and applied research.
- **Basic or 'pure' research:** Basic or 'pure' research is also called as the fundamental or the theoretical research. It is basic and original. Here pursuit of knowledge or finding truth can

Table 1.1: Difference between problem-solving and research.

Sl. No.	Problem-solving	Research
1.	Individualized	Mass
2.	Overcoming felt difficulties	Based on principles and facts and theories
3.	Depends on individuals own experiences on problem	Depends on individuals own experiences on problem
4.	Traditional	Scientific
5.	Counselee consults counselor	Researcher consults experts
6.	Short time	Long waiting
7.	Economical	Costly
8.	Information gathering	Review of literature
9.	No theory	Theory/concept
10.	Solution suggested	Hypothesis
11.	Outcome considered	Methodology
12.	Solution chosen	Data collected and analyzed
13.	Solution implemented and evaluated	Findings interpreted and conclusions drawn

lead to the discovery of a new theory. Basic research is usually considered to involve a search for knowledge without a defined goal of utility or specific purpose. Fundamental research is mainly concerned with generalizations and with the formulation of a theory. "Gathering knowledge for growing knowledge's is termed 'pure' or 'basic' research." Basic or 'pure' research can result in the development or refinement of a theory that already exists research studies, concerning human behaviors carried on with a view to make germanizations about human behavior, are also examples of fundamental research. It can helps in getting knowledge without thinking formally of implementing it in practice based on the honesty, love and integrity of the researcher for discovering the truth. Often uses laboratory setting findings may not be directly useful in practice may be used later in development of treatment/drug/theory.

- **Applied research:** Applied or 'practical' research based on the concept of the pure research. Applied research is problem-oriented, and is directed towards the solution of an existing problem. It directed toward generating knowledge that can be used in the near future and often conducted to seek solutions to existing problems (Burns and Grove, 2005; Kerlinger, 1986; Polit and Beck, 2004) generally applied research is problem oriented. Applied research aims at finding a solution for an immediate problem facing a society, an industry or business or any organization which is conducted in actual practice conditions which helps in finding results or solutions for real life problems and make decisions, predict/control outcomes. It also provides evidence of usefulness to society, evaluate interventions helps in testing empirical content of a theory and helps in testing the validity of a theory but under some condition. Knowledge intended to directly influence clinical practice. The research findings contribute to some modifications of present practices, i.e., patient care, education, administration.

Qualitative versus Quantitative

- **Qualitative research:** Qualitative research concern with qualitative phenomenon which focus on the whole of the human experience and the meaning given by the individuals experiencing it. It gives a broader understanding and deeper insight into the complex human behavior qualitative research is local, concrete. Motivation Research', an important type of qualitative research which aims at discovering the underlying motives and desires, using in depth interviews for the purpose. The tools recommended for of such research are word association tests, sentence completion tests, story completion tests and similar other projective techniques. Attitude or opinion research, i.e., research designed to find out how people feel or what they think about a particular subject or institution is also qualitative research. Qualitative research is especially important in the behavioral sciences where the aim is to discover the underlying motives of human behavior. Observations and findings depend on understanding contexts and the meanings held by the people in those contexts and the meanings of the things in those contexts. Qualitative research generally possesses loosely structured research process analysis is thematic and research process is inductive.

- **Quantitative research:** Quantitative research is based the measurement of quantity. It is applicable to phenomena that can be expressed in terms of quantity. It is formal, objective, systematic process to describe, test the relationships and examine the cause-effect interaction among variables. It is applicable to phenomenon that can expressed in terms of quantity. Quantitative research generally possesses highly structured research process statistical analysis research process is deductive.

Experimental versus Nonexperimental

- **Experimental:** Experimental research design concerned with testing a hypothesis and finding the cause-effect relationship between variables in which the researcher makes changes by independent variables and studies its effect on dependent variables under controlled conditions. It may be conducted in laboratory setting or at actual field experiment. There are three criteria in experimental design which are:
  1. **Manipulation:** Researcher manipulates some of the subjects.
  2. **Control:** Researcher introduces one/more control over the experimental situation including the use of control group.
  3. **Randomization:** Researcher assigns subjects to a control/experimental group on a random basis.
- **Nonexperimental:** Researcher collects data and describes a phenomena as they exist without any intervention. It describes or looks at relationships(s) or correlation between variables. The three characteristics of experimental research, such as manipulation, randomization and control are absent here.

Descriptive versus Analytical

- **Descriptive research:** Descriptive research includes surveys and fact-finding inquiries of different kinds. The major purpose of descriptive research is description of the state of affairs as it exists at present. It is used to gain more information about characteristics with in a particular field of study. This research is a simplest form of research which helps in identifying various features of a problem. It is generally restricted to the problems that are describable and not arguable and the problems in which valid standards can be developed for standards. Existing theories can be easily put under test by empirical observations through this research and underlines factors that may lead to experimental research. It is not directed by hypothesis.

* **Analytical research:** Analytical research is a specific type of research that involves critical thinking skills and the evaluation of facts and information relating to the research being conducted. In analytical research researcher uses the facts, information already available. From analytical research, a person finds out critical details to add new ideas to the material being produced within analytical research articles, data and other important facts that pertain to a project is compiled, after the information is collected and evaluated, the sources are used to prove a hypothesis or support an idea. Analysis is made to study the relationship between disease and other condition with different variables.

Conceptual versus Empirical

* **Conceptual research:** Conceptual research is that related to some abstract idea(s) or theory. It is generally used by philosophers and thinkers to develop new concepts or to reinterpret existing ones. The qualitative studies are mainly based on abstracts and ideas. These are otherwise called as conceptual research.
* **Empirical research:** Empirical research relies on experience or observation alone, often without due regard for system and theory. It is data-based research, coming up with conclusions which are capable of being verified by observation or experiment. Empirical means practical which is to be proved. We can also call it as experimental type of research. In such a research, it is necessary to get at facts firsthand, at their source, and actively to go about doing certain things to stimulate the production of desired information. In such a research, the researcher must first provide himself with a working hypothesis or guess as to the probable results. He then works to get enough facts (data) to prove or disprove his hypothesis. He then sets up experimental designs which he thinks will manipulate the persons or the materials concerned so as to bring forth the desired information. Such research is thus characterized by the experimenter's control over the variables under study and his deliberate manipulation of one of them to study its effects. Empirical research is appropriate when proof is sought that certain variables affect other variables in some way.

Retrospective versus Prospective

* **Retrospective:** Retrospective means observe the past, retrospective studies examines the data already collected in the past. Here the outcomes have all occurred before the starting of the investigation. This type of study is known by a variety of names. Retrospective studies are generally more economical and produce results more quickly than prospective study. In these studies a phenomena existing in present is linked to the phenomena that occurred in past before the study was initiated. For example, review of medical records to assess the previous history of cholesterol levels in myocardial patients, in this type of study sometimes we move from effects which had already occurred to identify its cause. To identify predisposing factors of any diseases are the examples of retrospective studies.
* **Prospective:** The study starts with a presumed cause and then goes forward in time to the presumed effect. Independent variables is in present and its effect on dependent variables is studied in forward, i.e., in future to test the association. These studies are more costly than retrospective study but these studies are stronger than the other. For example, study describing social support and coping mechanisms of women with ovarian CA. Cohort studies are also the examples of prospective studies.

Empirical and Theoretical Research

The philosophical approach to research is basically of two types: empirical and theoretical. Health research mainly follows the empirical approach, i.e., it is based upon observation and experience more than upon theory and abstraction. Empirical and theoretical research complement each other in developing an understanding of the phenomena, in predicting future events, and in the prevention of events harmful to the general welfare of the population of interest.

- **Empirical research:** Empirical research relies on experience or observation alone, often without due regard for system and theory. It is data-based research, coming up with conclusions which are capable of being verified by observation or experiment. Empirical means practical which is to be proved. We can also call it as experimental type of research. In such a research, it is necessary to get at facts firsthand, at their source, and actively to go about doing certain things to stimulate the production of desired information. In such a research, the researcher must first provide himself with a working hypothesis or guess as to the probable results. He then works to get enough facts (data) to prove or disprove his hypothesis. He then sets up experimental designs which he thinks will manipulate the persons or the materials concerned so as to bring forth the desired information. Such research is thus characterized by the experimenter's control over the variables under study and his deliberate manipulation of one of them to study its effects. Empirical research is appropriate when proof is sought that certain variables affect other variables in some way.
- **Theoretical research:** It is related to some abstract idea(s) or theory. It is generally used by philosophers and thinkers to develop new concepts or to reinterpret existing ones. The qualitative studies are mainly based on abstracts and ideas. These are otherwise called as conceptual research.

NURSING RESEARCH

Research on nursing practice began slowly, but since 1950 has been accelerating rapidly. The ultimate purpose of nursing is to provide high quality patient care. Nursing research must address questions relevant to the profession of nursing. It grow the body of literature which means body of knowledge related to nursing profession. Clinical nursing practice without research is based on tradition without empirical evidences. Research is needed to evaluate the effectiveness of nursing treatment modalities, to determine the impact of nursing care on the health of the patients or to test theories.

Definitions of Nursing Research

According to International Council of Nurses (1986)—'Nursing research is a way to identify new knowledge, improve professional education and practices and use of resources effectively.'

According to ANA, 1981 'nursing research develops knowledge about health and promotion of health over the full life span, care of person with health problems and disabilities to respond effectively to actual or potential health problems.'

Polit and Beck (2004) have broadly defined nursing research as 'systematic inquiry designed to develop knowledge about issues of importance to the nursing profession, including nursing practice, education, administration, and informatics'.

Burns and Grove (2005) have more narrowly defined nursing research as 'a scientific process that validates and refines existing knowledge and generates new knowledge that directly and indirectly influences clinical nursing practice'.

Importance of Nursing Research

Nursing research has a tremendous influence on current and future professional nursing practice, thus rendering it an essential component of the educational process. Nurses need research because it helps them to be advance in their field, stay updated and offer better patient care. Information literacy skills can help nurses use information more effectively to develop their own conclusions. Research in nursing promotes lifelong professional development of the discipline of nursing and supports the fact that nursing is a professional discipline. Nursing research improves clinical expertise and personal knowledge, helps to implement changes to provide excellence in nursing practice, education and in administrative field.

- **To develop more evidence-based practice skill in nursing:** Evidence-based practice is integrating research findings into clinical decision-making. It is the conscientious use of current best evidence in making decisions about patient care. Development of evidence-based practice, among the nurses using the current, best research findings in their delivery of care is very much essential. It is a problem-solving approach to clinical practice that integrates, a systematic search for and critical appraisal of the most relevant evidence to answer a burning clinical question.
- **Improve the knowledge of nurses:** Use of research in nursing can helps the nurses in updating them with the new knowledge. A knowledge base is necessary for the recognition of nursing as a science by health professionals, consumers, and society. By conducting research nurses can acquire new knowledge to improve patient care. She will review different literatures and she will develop herself as a knowledge based for conducting research.
- **Improve decision-making:** The researches can helps the nurses to take proper decision because by using researches the nurse can come-out from their traditional system of nursing practices and move towards more evidence based practice. Research means evidence-based practice by which it improve accountability for care-related decisions and expands nursing practice. The nurse can take decision independently by using research.
- **Changes in the conceptualization of nursing and increase the values:** The science of nursing practice is one that is—soundly grounded in fundamental scientific concepts, theories and facts relevant to nursing. We have moved towards a more scientific definition of nursing practice, which is compatible with increased use of research findings by clinicians and practice research is now regarded as a fruitful source of practice theories. Nurse researchers are now feeling more of a responsibility to go beyond just reporting their findings. They are sharing the responsibility for transmitting their results into practice. By using research the meaning of nursing changed, they are not simply obeying doctor's order and following the principles of evidence-based practice. The value of nursing has been increased.
- **Reinforce identity of nursing as a profession:** Nursing research can helps the nurse to take decision independently. The nurse can modify her care and improving the professional standards by using research. Research can improve the professional identities of nurses. Professions are those occupations possessing a particular combination of characteristics generally considered to be the expertise, autonomy, commitment, and responsibility. Using of research in the field of nursing can fulfil all the criteria. It will helps in intellectual growth, improving the body of knowledge in nursing and makes the identity of nursing profession.

- ❖ **Advances in the preparation of nurses to use research:** The National League for Nursing (NLN) has endorsed the position that the preparation of nurses to conduct research generally belongs at doctoral level. However students in baccalaureate program should acquire an understanding of the research process and its contribution to nursing practice as well as the ability to evaluate research findings for applicability to nursing practice.
- ❖ **To change healthcare environment:** Research also helps nursing respond to changes in the healthcare environment. The nurses can able to make changes in care and cure process through research. Quality in care is determined by research only. Through the research the nurses are able to modify the traditional care system and can protect the clients from emerging potential complications. Overall through research the standards of practice will be change and also government regulations will be changed.
- ❖ **To deliver the highest possible quality care:** nurses are expected to deliver the highest possible quality of care in a compassionate manner, while also being mindful of costs. To accomplish these diverse (and sometimes conflicting) goals, nurses must access and evaluate extensive clinical information, and incorporate it into their clinical decision-making. In today's world, nurses must become lifelong learners, capable of reflecting on, evaluating, and modifying their clinical practice based on new knowledge. And, nurses are increasingly expected to become producers of new knowledge through nursing research.

Scope and Areas of Nursing Research (Fig. 1.4)

- ❖ The scope of nursing research is to strengthen the body of knowledge in clinical nursing practices, education, administration and health systems and outcomes research.
- ❖ Clinical research or practices, based on biological, behavioral, and others types of investigations, provides the scientific basis for the care of individuals across the life span and occurs in any setting where nursing care is provided.
- ❖ Health systems and outcomes research examines the availability, quality, and costs of health care services as well as ways to improve the effectiveness and appropriateness of clinical practice.
- ❖ The nursing administration research focuses on issues related to management of nursing personnel, recruitment, placement, retention, attrition, nurse patient ratio, nurse's satisfaction, etc.
- ❖ Finally, nursing education research focuses on how students learn the professional practice and discipline of nursing as well as how to improve educational strategies to prepare clinicians and scientists.
- ❖ Therefore, the areas or scope of nursing research may be classified in the following four broad categories:
  1. Research in clinical nursing practices
  2. Research in nursing education
  3. Research in nursing administration
  4. Research in health systems and outcomes of care

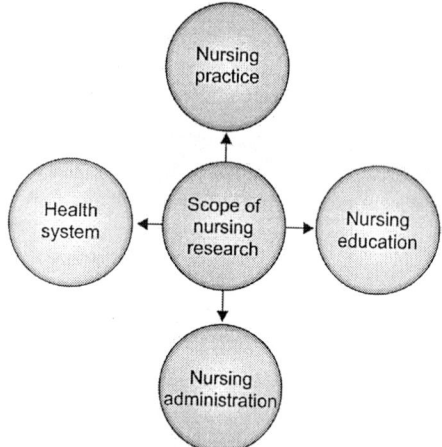

Fig. 1.4: Scope and areas of nursing research.

Research in Clinical Nursing Practice

The scope of nursing practice describes the 'who,' 'what,' 'where,' 'when,' 'why,' and 'how' of nursing practice. Each of these questions must be answered to provide a complete picture of the dynamic and complex practice of nursing and its evolving boundaries and membership. The profession of nursing has one scope of practice that encompasses the full range of nursing practice, pertinent to general and specialty practice. The depth and breadth in which individual registered nurses engage in the total scope of nursing practice is dependent on their education, experience, role, and the population served.

The scope of clinical nursing research may range from examining nursing interventions and experiences for health promotion, illness prevention, and care for individuals, families and communities in diverse setting. Nursing research is different from biomedical research because it focuses on examining and expanding the view of health, which emphasizes on health promotion, restoration and rehabilitation, as well as a commitment to caring and comfort. However, the focus of biomedical science on the discovery of diseases causation and cure is essential but not solely sufficient to improve health. Thus, it is better to obtain an expanded view of human health and illness with broader context of lifestyle, culture, and socioeconomic status. Complex problems in human health require interprofessional approaches. Nurses are uniquely qualified to lead and participate in interdisciplinary research teams because their education includes courses from all health related discipline (e.g., physiology, pharmacology, psychology, and sociology), and they focus on the integration of these disciplines in providing comprehensive care. Some of the common areas in clinical nursing practices are given below:

Evidence-based nursing care practices are in greater need to improve the quality of patient care. High quality and high cost-effective nursing care is only possible through research in this area of nursing profession. Nursing practices are the most researched field in nursing science, where nurse researcher regularly make modest attempts to generate or refine the nursing interventions for the following subareas:

- Health promotion, maintenance and disease prevention.
- Patient safety and quality of health care.
- Promotion and risk reduction interventions of health of vulnerable, minority groups and marginalized community.
- Patient-centered care coordination.
- Promotion of health and well being of older people.
- Palliative and end of life care.
- Development of evidence-based practices and translational research.
- Care implication of genetic testing and therapeutics.
- Nurses working environment.
- Home care and community health nursing care practices.
- Treatment compliance and adherence to treatment.
- Description of holistic nursing situations—social, cultural, religious, traditional and family practices, which have health implications and fall under the nursing care.

Tenets Characteristic of Nursing Practice
- **Nursing practice is individualized:** Nursing practice respects diversity and is individualized to meet the unique needs of the healthcare consumer or situation. Healthcare consumer is defined to be the patient, person, client, family, group, community, or population who is the focus of attention and to whom the registered nurse is providing services as sanctioned by the state regulatory bodies. The service to

be provided to the individual family and community will be valid by proving it through research. What type of service will be more effective for individual? and how the family is a one unit in providing care will be determined by research?

- ❖ **Nurses coordinate care by establishing partnerships:** The registered nurse establishes partnerships with persons, families, support systems, and other providers, utilizing in-person and electronic communications, to reach a shared goal of delivering health care. Health care is defined as the attempt 'to address the health needs of the patient and the public' (ANA, 2001, p. 10). Collaborative interprofessional team planning is based on recognition of each discipline's value and contributions, mutual trust, respect, open discussion, and shared decision-making. Previously there are no participation of family members in patient care which concept was now changed and research proved that the involvement of people in care of patient or in community can generate cost effective care and there will be a psychological satisfaction of patient and family members. This is only possible through by research.

- ❖ **Caring is central to the practice of the registered nurse:** Professional nursing promotes healing and health in a way that builds a relationship between nurse and patient (Watson, 1999, 2008). 'Caring is a conscious judgment that manifests itself in concrete acts, interpersonally, verbally, and nonverbally' (Gallagher-Lepak and Kubsch, 2009, p. 171). While caring for individuals, families, and populations is the key focus of nursing, the nurse additionally promotes self-care as well as care of the environment and society (Hagerty, Lynch-Sauer, Patusky and Bouwseman, 1993). Florence Nightingale through research proved that the proper use of fresh air, light, warmth, cleanliness, quiet, and the proper selection and administration of diet—all at the least expense of vital power to the patient.

- ❖ **Registered nurses use the nursing process to plan and provide individualized care to their healthcare consumers:** Nurses use theoretical and evidence-based knowledge of human experiences and responses to collaborate with healthcare consumers to assess, diagnose, identify outcomes, plan, implement, and evaluate care. Nursing interventions are intended to produce beneficial effects, contribute to quality outcomes, and above all, do no harm. Nurses evaluate the effectiveness of their care in relation to identified outcomes and use evidence-based practice to improve care (ANA, 2010). Critical thinking underlies each step of the nursing process, problem-solving, and decision-making. The nursing process is cyclical and dynamic; interpersonal and collaborative; and universally applicable which is validated through research.

- ❖ **A strong link exists between the professional work environment and the registered nurse's ability to provide quality health care and achieve optimal outcomes:** Professional nurses have an ethical obligation to maintain and improve healthcare practice environments conducive to the provision of quality health care (ANA, 2001). Extensive studies have demonstrated the relationship between effective nursing practice and the presence of a healthy work environment. Mounting evidence demonstrates that negative, demoralizing, and unsafe conditions in the workplace (unhealthy work environments) contribute to medical errors, ineffective delivery of care, and conflict and stress among health professionals which is also proved through research.

Research in Nursing Education

Nursing education is another important area of nursing research where nurse researchers try to generate or refine the knowledge, which is useful to improve the teaching learning methods and environment in nursing discipline. The main aim of nursing education is to continuously provide skilled nursing manpower to country, which is the need of hour for a country like India. There are several issues and subareas of nursing education on which nursing research may focus they are:

- Testing the effectively and efficiency of the old teaching methods or techniques, and generating newer effective teaching tools and techniques.
- Curriculum taught and learning experiences of nursing students at undergraduate and postgraduate level.
- Enhancing the psychometric domain of learning among nursing students in clinical practices.
- Extent of strict discipline required for the nursing students to improve their learning and education.
- Promoting clinical and classroom learning among nursing students.
- Refining and generating evaluation methods to judge the efficiency of the teaching-learning process.
- Identifying and managing problems of absenteeism and lack of motivation among nursing students.
- Resolving any issue or phenomenon related to the teaching-learning process of the nursing students.

Research in Nursing Administration

Administration is one of the most difficult disciplines to manage. Similarly, nursing administration also encounters several problems and issues that require solution and a solution may be obtained through research. Therefore, there are several main subareas of nursing administration which requires investigation such as:

- Assessing existing organizational structure, span of control, communication, staffing pattern, wages, benefits, performance evaluation practices, etc., and their effectiveness. In addition, developing new knowledge or refining the old knowledge regarding nursing administrative phenomena.
- Developing and testing different administrative model to enhance swift administration, employees, and customer satisfaction.
- Retention and effective use of nursing personnel in providing the quality of nursing care.
- Furthermore, research can be conducted on any phenomenon related to nursing administrative issues.

Research in Health Systems and Outcomes of Care

Research in health system and outcome of care is one of the important areas of nursing research, where nurse scholars may identify the success of presently existing healthcare delivery systems and models in country and to identify the ways and means to develop affordable quality of health care to individual, families and communities of the country.

Nursing research has a great impact on healthcare delivery and overall health system. It can help in modifying health environment. Florence Nightingale the first Nurse researcher who proved that good environment (lighting, ventilation, cleanliness, etc.) have a great influence on health and illness. Nursing research is not separated completely from biomedical research rather a part of it. A Nurse can be conduct on research on present healthcare delivery system for example, "A study to assess utilization of ASHA service on MCH care". Nursing research is integrated with health service research regarding issues organization and delivery of health service, it's utilization and effectiveness, etc. A study can be conducted on patient's satisfaction on the care provided at any setup which can be considered as an input to modify health system. Through research a nurse can make the evidence to change health policies for modification of health services. The healthcare delivery system is changing from time to time based on the research studies. First majority healthcare services are provided by doctors and nurses only but after that it was proved if we involve more para professional and semiprofessional health workers it will be more fruitful. So involvement of trained Dais, Anganwadi workers ASHA worker is essential to reduce infant mortality rate (IMR) and maternal mortality ratio (MMR) the government take initiative. Changes in healthcare delivery system is possible through only research nursing research is integrated with health services research regarding issues of organization, delivery, financing, quality, patient and provider behavior, informatics, effectiveness, cost, and outcomes.

Some of the common examples that require investigation in this area are as follows:
- Developing models of health care, which are affordable and accessible to people located in remote and hilly areas.
- Developing cost-effective model of healthcare for rural and deprived communities.
- Effective use of information and technology to provide health care services from tertiary care centres to the remote and outreach areas.
- Evaluate the effectiveness of existing policies and programmes for health care of people, such as NHRM, etc.

History of Nursing Research

If analyzed properly, historical knowledge can provide insight into the past, leading to resolution of present and future issues in nursing. The history of nursing comprises many changes and developments. The historical evolution of research in nursing can be traced back to Florence Nightingale, who made detailed records of observations about the effects of nursing actions. During 1970s and 1980s, numerous studies were conducted that focused on clinical practice.

Contribution of Florence Nightingale (1820–1910)

Florence Nightingale was one of the founder of professional nursing and is considered as the first nurse researcher. During the Crimean war, she kept a meticulous record and statistics of mortality rates among the sick and the wounded.

Nightingale initiated nursing research nearly 150 years ago. Her notes on nursing (1859) describe her initial research activities, which focused on the importance of healthy environment in promoting patient physical and mental well-being. She mostly carried out her data collection and statistical analysis during the Crimean war. She gathered data on soldier morbidity and mortality. Her research enabled her to instigate attitudinal, organizational, and social change.

Major Milestones of Nursing Research in Western Countries

- **1950:** There was an increase in federal funding for research in nursing. American Nurses foundation was devoted exclusively to the promotion of research in nursing.
- **1952:** For the first time, there was publication of nursing research.
- **1953:** The institute of Research and services in Nursing Education was lunched at Colombia University.
- **1954:** PhD program was introduced in nursing education.

- **1955:** American Nursing Association (ANA) established American Nurses Foundation as an independent organization for the purpose of development of nursing research by conducting and supporting research projects.
- **1957:** A department of nursing research was established at Walter Reed Army Institute.
- **1960:** The 1960s brought reordering of nursing research. The focus was to target practice oriented research to improve the quality of patient care.
- **1965:** The ANA took an official position in educational preparation of licensed nurses in which the need for research in nursing and for educating nurse researches was recognized.
- **1970:** A content analysis of articles published in nursing research from 1970 to 1978 shaved a shift from research in nursing being conducted by a large group of members of other disciplines, especially social sciences which served as the basis for much of what nurses do in practice today.
- **1976:** The ANA commission on nursing research published guidelines for the academic preparation of nurses in participation in research and its utilization.
- **1986:** National Centre for Nursing Research (NCNR) was established at National Institute of Health (NIH) under the Health Research Extension Act, 1985.
- **1990:** The 1990s brought the promise of reducing the gap between practice and research. The publication **healthy people 2000 in 1992** by the US Department of Health and Human services laid the national health agenda for the future.
- **1993:** National Centre for Nursing Research was renamed National Institute for Nursing Research (NINR). The Cochrane collaboration was established. In addition **Journal of Nursing** measurements started being published.
- **1994:** The journal **Qualitative Research** started being published.
- **1995:** The Joanna Biggs Institute, an international EBP collaboration, was established in Australia.
- **1997:** Canadian Health Services Research foundation was established with federal funding.
- **1999:** US Agency for Health Care Policy and Research (AHCPR) was renamed as Agency for Health Care Research and Quality (AHCRQ).
- **2000:** NINR issued funding priorities for 2000–2004; annual funding exceeded US $100 million. The Canadian Institute of Health Research was launched. The journal Biological Research for Nursing started being published.
- **2004:** The journal world views on Evidence Based Nursing started being Published.
- **2005:** Sigma Theta Tau International issued a position paper on nursing research priorities that incorporated priorities from nursing.

Major Milestones of Nursing Research in India

Research related to nursing in India has its roots in the philosophy of Florence Nightingale which stated that the profession is committed to the task enlarging professional body of knowledge through systematic approach to solve problems in nursing.

The statistics on the unsanitary conditions in the Indian army prepared by Florence Nightingale may be starting point of nursing research in India.

Some of the main historical milestones that influenced the development of nursing research in India are as follows:
- **1946:** Bhore Committee (1943) submitted a report in which recommendations were made for the improvement of various aspects of nursing profession, nursing education, nursing research, working condition, nursing services in both hospital and community, sending nurses for higher education to abroad, etc.

- **1953:** MS Edith Buchanan, Vice-Principal Rajkumari Amrit Kaur (RAK), College of Nursing, New Delhi, was the first nurse from India who was sent to Columbia University to earn her Doctorate in Education (DEd) under a World Health Organization (WHO) fellowship programme.
- **1955:** MS Margaretta Craig, Principal, College of Nursing, New Delhi, attended International Council of Nurses (INC) meet in France to present a paper on the need for nursing research.
- **1960:** First two years master degree programme in nursing was started by RAK College of Nursing, New Delhi, which influenced nursing research as a full subject with a thesis work on nursing topics.
  - Nursing research commenced on an all-India basis along with a master's programme in nursing in an intensive manner, although nurse leaders had been already participating in research at various levels.
  - Clinical studies were even being carried out on short-term basis by the beginning level postgraduate nursing students.
- **1963:** A study of health services was carried out in connection with the revision of syllabus of General Nursing and Midwifery by the Indian Nursing Council in 1963. The study provided valuable insights into the trends in the health services and complication of nursing.
- **1964:** Dr Marie Ferguson, a public health nurse who joined RAK College of Nursing, New Delhi, was able to create greater appreciation and understanding and value of the research in nursing for nursing practices, administration and education. With senior nursing leaders of the country, she conducted a research study titled Activity Study to Define Nursing and Non-Nursing Functions of Nurses in selected health institutes of India.
- **1966:** Trained Nurses Association of India (TNAI) established a research section under the guidance of chairman MS Anna Gupta, Principal, RAK College of Nursing, under supervision of Dr Sulochana Krishnan.
- **1971:** TNAI conducted a study on the socioeconomic status of nurses in India.
- **1976:** Dr Marie Farrell and Dr Aparna Bhaduri of RAK College of Nursing, New Delhi, conducted seminars on nursing research for educationists at Delhi, Mussoorie (Uttarakhand) and Yercaud (Tamil Nadu) to strengthen the nursing research in India.
- **1981:** Dr Farrell and Dr Bhaduri's book health research—a community based approach was published by the World Health Organization (WHO).
- **1982:** During October a national conference titled nursing research in India. Prospect and retrospect was organized, which was the first conference in India related to nursing research, and was held at College of Nursing, Bengaluru. Some of the recommendations of the participants of the conference were as follows:
  - Each college of nursing should have a research cell.
  - The faculty at nursing colleges should encourage students and provide them time for conducting research.
  - Colleges of nursing should foster research attitude among nursing students.
  - Central and state governments and private organizations should include nursing research in their budget.
  - Opportunities should be provided for faculty to visit foreign countries on short-term basis to learn about nursing research.
  - Efforts should be taken to establish collaborative activities in the area of research and scholastic interactions with the nursing colleges in the other countries.
- **1984:** A nursing research workshop was conducted titled **Teaching Nursing Research to Nursing College Teachers at Bangalore**, which was sponsored by the University Grants Commission. This workshop was open to all the teachers of all nursing colleges in India.

- A workshop was conducted on 'Nursing Process' by Dr Marie Farrell at Leelabai Thackersey College of Nursing, SNDT Women University, Mumbai, which was sponsored by the WHO.
- **1986:** The Nursing Research Society of India (NRSI) was established by Dr (Mrs) Inderjit Walia (President) and Mrs Uma Handa (Secretory) to promote research within and related to nursing.
    - For the first time, MPhil program in nursing started at RAK College of Nursing, University of Delhi, New Delhi.
    - All undergraduate and postgraduate nursing student taught the uniform nursing research course developed by INC.
    - PhD in Nursing started in College of Nursing, PGIMER, Punjab University, Chandigarh.
- **1998:** Nursing Research Interest Section was organized by Mr R Rajarathnan (senior Nursing Tutor–NIMHANS)
- **2002:** Revised syllabus of GNM and PBBSc by INC has included nursing research as a full subject.
- **2004:** Publication of Nightingale Nursing times was started by Jain and Co., Noida, Uttar Pradesh.
- **2005:** Publication of research based journal titled Nursing and Midwifery Research journal was started at PGIMER, Chandigarh.
- **2006:** National Consortium PhD Nursing has been constituted by INC under the ledership of Shri T Dileep Kumar (President) to promote research activities in various field of nursing.
- **2007:** Nursing Research Society of India has launched its official journal titled Journal of Nursing Research Society of India at College of Nursing, Bharati Vidyapeeth Deemed University, Pune.
- **2008:** Central institute of Nursing and Research (CIN) was brought in existence under control of Trained Nurses Association of India in New Delhi.
- **2009:** Indira Gandhi National Open University (IGNOU) started PhD in Nursing.
- **2010:** Faculty of nursing sciences started PhD in nursing.
- **2011:** Publication of several nursing scholarly journals started in India, such as Kerala Nursing Forum, Indian Journal of Nursing Studies, trends in Nursing Administration and Education, Indian Journal of Holistic Nursing, the nurse, etc. Thus increasing no, of nurses started publishing their research work in these journals, and these journals helped nurses to disseminate the research evidences generated by them.
- **2012:** Postgraduate and doctoral nurses use the database of thesis abstract for nursing research created by Nursing Research Society of India.
- **2013:** Ministry of Health and Family Welfare, Government of India constituted an expert Advisory Committee of Nursing Education and Research to work and provide recommendation on starting the Doctoral Nursing programs in addition to undergraduate and postgraduate nursing programs in new six AIIMS started by the Government of India at Bhopal, Bhubaneswar, Jodhpur, Patna, Raipur and Rishikesh.

Use of Nursing Research in Practice

The use of research in nursing practice is a topic of pressing concern to the profession. Some would argue that the development of practice relevant research and the use of research findings into delivery of health care is unimportant. The amount of current literature devoted to topics related to use of research, the strong endorsement of the professional organization and the nature of federally funded projects all attest that the use of research findings in practice is a significant professional objective.

Barriers of Using Nursing Research

Barriers to the use of research findings by practicing nurses can be organized into three categories:

Values and Qualification of Practicing Nurses

- Most nurses lack the preparation necessary to evaluate and implement research in their own environment. Although many baccalaureate programs now include some orientation to research, more course content is needed. Most practicing nurses have not had courses in nursing research and may not be qualified to understand, critically evaluate and implement research findings.
- Most nurses depends on few journals, i.e., AJN, for their continuing education.

Process of Implementing Research

The CURN (conduct and utilization of research in nursing) suggests that in order to incorporate research based knowledge into the delivery of patient care, nurses must be able to:
- Identify and synthesize results from many studies into a common research base
- Transform knowledge into clinical protocols
- Create specific nursing actions from the protocols
- Evaluate the innovation

Institutional Factors

- Organizational structures are also related to the use of research in nursing practices. Many staff nurses lack authority and control over their practices. They may feel powerless to effect changes in their clinical settings. In sufficient time and money can also prohibit involvement in nursing research.
- Institutional factor is a critical factor in the conduct and use of research and the nurse administrator is in a particularly influential role.

Problems Faced by Nurse Researcher in Conducting Research

Lack of a Scientific Training in the Methodology of Research

The lack of a scientific training in the methodology of research is a great impediment for nurse researchers in our country. Generally when a nurse researcher wants to do a research she may not be know how to conduct it. If she had completed graduation or postgraduation in nursing she may had a little knowledge during study time which may erase from her mind. If in every tertiary level hospitals or medical college hospitals there should be provision of short duration intensive courses on research methodology and it's implication in nursing with free of cost for meeting the requirement of nurse researchers might be helpful.

Lack of Funding

Nowadays nurses are interested in conducting research not only to modify care by themselves but also to change the protocol and policies of hospital but lack of funding plays a major barrier in conducting research. There are few funding agencies which can provide fund to conduct nursing research which is very difficult to avail by a nurse. With limit salary a nurse take a step back to conduct research from her own money even though she/he has interest in conducting research.

Lack of Study Subjects

For conducting a research outside of the laboratory at least 30 (large study) are needed. Thirty or more similar type of patient at same time is very difficult to get in a hospital. Even though the nurse started a study when the patient admitted in hospital in mean time the patient may be transferred or left the hospital due to any cause which may result lack of sample subjects to conduct a study. This is a major problem face by a nurse in conducting study.

Lack of Time

Contributing time for conducting research is a very difficult task for a nurse researcher. In a hospital among all healthcare providers nurses contributes maximum time to take care of patients. In emergency situations she contribute extra time to save life of the peoples even their duties over. Not only this during charge handover she use to contribute extra time with explained details about patients to her next colleague. So creating extra time for conducting research is very difficult for them. So many nurses unable to complete their studies due to time factor.

Lack of Administrative Support and Cooperation

Due to lack of administrative support & cooperation the nurses may left out from their own research studies. The nurse researcher may find it very difficult to conduct research independently. Research projects require administrative support for getting permission, ethical consideration, funding and overall in conducting research.

Lack of Standardized Tools

A standardized tool can help the researcher directly to conduct a research otherwise a researcher will prepare a tool by taking the guidance of a group of experts, check it's validity and reliability by applying a small sample subjects is very difficult task and time consuming procedure. So many times it is very difficult for a nurse researcher to search a group of experts to check the validity and reliability of the tools.

Lack off Accessibility to Books and Journals

Library management and functioning is not satisfactory even not available for nurses at many places and much of the time and energy of nurse researchers are spent in tracing out the books, journals, reports, etc., rather than in tracing out relevant material from them.

Difficulties to Control External Variables

In nursing and other social studies generally deals with the phenomenon related to human where ethically as well as practically it is impossible to conduct such studies in laboratories. Due to minimal possibility of laboratory research it is very difficult to control external variables which variables can change the study results. So the nurse researcher has to work hard to control such variables and sometimes it is impossible to do so.

Ethical Barriers

As nursing deals with human being safe guarding their right also big issues. The ethical constraint is more when conducting experimental studies. So many research problems are not consider for conducting research studies due to ethical issues.

Strategies for Increasing use of Research in Practice

Nursing profession is acutely aware of the problems discussed above and a number of ways to facilitate the translation of nursing research into practice have been advanced.

1. Planned Changes

Lewin's three phases of planned changes:

Unfreezing

It involves breaking down to old traditions and customs to make way for new alternatives. This might entail motivating nurses to abandon their usual approach to practice based on intuition and to substitute a desire to provide patient care based on tested theories and knowledge about human responses to health and illness.

Changing

It requires new patterns of behaviors acquired through the mechanism of identification and internalization.

Refreezing

It is the process by which the newly acquired behaviors become integrated into the nurse's personality and work role.

The CURN project which focused on transferring research based knowledge into protocols for nursing practices has identified seven specific steps in the research use process that must be incorporated into any planned change effort:
- Systematically identifying patient care problems.
- Identifying and assessing research based knowledge to solve identified patient care problems.
- Designing a nurse practice innovation to meet the needs of the clinical problems.
- Conducting clinical trials and evaluating the innovations.
- Deciding whether to adopt, alter or reject the innovation.
- Developing means to extend the new practice to other units.
- Developing mechanisms to maintain the innovation over time.

2. Conceptualization of Nursing Research and Nursing Science

Nature of Nursing Science

Nursing research focuses on the role of nursing care in the prevention of illness, care of sick and the promotion and restoration of health. Although it relies upon and utilizes the substantive scientific information and methodology provided by the other biological and behavioral sciences, it differs from those other scientific areas in that it focuses on their relevance to nursing rather than other aspects of health care. The product of research is knowledge or science (National Academy of Sciences, 1977).

Model for Conceptualization of Nursing Research and Nursing Sciences
- The model is designed to enhance nursing exploration, it incorporates parallel conceptualization of medical research and the practice research of other healthcare professionals.
- An important feature of the model is that it aids in the identification of two types of research, namely fundamental research and practice research and helps underscore the view that there are two categories of sciences: fundamental sciences and science of professional practice.

- ❖ One of the most crucial aspects of the model is its recognition that the broad structure of fundamental science is not specific nor is it limited to the use of any particular category of healthcare professional. It recognizes that the theories and facts produced by fundamental research constitute a vast communal pool, and that from this pool each health professional group may selectively draw professionally relevant facts and theories.

Fundamental Research and Science
- ❖ Traditionally 'basic research' has been understood as a way to establish fundamental theories, facts or statements of relationships among facts in some area of knowledge that are not intended for immediate use in some real life situations. The aim of basic research is to advance scientific knowledge and to facilitate further research in the area of knowledge.
- ❖ The term fundamental research includes both the traditional basic or non problem oriented research and the more problem oriented research, which only recently has been recognized to have fundamental qualities.
- ❖ Knowledge produced by fundamental research cannot be introduced into practice without translation into some sort of intervention.

Practice Research and the Science of Practice
- ❖ Nursing practice research requires relevant facts and theories from the communal pool of fundamental scientific knowledge, to bring these knowledge elements to bear upon a problem derived from professional practice.
- ❖ The science resulting from nursing practice research, which is soundly grounded in fundamental science concepts, theories and facts relevant to nursing, is defined as the science of nursing practice.
- ❖ The categories of research are:
  - Fundamental research (focus on fundamental process of biology and behavior)
  - Nursing practice research (focus on nursing process, nursing intervention)
  - Nursing profession research (focus on practitioner)
  - Delivery of nursing services research (focus on the provision of services)
  - Nursing education research (focus on the process of education)

NURSING RESEARCH AND EVIDENCE-BASED PRACTICE

The purpose of conducting research is to generate new knowledge or to validate existing knowledge based on a theory. Research studies involve systematic, scientific inquiry to answer specific research questions or test hypotheses using disciplined, rigorous methods. While research is about investigation, exploration, and discovery, it also requires an understanding of the philosophy of science. For research results to be considered reliable and valid, researchers must use the scientific method in orderly, sequential steps.

The process begins with burning (compelling) questions about a particular phenomenon, such as: What do we know about the phenomenon? What evidence has been developed and reported? What gaps exist in the knowledge base?

The first part of investigation involves a systematic, comprehensive review of the literature to answer those questions. Identified knowledge gaps typically provide the impetus for developing a specific research question (or questions), a hypothesis or hypotheses, or both. Next, a decision can be made on the underlying theory that will guide the study and aid selection of type of method to be used to explore the phenomenon.

The impact of evidence-based practice (EBP) has echoed across nursing practice, education, and science. The call for evidence-based quality improvement and health care transformation underscores the need for redesigning care that is effective, safe, and efficient. In line with multiple direction-setting recommendations from national experts, nurses have responded to launch initiatives that maximize the valuable contributions that nurses have made, can make, and will make, to fully deliver on the promise of EBP. Such initiatives include practice adoption; education and curricular realignment; model and theory development; scientific engagement in the new fields of research; and development of a national research network to study improvement.

Understanding EBP

Evidence-based practice (EBP) is a problem-solving approach to patient care that integrates the best evidence from well-designed studies with clinician's expertise, patient assessments, and patient's own preferences leads to better and safer care, better outcomes and lower health care costs. Unlike research, EBP is not about developing new knowledge or validating existing knowledge. It is about translating the evidence and applying it to clinical decision-making. The purpose of EBP is to use the best evidence available to make patient-care decisions. Most of the best evidence stems from research. But EBP goes beyond research use and includes clinical expertise as well as patient preferences and values. The use of EBP takes into consideration that sometimes the best evidence is that of opinion leaders and experts, even though no definitive knowledge from research results exists. Whereas research is about developing new knowledge, EBP involves innovation in terms of finding and translating the best evidence into clinical practice.

Concept of EBP and Research Utilization

Research utilization (RU) is the process of synthesizing, disseminating and using research generated knowledge to make an impact or change in the existing practice in society. The time lag between generating and using new knowledge by society has been a concern for many years. For example, the time lag between the discovery of citrus as a preventive measure for scurvy and its use on British ships was 264 years (Glaser, Abelson and Garrisons, 1983).

So to fill the gap between research theory and practice EBP was developed. The roots of EBP in nursing can be traced in Florence Nightingale's era of nursing practice. Her concept of promoting health, prevention of diseases and care of sick were central ideas for her system.

During past decade research utilization term was used only to implement the research study. But later on it was expanded and termed as 'evidence-based practice' in nursing. Evidence-based nursing practice means utilization or implementation of best research evidence in our clinical practice to provide quality care to individual or groups and needs delivery quality and cost-effective also.

Best research evidence is produced by the conduct and synthesis of numerous high-quality studies in a specific health care. In nursing the best research evidence is focused on health promotion, illness prevention, diagnosis and management of acute and chronic illness (American Nurses Association, 2004).

Evidence-based practice (EBP) has been emphasized in medicine for many years and is now is a measure focus of nursing. The goal of EBP is the implementation of high quality, cost-effective care to promote positive outcomes for patients, providers and healthcare agencies. So, EBP has a broader focus than that of high quality health care delivery.

Evidence-based care concerns the incorporation of evidence from research, clinical expertise, and patient preferences into decisions about the health care of individual patients. Most professionals seek to ensure that their care is effective, compassionate, and meets the needs of their patients. Therefore sound research evidence which tells us what does and does not work, and with whom and where it works best, is good news. Maximum use must be made of scientific and economic evidence, and the products of initiatives, such as the Cochrane Collaboration. However, nurses and consumers of health care clearly need other evidence, arising from questions which cannot be framed in scientific or economic terms. Nursing could spark some insightful debate concerning the nature and contribution of other types of knowledge, such as clinical intuition, which are so important to practitioner.

Meaning of EBP

- It is the conscientious, explicit and judicious use of theory derived research base information in making decision about care of delivery of individual or group of patients and in the consideration of individual needs and preferences. —*Ingersoll, 2000*
- It is the using of best available to guide clinical decision making. —*Benefield, 2002*
- It is the use of evidence to support decision-making in health care. —*Green Berg and Pyle, 2004*
- It is an integration of the best evidence available, nursing expertise and the values and preference of the individual, families and communities who are served. —*Sigma Theta Tau, 2005*
- It is an integration of the best research evidence with clinical expertise and patient value to facilitate clinical decision-making. —*Di Censo et al. 2005*
- Evidence-based nursing is an approach to health care practice that enables nurses to provide the highest quality care based on the best evidence available to meet the needs of their patients. —*Melnyk and Fineout-Overholt, 2005*
- The integration of the best research evidence with clinical expertise and patient values.

Steps in the EBP Process

The EBP process has seven critical steps (**Fig. 1.5**):
1. Cultivate a spirit of inquiry
2. Ask a burning clinical question
3. Collect the most relevant and best evidence
4. Critically appraise the evidence
5. Integrate evidence with clinical expertise, patient preferences, and values in making a practice decision or change
6. Evaluate the practice decision or change
7. Disseminate EBP results

Cultivate a Spirit of Inquiry

Cultivating a spirit of inquiry means that individually or collectively, nurses should always be cultivating a spirit of inquiry how to improve healthcare delivery. For this the nurse should develop her own attitude to learn new things or attitude to enquiry what are the lacunas. By this the nurse can get different issues and problems in healthcare delivery.

Ask a Burning Clinical Question

The burning clinical question commonly is triggered through either a problem focus or a knowledge focus. Problem-focused triggers may arise from identifying a clinical problem or

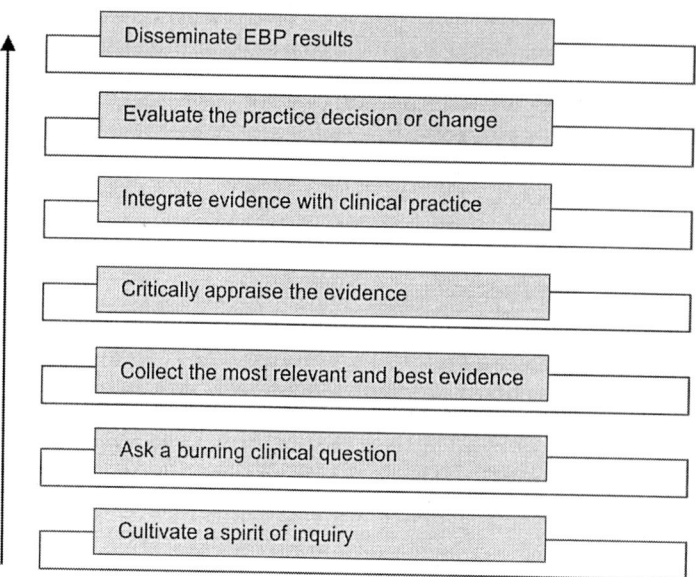

Fig. 1.5: Steps of evidence-based practice.

from such areas as risk management, finance, or quality improvement. Knowledge-focused triggers may come from new research results or other literature findings, new philosophies of care, or new regulations. Sometime during giving care the nurse can face different challenges which can act as a base to go to next step.

Hierarchy of Evidence

Regardless of the origin, the next step in the EBP process is to review and appraise the literature. Whereas a literature review for research involves identifying gaps in knowledge, a literature review in EBP is done to find the best current evidence. Here the nurse researcher has to collect the most relevant and best evidence. In searching for the best available evidence, nurses must understand that a hierarchy exists with regard to the level and strength of evidence. All of the various hierarchies of evidence are similar to some degree. The highest (strongest) level of evidence typically comes from a systematic review, a meta-analysis, or an established evidence-based clinical practice guideline based on a systematic review. Other levels of evidence come from randomized controlled trials (RCTs), other types of quantitative studies, qualitative studies, and expert opinion and analyses.

Critical Appraisal

Once the evidence is gathered, the researcher must critically appraise each study to ensure its credibility and clinical significance. Critical appraisal often is thought to be tedious and time-consuming. But it's crucial to determine not only what was done and how, but how well it was done. An easy method for conducting critical appraisal is to answer these three key questions:
- ❖ What were the results of the study? (In other words, what is the evidence?)
- ❖ How valid are the results? (Can they be trusted?)
- ❖ Will the results be helpful in caring for other patients? (Are they transferable?)

Final Steps of EBP

The final steps of the EBP process include integrating the evidence with one's clinical expertise, taking into account patient preferences, and evaluating the effectiveness of applying the evidence. Disseminating or reporting the results of EBP projects may help others learn about and apply the best evidence. Examples of potential EBP projects include implementing an evidence-based clinical practice guideline to reduce or prevent urinary tract infections (UTIs), evaluating an evidence-based intervention to improve wound healing, and applying an EBP to improve compliance with a specific treatment for a chronic disease.
- Evaluate the practice decision or change
- Disseminate EBP results

Melnyk and Fineout-Overhott (2011) suggest that EBP involve five critical steps.

Select a Clinical Research Problem or Question

The first step of EBP is to select a research question from clinical area. The selection of clinical research problem can be result following triggers:
- **Knowledge focused triggers:** These triggers come from advancement of knowledge of healthcare professionals though reading literature or attending professional conferences for, e.g., implementing of revised guidelines or standard to improve the healthcare practice.
- **Problem focused triggers:** These triggers are identified by the healthcare professionals in response to clinical problem, barriers or any other difficulties face in day-to-day life in clinical area.

The clinician should appropriately frame clinical research question by using following acronym called PICO. It stands for:

P = Who is patient population?
I = What is the potential intervention?
C = Is there a comparison of intervention and status?
O = What is the desired outcome?

For example, 'are self-management strategies more effective than medical care alone for improving health status, quality of life and occupational functioning among adult with coronary heart disease'?

Use of PICO approach:
P = Adult with coronary heart disease
I = Self-management strategies
C = Medical care
O = Health status, quality of life and occupational functioning

Search Relevant Literature Review

Once the clinical question selected, the researcher should explore the relevant literature review through clinical studies, expert opinions or existing EBP guidelines.

Critically Appraise the Evidences

- The available evidences should be evaluated for their strengthen and weakness.
- It should be focused for evaluation of their feasibility like in term of cost, duration, need of manpower and other sources, etc.

Implement the Best Evidence in Practice

- After critical appraisal of the evidence, the researchers should decide to implement the best available evidence in clinical setting.
- The final evidences must be extensively discussed among the users with risk-benefit ration of evidences.

Evaluate the Efficacy of the Evidence

Finally after the implementation of the useful findings for the clinical practice; the researcher must determine the expected change in practice and the benefits of the evidence used.

'A's of the Steps of EBP

- **Ask:** Formulate the question
- **Acquire:** Evidence search for answers
- **Appraise:** The evidence for quality and relevance
- **Apply:** The results
- **Assess:** The outcome

Strategy to Expand Research Use in Practice: Rogers' Theory of Diffusion of Innovation

Most people believe that a good idea generated through research will spread rapidly and the idea will quickly be used. But this is seldom true. During most of the 20th century research findings where seldom used by nurses to improve practice.

So to address this problem Rogers (1995) studies the processes for using research findings in society and developed a theory for communicating innovations or new ideas developed through research.

Roger's theory of diffusion of innovations includes a five stage process:

Knowledge Stage

This is the first stage of awareness of the existence of an innovation or a new ideas for use in practice. Knowledge of research finding can be obtained by formal communication through conference presentation, publications in clinical and research journal. Internet sites, news releases on television and in newspaper. In addition, informal communication within an agency from one nurse to another or among different health professionals can be effective in increasing awareness of research knowledge.

Persuasion Stage

In this stage, an individual or a group is motivated to adopt the innovation. Innovations with highly relative advantages and beneficial result will be easily and rapidly adopted. In this stage, the proposed change is best communicated in small group or one-to-one interaction.

Decision Stage

All this stage, the innovation is either adopted or rejected. Adoption involves full acceptance and implementation of the innovation or intervention in practice.

Implementation Stage

In this stage, the intervention is put to use by an individual, a clinic a hospital unit, many units or a group of hospitals. A detailed plan for implementation that addresses the risk and benefits of the intervention will facilitate change.

Confirmation Stage

During this stage nurses evaluate the effectiveness of the change in practice and decided to either continue or discontinue it. After using the new interventions one-two month onwards, data must be collected about the effectiveness if any advantages evaluated then the innovation can be adopted easily. If there is no benefit occurred then intervention may be discontinued.

An Example for Research-based Protocol for Decreasing Discomfort with Intramuscular Injection

- Wash hands, gather necessary equipment for the injection and put on gloves.
- Explain to the patient that you will position him/her to decrease the discomfort of the intramuscular (IM) injection based on research.
- Position the patient in the prone position or lying face down.
- Identify the ventrogluteal (VG) site.
- Have the patient turn his/her toes inward. This internal rotation of the femur causes relaxation of the gluteal muscle which decreases the discomfort from the injection.
- Give the injection and reposition the patient for comfort after the injection.
- Document how the injection was given and patient's response or perceived level of comfort.

Importance or Purpose of EBP

- It improve patient care.
- It increases confidence in decision-making.
- It improves nurses and other healthcare professional's job satisfaction and reduce employees turnover in an organization.
- EBP keeps practice current and relevant.
- It improves the consumers (patient and their family) satisfaction in healthcare services.
- Integration of EBP into nursing practice is essential for high quality patient care and most cost-efficient care.
- EBP eliminates unsound or excessively risky practice in favor of those that have better outcomes.

Iowa Model of Evidence-based Practice in Nursing

The Iowa model of evidence-based practice provides direction for the development of EBP in a clinical agency. This EBP model was initially developed by Titler and colleagues in 1994 and revise in 2001.

In a healthcare agency a clinical problem may arise by knowledge trigger or by problem base trigger.

If a trigger is considered an agency priority, then a group is formed to search for the best evidence to manage the clinical concern (Titler, 2001). Then the review of previous theory, scientific principles, expert opinion and case reports also review of literature are done to provide fairly strong evidence for use in practice. The strongest evidence is generated from meta-analysis of several controlled clinical trials.

Then this evidence would be pilot tested on a particular unit and then evaluated to determine the impact on patient care. If the outcomes are favorable from the pilot test, then the change would be made in practice and monitored over time to determine its impact on the agency environment, staff costs and the patient and family (Titler et al. 2001). If an agency strongly support the use of the Iowa model, implements patient care based on the best research evidence and monitors change in practice to ensure quality care, then the agency is promoting EBP.

An Example of the Iowa Model of Evidence-based Practice

- ❖ The steps of Iowa model were used as a guide for implementing a research-based protocol for saline flush irrigation of peripheral venous catheters rather than heparin flush in adult patient.
- ❖ Goode and colleagues (1991) conducted a meta-analysis 'to estimate the effects of heparin flush and saline flush solutions on maintain patency, preventing phlebitis and increasing duration of peripheral heparin locks (peripheral venous catheters)'.
- ❖ The meta-analysis was conducted on 17 high-quality studies having total sample 4,153 and the samples were included a variety of medical-surgical and critical care units (only adult patients).
- ❖ It was concluded, that saline is as effective as heparin in maintaining patency, preventing phlebitis and increasing duration in peripheral heparin locks of adult patients.
- ❖ Quality care can be enhanced by using saline as the flush solutions, thereby eliminating problems associated with anticoagulant effects and drug incompatibilities.
- ❖ Clinical relevance is evident that the use of saline to flush peripheral venous catheters promote quality outcomes for the patient (i.e., patent heparin lock, fewer problems with anticoagulant effects and fewer drug incompatibilities); the nurse (decreased time to flush the catheter); the agency (extensive cost saving and quality patient care).
- ❖ A decision at one level may lead to contact with another official who must approve the action.
- ❖ In addition, early savings could be attained. After that the change requires institutional approval and approval of nurses managing patients' peripheral venous catheters. So the change from heparin flush to saline flush will involve:
  - Physician's ordering saline for flushing
  - Pharmacy will have to package saline for use a flush
  - The nurses also need the support to sue the saline flush and communicate the other health personals.

Stetler Model of Evidence-based Practice

The Stetler model of research utilization helps practitioners assess how research findings and other relevant evidence can be applied in practice. This model examines how to use evidence to create formal change within organizations, as well how individual practitioners can use research on an informal basis as part of critical thinking and reflective practice. The model links research use, as a first step, with evidence-informed practice. The Stetler model provides a way to think about the relationship between research use and evidence-informed practice. These two concepts are not the same. Integrating both concepts enhances the overall application of research. The Stetler model first developed in 1976 and refined in 1994 and once again update in 2001.

This model consists of five phases:
1. Phase I: Preparation
2. Phase II: Validation
3. Phase III: Comparative evaluation/decision-making
4. Phase IV: Translation/application
5. Phase V: Evaluation

Phase I: Preparation—Purpose, Context and Sources of Research Evidence

This step include the identification of the purpose of consulting evidence (such as need to solve a problem and recognize the need to consider important contextual factors that could influence implementation). The researcher should note that the reasons for using evidence will also identify measurable outcomes.

Phase II: Validation—Credibility of Findings and Potential for/Detailed Qualifiers of Application

This step include critiquing and synthesizing of the evidence. When using the evidence the nurse has to assess each source of the evidence for its level of overall credibility, applicability and operational details, with the assumption that a methodologically weak study may still provide useful information in light of additional evidence and determine whether a given source has no credibility or fit and thus whether to accept or reject it for synthesis with other evidence and lastly summarize relevant details regarding each source in an 'applicable statement of findings' to look at the implications for practice.

Phase III: Comparative Evaluation/Decision-making—Synthesis and Recommendations per Criteria of Applicability

This step include:
- Logically organize and display the summarized findings from across all validated sources in terms of their similarities and differences.
- Determine whether it is desirable or feasible to apply these summarized findings in practice, based on applicability criteria, i.e., substantiating evidence, in terms of the overall strength of the accumulated findings. The criteria are fit to the targeted setting; current practice; and feasibility.
- Based on the comparative evaluation, the user makes one of four choices:
    1. Decide to use the research findings by putting knowledge into effect and moving forward in terms of the appropriate types of uses (instrumental, conceptual, symbolic).
    2. Consider use by gathering additional internal information before acting broadly on the evidence.
    3. Delay use since more research is required which you may decide to conduct based on local need (no further action is considered with the information available at this point).
    4. Reject or not use (no further consideration).

Phase IV: Translation/Application—Operational Definition of Use/Actions for Change

When the nurse is using evidence-based practice she should be, write generalizations that logically take research findings and form action terms:
- Identify type of research use.
- Identify level of use (individual, group, organization).
- Assess whether translation or use goes beyond actual findings/evidence.
- Consider the need for appropriate, reasoned variation in certain cases.
- Plan formal dissemination and change strategies and pilot project may be conducted.

Phase V: Evaluation

In this last stage of utilizing research evidence the nurse has to evaluate change strategies and pilot project.
- Clarify expected outcomes relative to purpose of seeking evidence and whether the evaluation is related to a direct use or consider use decision.
- Differentiate formal and informal evaluation of applying findings in practice.
- Consider cost-benefit of various evaluation efforts.
- Use research utilization as a process to enhance the credibility of evaluation data.

Barriers to EBP in Nursing

- Lack of knowledge regarding EBP strategies.
- Contradictory finding between research studies and literature create confusion among practitioners.
- Lack of belief that EBP will result in more positive outcomes than traditional care.
- Lack of time and resources to change the practice.
- Lack of support from professional colleagues and organizations.
- Overwhelming patient load.
- Peer pressure to continue with practices that are steeped in tradition.
- Lack of continuing education programs for nurses.
- Lack of initiatives among nursing leaders and mangers to create the environment of EBP.
- Physician's dominance in clinical practice, thus nurses are not given autonomy to implement newer evidences.
- Demands for certain types of treatment from patient side.
- Lack of motivation to do new things in nursing's.
- Fear of rejection or to change.

SUMMARY

- Research is diligent, systematic inquiry or investigation to **validate** and refine existing knowledge and generate new knowledge with some specific goals.
- Nursing research is systematic inquiry to develop knowledge about issues of importance to nurses.

- Nurses in various settings are adopting an evidence-based practice that incorporates research findings into their decisions and their interactions with clients.
- General aims of research are observe and describe, predict, explore.
- The problem-solving method aims at presenting the knowledge to be learned in the form of a problem. It beings with a problematic solution and consists of continues, meaningful, well integrated activity.
- The problem-solving process consists of a series of steps that are followed depending on the type of problem to be solved.
- The scientific method is a logical and rational order of steps by which scientists come to conclusions about the world around them. The scientific method is the research.
- Research can be classified based on their origin as Basic vs Applied, based on their approach & design Qualitative vs Quantitative, Experimental vs Nonexperimental, Based on the description it is classified as descriptive verses analytical, based on the time taken it is Retrospective vs Prospective and so on.
- According to ANA, 1981 'nursing research develops knowledge about health and promotion of health over the full life span, care of person with health problems and disabilities to respond effectively to actual or potential health problems'.
- Nursing research has a tremendous influence on current and future professional nursing practice, thus rendering it an essential component of the educational process.

QUESTIONS TO TEST YOUR KNOWLEDGE

Q1. What do you mean by problem solving? Write down it's purposes. Explain the problem solving process in detail. Write how it is differ from research. (15)

Q2. Enumerate the concept of research. Describe the characteristics and aims of research. (3 + 3 + 4)

Q3. Explain different types of research briefly. (10)

Q4. Write short notes on: (5 × 4)
   a. Importance of nursing research
   b. Tenets characteristic of nursing practice
   c. Scope of nursing research
   d. Problems faced by nurse researcher

Q5. State True or False (T/F) (1 × 5)
   a. A careful enquiry or examination in seeking facts or principles is termed as research.
   b. The study starts with a presumed cause and then goes forward in time to the presumed effect is termed as retrospective studies.
   c. Applied research pursuit of knowledge or finding truth can lead to the discovery of a new theory.
   d. The most objective mean of obtaining nursing knowledge is through scientific research.
   e. Inductive reasoning is the process of drawing specific conclusion from a set of premises.

> **Ans.** a. True   b. False   c. True   d. True   e. False

Q6. Multiple choice questions:
   I. _____ is a specific type of research that involves critical thinking skills and the evaluation of facts and information relative to the research being conducted.
   a. Descriptive research   b. Analytical research
   c. Pure research   d. Applied research

Essentials of Nursing Research and Biostatistics

II. Qualitative methods of research include:
   a. Ethnography
   b. Descriptive studies
   c. Focus groups
   d. Both a and c

III. Gaining knowledge through problem solving method is an example of:
   a. Unstructured methods of acquiring the knowledge
   b. Structured methods of acquiring the knowledge
   c. Trial and error method
   d. Logical reasoning method

IV. Information acquired through experience is:
   a. Logical
   b. Empirical
   c. Scientific
   d. Facts

V. A researcher investigates the effect of frequency of position change on healing of decubitus ulcers. The study would be described as:
   a. Applied research
   b. Basic research
   c. Descriptive research
   d. Phenomenological research

VI. Development of theory is based on which of the following types of research:
   a. Applied research
   b. Basic research
   c. Descriptive research
   d. Phenomenological research

VII. Which of the following is not the purpose of problem solving?
   a. Give practical knowledge
   b. Discover new knowledge
   c. Solve a puzzling problem
   d. Solve the problems of mass people

VIII. Which of the following is not the purpose of evidence based practice?
   a. To provide high quality care
   b. To obtain more research funds
   c. To eliminate un-sound practice.
   d. To modify nursing curriculum

IX. A reasoning process that proceeds from the general to the specific is_____.
   a. Empirical generalization
   b. Empirical reasoning
   c. Inductive reasoning
   d. Deductive reasoning

X. Which of the following is not a phase in Lewin's three phases of planned changes?
   a. Unfreezing
   b. Freezing
   c. Refreezing
   d. Changing

XI. Research is an organized and systematic enquiry defined by:
   a. Emory
   b. Marshall
   c. PV Young
   d. Kerlinger

XII. Gaining knowledge through problem solving method is an example of:
   a. Unstructured methods of acquiring the knowledge
   b. Structured methods of acquiring the knowledge
   c. Trial and error method
   d. Logical reasoning method

ANSWERS

I. b	II. d	III. b	IV. b	V. a
VI. b	VII. d	VIII. b	XI. d	X. b
XI. a	XII. b			

Chapter 2

Research Process

Learning Objectives

After completion of this chapter, the students will be able to:
- Describe major phases in the quantitative research process.
- Enumerate the different steps of each phase in quantitative research process.
- Explain the qualitative research process steps.
- Define common research terms.

INTRODUCTION

Scientific research involves a systematic process that focuses on being objective and gathering a multitude of information for analysis so that the researcher can come to a conclusion. This process is used in all research and evaluation projects, regardless of the research method (scientific method of inquiry, evaluation research, or action research). The process focuses on testing hunches or ideas in a park and recreation setting through a systematic process. In this process, the study is documented in such a way that another individual can conduct the same study again. This is referred to as replicating the study. The research process is the step-by-step procedure of developing one's research—and research paper however, one can seldom progress in a step-by-step fashion as such and such activities overlap continuously rather than following a strictly prescribed sequence. At times, the first step determines the nature of the last step to be undertaken. If subsequent procedures have not been taken into account in the early stages, serious difficulties may arise which may even prevent the completion of the study. Any research done without documenting the study so that others can review the process and results is not an investigation using the scientific research process. The scientific research process is a multiple-step process where the steps are interlinked with the other steps in the process. If changes are made in one step of the process, the researcher must review all the other steps to ensure that the changes are reflected throughout the process. The research process involves identifying, locating, assessing, analyzing, and then developing and expressing researcher ideas. It must be remember that the various steps involved in a research process are not mutually exclusive; nor they are separate and distinct. They do not necessarily follow each other in any specific order and the researcher has to be constantly anticipating at each step in the research process the requirements of the subsequent steps. The following five phases outline a simple and effective strategy for conducting effective research especially for conducting quantitative research.

MAJOR PHASES IN THE QUANTITATIVE RESEARCH PROCESS (FIG. 2.1)

1. Conceptual phase
2. Phase of construction of research design

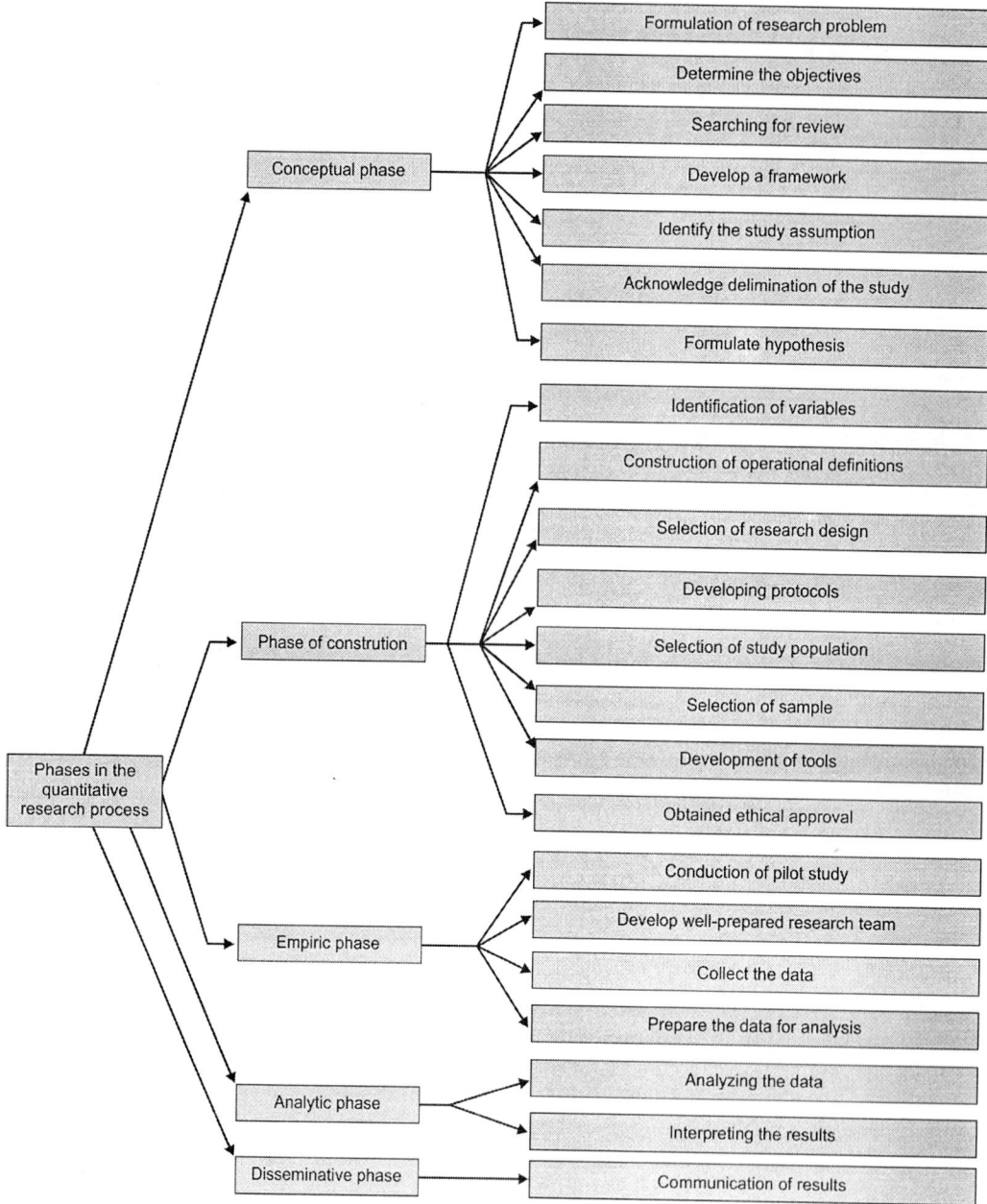

Fig. 2.1: Phases in the quantitative research process.

3. Empiric phase
4. Analytic phase
5. Disseminative phase

Phase of Conception

According Brink et al. (2006) this phase of research involves activities with a strong conceptual element. Conceptualization refers to the process of developing refining abstract ideas. During this phase, the researcher categorizes and labels his/her impressions. Thus, the activities include thinking, rethinking, theorizing, making decision, and reviewing ideas with colleagues, research partners or mentors/supervisors. The researcher also needs to draw on the skills and abilities of creativity, analysis and insight, as well as on the firm grounding of existing research on the topic of interest.

Phase of conception is the first phase of original research. In this phase created content and structure of the planned research. Creation of conception of new research project is structured process. It can be divided into seven steps as follows:

Formulation of Research Problem

In research the first step is the identification of research problems. Good research depends to a great degree on good question. In research process, the first and foremost step is selecting and properly defining a research problem. A researcher must find the problem and formulate it when he/she is interested to make a research study and a research problem is one which requires a researcher to find out the best solution for the given problem. A research problem, in general refer to some difficulty which a researcher experience in the contest of either a theoretical or practical situation and wants to obtained a solution for the same. The problem section justifies the need for the researcher. In quantitative research the researchers usually proceed from the selection of a broad problem area to the development of specific questions that are necessary to empirical inquiry. The initial justification of the research is generally only the beginning in the developing and understanding of the research problem. All research activities should be couched within 'further understanding the problem or problems'. Without this concept, research programs run the high risk of failure from investing in solutions searching for problems, or allocating resources to problems. There are two types of research problems, viz., those which relate to states of nature and those which relate to relationships between variables. At the very outset the researcher must single out the problem he wants to study, i.e., he must decide the general area of interest or aspect of a subject-matter that he would like to inquire into. There are so many sources to get a research problem they are curiosity, new personal experience, development of technology, research reports, gaps in the literature, theoretical and practical experiences. During selection of problems the researcher should be conscious regarding feasibility of research problems. The overdone and controversial problems should be avoided. The best way of selecting the research problem is to discuss it with one's own colleagues or with those having expertise in the research. In an academic institution the researcher can seek the help from a guide who is usually an experienced man and has several research problems in mind. First the researcher puts forth the problem in general terms and then narrow it down and phrase the problem in operational terms.

Determine the Objectives of the Study

The problem statements formulated based on the objectives of the study. Once problem statement formulated the objectives of the study must be stated with the problem statements and it should be stated very clearly. The objective is what products are expected from the research. The ability to define products that will resolve the problems are attainable, can be implemented and has a major impact on the likelihood of success. Research objectives are clear concise declarative statement expressed in the present tense and measure through statistical method which is the specific accomplishment of the researcher that hopes to achieve by conducting

the study. The objectives include obtaining answer to research questions or testing research hypothesis. The objectives are generally classify into two types:
1. **General objectives** are corresponding to the function of researcher/learner after completion of study. That means according to the problem how achievement was gain by researcher.
2. **Specific objectives** are arrived by breaking down the professional activities which together indicate the nature of these functions and corresponding from precise professional task whose result are observable and measurable against given criteria.

Searching and Review the Literature Relating to the Research Problem

Though literature review started before selecting a problem statement in some cases but after selecting problem statement it is compulsory to undergone a literature review to identify the strength and weakness of problem statements. A literature review surveys books, scholarly articles, and any other sources relevant to a particular issue, area of research, or theory, and by so doing, provides a description, summary, and critical evaluation of these works in relation to the research problem being investigated. Conducting a literature review will help researcher to see if his/her topic has already been researched, help him to see how to revise his/her research idea, and show methodological techniques and problems specific to the research problem that will help in designing a study. Most importantly, after conducting a thorough literature review, specific research questions and hypotheses will become clearer to the researcher. Literature reviews are designed to provide an overview of sources explored while researching a particular topic and to demonstrate to the readers how the research fits within a larger field of study. A literature review may consist of simply a summary of key sources, but it usually has an organizational pattern and combines both summary and synthesis, often within specific conceptual categories. A summary is a recap of the important information of the source, but a synthesis is a reorganization, or a reshuffling, of that information in a way that informs how researcher is planning to investigate a research problem. The analytical features of a literature review might:

* Give a new interpretation of old material or combine new with old interpretations.
* Trace the intellectual progression of the field, including major debates.
* Depending on the situation, evaluate the sources and advise the reader on the most pertinent or relevant research.
* Usually in the conclusion of a literature review, identify where gaps exist in how a problem has been researched to date.

Develop a Theoretical or Conceptual Framework

A theory is a systematic, abstract explanation of some aspect of reality. In a theory, concepts are knitted together into a coherent system to describe or explain some aspect of the world. At the start of any research study, it is important to consider relevant theory underpinning the knowledge base of the phenomenon to be researched. In a quantitative study, it is essential for a researchers to start the study with the help of a theoretical framework, or conceptual model. By addressing simple questions, the researcher can begin to develop a loosely-structured theoretical framework or concept to guide them. The following questions have been adapted:

* What do I know about the phenomenon that I want to study?
* What types of knowledge are available to me (empirical, nonempirical, tacit, intuitive, moral or ethical)?
* What theory will best guide my research study?
* Is this theory proven through theory-linked research?
* What other theories are relevant to this practice?

Theoretical framework present a broad general of relationship of research study by based on an existing theory but conceptual framework can be developed by the researcher by following more than one theory. On the basis of theory, researchers make predictions about how phenomena will behave in the real world if the theory is true. In other words, researchers use deductive reasoning to develop from the general theory specific predictions that can be tested empirically. It is the researcher's own position on the problem and gives direction to the study. It may be an adaptation of a model used in a previous study, with modifications to suit the inquiry aside from showing the direction of the study. The researcher has to develop any type of framework for her study.

Identify the Study Assumption

An assumption is a realistic expectation which is something that we believe to be true. However, no adequate evidence exists to support this belief. In other words, an assumption is an act of faith which does not have empirical evidence to support. Assumption provide a basis to develop theories and research instrument and therefore, influence the development and implement of research process. Assumptions in research study are things that are somewhat out of your control, but if they disappear the study would become irrelevant. If a researcher is conducting a survey he/she need to assume that people will answer truthfully. In choosing a sample, a researcher need to assume that this sample is representative of the population. Assumption cannot be stated without justification. The researcher will justify that each assumption is 'probably' true, otherwise the study cannot progress. To assume, for example, that participants will answer honestly. The researcher can explain how anonymity and confidentiality will be preserved and that the participants are volunteers who may withdraw from the study at any time and with no ramifications. To assure the researcher that a research will be fruitful and enable the researcher to answer the research questions, a pilot study is often performed. Even though assumptions are the statements that are taken for granted or are considered true and not been scientifically tested but the principles those are accepted as being true based on logic or reasons. That's why during research the researcher has to identify assumptions intelligently.

Acknowledge the Limitation of the Study

The limitations of the study are those characteristics of design or methodology that impacted or influenced the interpretation of the findings from your research. They are the constraints on generalizability, applications to practice, and/or utility of findings that are the result of the ways in which you initially chose to design the study and/or the method used to establish internal and external validity. Limitations are restrictions of the study due to theoretical or methodological reasons which may decrease the credibility and generalizability of the research findings. Usually, there are two types of limitations in research studies which may reduce the credibility and generalizability of the research findings they are: theoretical limitations and methodological limitations.

- **Theoretical limitations:** They restrict the ability of research findings to generalizes due to the use of specific theoretical concepts in study, or limiting the study of variables through operational definitions.
- **Methodological limitations:** Methodological limitations usually result from some of the methodological factors, such as unrepresentative sample, weak design, single setting, limited control over extraneous variables, poor data collection procedure, ineffective use of statistical

analysis, etc. Therefore, researchers usually mention limitations of their study, so that the readers can have idea about the credibility and generalizability of the research finding.

Formulate Hypothesis

Hypothesis is proposition, condition or principle which is assumed, perhaps without belief, in order to draw its logical consequences and by this method to test its accord with facts which are known or may be determined (Webster's New International Dictionary of English). Hypotheses, in other words, are predictions of expected outcomes; they state the relationships researchers expect to find as a result of the study. A tentative statement about something, the validity of which is usually unknown hypothesis is proposition that is stated is a testable form and that predicts a particular relationship between two or more variable. In other words, if we think that a relationship exists, we first state it is hypothesis and then test hypothesis in the field. The research question identifies the concepts under investigation and asks how the concepts might be related; a hypothesis is the predicted answer. In research process it is a major step here we predict what we expect from a research problem and it is tested to prove whether true or false. Hypothesis should be very specific and limited to the piece of research in hand because it has to be tested. The role of the hypothesis is to guide the researcher by delimiting the area of research and to keep him on the right track. It sharpens his thinking and focuses attention on the more important facets of the problem.

There are different types of hypothesis:
- Null/alternative hypothesis
- Simple/complex
- Directional/nondirectional
- Casual/associative

Phase of Construction of Research Design

The aim of this phase of research is to prepare general plan of real research. This phase is composed of following parts:

Identification of Variables

Every research study has some variables which should be identified. A variable is defined as anything that has a quantity or quality that varies. In every research problem statements there are different types of variables like:
- Dependent variables (responses, outcome or criterion variables)
- Independent variables (explanatory or predictor variables)
- Extraneous and confounding variables
- Control variables
- Intervening variables

The researcher has to identify what the different variables are and how they are influencing the study. The researcher here identify the variables in his/her studies like dependent variables and independent variables which variable is be going to change by what, how he/she will be manipulate the dependent variables through independent variables, etc.

Construction of Operational Definitions

An operational definition is a result of the process of operationalization and is used to define something (e.g., a variable, term, or object) in terms of a process (or set of validation tests) needed to determine its existence, duration, and quantity. After development of problem statement, hypothesis, assumptions it is essential for the researcher to define different terms used in the study operationally means what is the meaning of different concepts/terms in present study which is differ from actual definitions. An operational definition in research is how we (the researcher) decide to measure the variables in study (variable is anything that can be measured). Operationalization also sets down exact definitions of each variable according to the study. Increasing the quality of the results, and improving the robustness of the design.

A study to assess the effectiveness of video-assisted teaching module (VATM) regarding prevention of malnutrition among under fives on knowledge of the mothers in a selected rural community. Here knowledge means we are understanding correct responses of mothers with under five children to the knowledge items listed in the interview schedule regarding prevention of malnutrition and mother means—a biological mother with one or more under five children and prevention refers to action taken to arrest the occurrence of nutritional deficiency disorders and early detection and treatment. These definitions are differ from the dictionary definitions, because it reflects actual situations and the definitions developed based on the actual situation.

Selection of Research Design

The research design is the overall plan for obtaining answers to the questions being studied and for handling some of the difficulties encountered during the research process. A research design is the framework or guide used for the planning, implementation, and analysis of a study and the arrangement of conditions for collection and analysis of data in a manner that aims to combine relevance to the research purpose with economy in procedure. It is the plan for answering the research question or hypothesis which is the end result of a series of decisions made by the researcher concerning how the study will be conducted. Different types of questions or hypotheses demand different types of research designs, so it is important to have a broad preparation and understanding of the different types of research designs available. Research purposes may be grouped into four categories, viz., (i) exploration, (ii) description, (iii) diagnosis, and (iv) experimentation. A flexible research design which provides opportunity for considering many different aspects of a problem is considered appropriate if the purpose of the research study is that of exploration. But when the purpose happens to be an accurate description of a situation or of an association between variables, the suitable design will be one that minimizes bias and maximizes the reliability of the data collected and analyzed. The design is also closely associated with the framework of the study and guides planning for the implementation decisions regarding what, where, when, how much, by what means concerning an inquiry or a research study constitute a research design. Logical and systematic plan, structure and strategy of investigation used to answer the research question and to control the variance. The function of a research design is to ensure that the evidence obtained enables us to answer the initial question as unambiguously as possible. There are a wide variety of research design from which the researcher can select for any research.

Developing Protocols

The research protocol forms an essential part of a research. A written protocol will help to formalize researcher's ideas and gain feedback from others through peer review. A well written protocol is also necessary for researcher's applications to funding bodies and ethics and research governance committees. The protocol can also act as a manual for members of the research team to ensure they adhere to the methods outlined, budget estimated and try to finish it within given time period. Protocol is the overall layout or written plan for the researches which contain detail steps of research process, starting from problem statements to tentative expectation of results. It also contain budget planning and the tentative time requirement to complete each task. The protocol contain all the steps of the research in its planning stage which prevent any deviation and helps in conducting smoothly. It is the essential step especially for experimental research. In experimental research, researchers actively intervene and create the independent variable, which means that people in the sample will be exposed to different treatments or conditions. Protocol will explain how the whole procedure of research will be conducted smoothly.

Selection of Study Population

Identifying the population helps the researcher to know what characteristics the study participants should possess, and clarify the group to whom study results can be generalized. Before selecting subjects, quantitative researchers need to know what characteristics participants should possess. Researchers and others using the findings also need to know to whom study results can be generalized. Thus, during the planning phase of quantitative studies, researchers must identify the population to be studied. A population is all the individuals or objects with common, defining characteristics. Detailed information regarding study subjects should be given. For example, the study population, including a rationale of why they were chosen where wills the research take place? The methods by which subjects will be identified and recruited and what inclusion and exclusion criteria will be used, etc.

Selection of Sample

Sample is the small collection of population which is actually observed and sampling is a process of selecting subjects who are representative of population events, behaviors or other elements with which to conduct study. The sample size should be justified by using sample size calculations technique to avoid sampling error. As the sample size is increasing the chance of error is going on decreasing. Two general approaches to sampling are used in social science research. With probability sampling, all elements, (e.g., persons, households) in the population have some opportunity of being included in the sample, and the mathematical probability that any one of them will be selected can be calculated. With nonprobability *sampling*, in contrast, population elements are selected on the basis of their availability (e.g., because they volunteered) or because of the researcher's personal judgment that they are representative. The consequence is that an unknown portion of the population is excluded (e.g., those who did not volunteer). One of the most common types of nonprobability sample is called a *convenience* sample—not because such samples are necessarily easy to recruit, but because the researcher uses whatever individuals are available rather than selecting from the entire population. Because some members of the population have no chance of being sampled, the extent to which a convenience sample—regardless of its size—actually represents the entire population cannot be known.

Development of Tools and Specifying Methods to Measure Variables

Before conducting the study the researcher has to develop and validate the tools that will be used to conduct the data and select the method of data collection will be followed. Quantitative researchers must develop or borrow tools to measure the research variables as accurately as possible. A variety of quantitative data collection approaches exist like interviews, observations, questionnaires and biophysiologic measurements. Similarly a variety of tool can be developed and used for collecting data, e.g., interview schedule, observation checklist, rating scales and questionnaires, etc. The task of measuring research variables and developing a data collection plan is a complex and challenging process.

Obtained Ethical Approval

Nursing research usually deals with the human being where implication of the ethics becomes very essential. Ethics ensure the fullest respect, dignity, privacy, disclose of information and fair treatment for the study subject and build the capability of subject to accept or reject participation in study. For ensuring that the study adheres to ethical principles each aspect of the study plan needs to be scrutinized to determine whether the rights of subjects have been adequately protected or not.

Empiric Phase

In this phase, the researcher implements all the plans that he/she made in first phase. In many studies empirical phase is the most time-consuming part of the investigation. The amount of time spent, however, varies from study to study. So, we can say that empiric phase is composed of all the activities related to gaining scientific results, to sort them, and to evaluate them.

Conduction of Pilot Study

Pilot study is the study carried out at the first step of the implementation phase of research, in order to explore and test the research elements. Pilot studies, although not an absolute requirement, are frequently worthwhile. A pilot study is a miniature version of the planned research, search to identify and correct problems, which could affect the research process. It is important that the phase of the pilot study should be carried out as carefully as the actual research. It is also important that the sample for the pilot study, be as representative of the entire research sample as possible, ideally the pilot sample should be selected at random from the research sample.

Develop Well-prepared Research Team

Conducting research is not so easy. For that a well-prepared research team should be kept ready. The researchers should be skilled in using research methods. The members who are going to assists researchers should be well trained. All the team members should be manually and mentally skilled and experienced.

Collect the Data

The collection of data is a critical step in providing the information needed to answer the research question. The actual collection of data in a quantitative study often proceeds according to a pre-established plan. Data can be collected in the form of words on a survey, with a questionnaire, through observations, or by a variety of methods available. In the obesity study, the programmers will be collecting data on the defined variables, such as weight, percentage of body fat, cholesterol levels. The researchers or well trained person can collect the data. The person who is going to collect data should know that what data should be collected, how to be collected when and where the data to be collected. There are a multitude of methods available to the nurse researcher who is going to collect data. The choice of method is determined by studying research questions, design of the study and the amount of knowledge available about the study. The method or methods of data collection will be selected in the planning phase.

Preparing the Data for Analysis

The researcher normally collects the data according to the pre-established plan, and collects actual information by using the instrument that has been developed and tested in the pilot study. First the researcher will check the control of data completeness and correctness before coding. Coding is the process of translating verbal data into numeric form (e.g., coding gender information as 'a' for females and 'b' for males). Another preliminary step involves transferring the data from written documents onto computer files for analysis. A statistician should be concerned at the early phase during development of the tools and also data coding and the data analysis phase.

Analytic Phase

Quantitative data subjected to analysis and interpretation, which occurs in the fourth major phase of a project. Analysis can help in testing hypothesis and drawing conclusion.

Analyzing the Data

To answer research questions and test hypotheses, researchers need to analyze their data in an orderly, coherent fashion. After coding the quantitative information is analyzed through statistical analyzes methods by the help of computer or scientific calculator. Now data analysis become easy by the help of the computer. Descriptive and inferential statistics can be applied in this step to analyze data in quantitative studies. The application of statistics include from simple procedure like calculation of central tendencies to complex and sophisticated procedure like calculation of ANOVA, MANCOVA, etc., by which the researcher can test the hypothesis. In this stage concerning of a statistician is very essential in order to be meaningful, the results obtained from data analysis require interpretation.

Interpreting the Results

In order to be meaningful, the results obtained from data analysis require interpretation. Interpretation reports to the researcher's act of drawing conclusions and making sense of the results. Interpretation is the process of making sense of study results and of examining their implications. Researchers attempt to explain the findings in light of prior evidence, theory, and their own clinical experience—and in light of the adequacy of the methods they used in the study and also make comparison with his/her analytical values with the value of other research studies and find out the cause of the difference. Interpretation also involves determining how the findings can best be used in clinical practice, or what further research is needed before utilization can be recommended.

Disseminative Phase

The job is not completed, however, until the researcher communicates the result of the study to others who may find it useful. Preparing a research report is also essential. A research report is a written or oral summary of a study. No research project is complete until the final report has been written. Even when a verbal presentation is planned, the research report should be written out in its entirety. So, dissemination means process when results of the research should be presented or published. Nurses have many opportunities to present their study results at research conferences and seminars. Nursing organizations, such as the American Nurses Association and Sigma Theta Tau sponsor research seminars. Many nursing schools and regional nursing associations sponsor research conferences. Some organizations make special provisions for presentations by students.

Potential participants are contacted through a call for abstracts, a request for a summary of a study that the researcher wishes to present at a conference. These requests are published in professional journals and distributed to educational institutions, healthcare agencies, and potential participants whose names have been obtained through the mailing lists of professional organizations. Notices of research conferences are generally distributed 6–12 months before the event. Each conference or seminar will provide special guidelines for presenters and deadlines for submission of abstracts. The required length of the abstract varies from 50 to 1,000 words, but many have a 200–300 word limit. Abstracts should contain the purpose, research question(s) or hypothesis(es), design, methodology, major findings, and conclusions. If the research is still in progress, the last two items are not required. Abstracts it is very important to know where is suitable to present your research results. A nurse researcher might begin by presenting study results to peers. She can write final research report from research project and submit for publication in the websites. Next, this researcher might attend a research conference at which study results are discussed in an oral presentation or in a poster session. As a next step, study results might be published in a journal article. If funding has been received for a research project, the researcher probably will be required to submit a written report of the study to the funding agency. Finally, many researchers are pursuing advanced degrees and will present their research results in the form of theses and dissertations.

Putting the Evidence into Practice

This the step which is not under control of the researcher. Ideally, the concluding step of a high-quality study is to plan for its use in practice settings. Although nurse researchers may not themselves be in a position to implement a plan for utilizing research findings, they can contribute to the process by developing recommendations regarding how the evidence could be incorporated into nursing practice, and encouraging others to implement it in practice, ensuring that adequate information has been provided for a meta-analysis, and by vigorously pursuing opportunities to disseminate the findings to practicing nursing.

QUALITATIVE RESEARCH PROCESS STEPS

In a world of methodological pluralism and mixed-methods, qualitative researchers can take a pathway of pragmatic curiosity by exploring their research interests and the possible design and methodology choices to create studies that not only allow them to pursue their investigative curiosities, but also result in coherent and effective systems of procedural choices. Qualitative research is a broad field of inquiry that uses unstructured data collection methods, such as observations, interviews, surveys and documents, to find themes and meanings to inform our understanding of the world. It tends to try to uncover the reasons for behaviors, attitudes and motivations, instead of just the details of what, where and when. Qualitative research can be done across many disciplines, such as social science, health care and business, and is a common feature of nearly every single workplace and educational environment. Though the qualitative research process planned less formally and does not have clearly defined boundaries still some researcher follow some steps to undergo the study that's are **(Fig. 2.2)**:

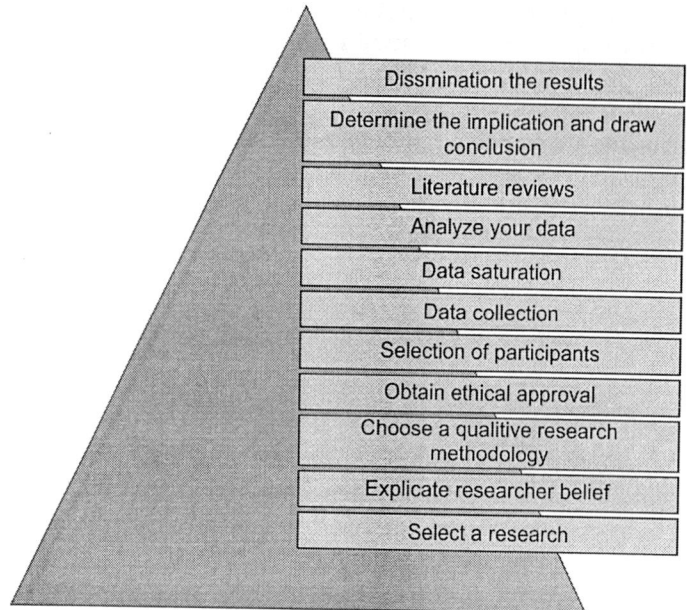

Fig. 2.2: Steps of quantitative research process.

Select a Research

To conduct qualitative research, it should explore reasons for why people do things or believe in something. What a researcher want to learn or understand and also helps to focus the study should be determined? For selecting good research a researcher can take the help of experts by acknowledging them his/her area of interest. First the researcher can select a broad area which will be making narrower later. During selection of research study researcher should explain why the topic is significant, relevant, and trust worthy. By doing so he/she begin to address the 'so what' question right away. During selection of research the researcher himself or herself may well known about among whom he want to study and from whose perspective do he want to learn about. What aspect, when would he focus on this phenomenon, where would he observe/interact this phenomenon why would he study this phenomenon (e.g., because he/she want to inform, perform, reform, transform, describe, interpret, explain, confirm, criticize, suggest, evaluate, or assess something)? and how will he generate data in order to study this phenomenon (e.g., administer a survey, conduct interviews, make observations, collect transcripts of online sessions, or gather student journals).

Explicate Researcher Belief

After selecting a research problem for qualitative study the researcher has to explicate researcher's own belief which may affect the study process. Bracketing is a method used in qualitative research to mitigate the potentially deleterious effects of preconceptions that may taint the research process. In the bracketing process, the researcher acknowledges his or her previous experience, attitude and beliefs, but tries to set them aside for the duration of the study to see the object of study anew. First, the author described his own experiences and thoughts related to virtual embodiment in order to set aside assumptions and beliefs of what virtual embodiment was about. As many authors have argued, it is something that cannot be fully achieved. Still, it proved to be useful to continuously reflect on how existing conceptual constructs tried to affect the analysis and descriptions of embodiment investigator keeps a diary of personal thoughts and feelings about the topic. Purpose is to make known to the researcher her/his beliefs about the topic so that the researcher may approach the topic honestly.

Choose a Qualitative Research Methodology

Here the researcher has to choose a qualitative research design. There are a number of accepted methodologies available. The researcher can choice any type of research based on his/her objectives. The different types of qualitative research studies are described as follows:

- **Action research:** Action research focuses on solving an immediate problem or working with others to problem solve and address particular issues.
- **Ethnography:** It is the study of human interaction and communities through direct participation and observation within the community you wish to study. Ethnographic research comes from the discipline of social and cultural anthropology but is now becoming more widely used.
- **Phenomenology:** It is the study of the subjective experiences of others. It researches the world through the eyes of another person by discovering how they interpret their experiences.
- **Grounded theory:** The purpose of grounded theory is to develop theory based on the data systematically collected and analyzed. It looks at specific information and derives theories and reasons for the phenomena.
- **Case study research:** This method of qualitative study is an in-depth study of a specific individual or phenomena in its existing context.

Obtain Ethical Approval

After selecting research study and research methodology in qualitative study the role of researcher is to obtain ethical approval of his/her research study. In qualitative studies the risk of exploitation may become especially acute because the psychological distance decline as the study progress. In ethical aspect of researches all researchers are responsible for ensuring that participants are:

- Well-informed about the purpose of the research they are being asked to participate.
- Understand the risks they may face as a result of being part of the research.
- Understand the benefits that might accrue to them as a result of participating.
- Feel free to make an independent decision without fear of negative consequences.
- The obligation to inform people that they are part of a research project is universal, no matter what is the methods of data collection.

Selection of Participants

Participant or informant refers to the individual among whom the study will be conducted. They are also called as subjects or respondents.

- They should be fulfils the study criteria.
- Must have 1st hand experience with research phenomenon.
- They want to help others understand their lives and the social contexts in which they live and create meaning. Participants must have first and experience with the research experience and be able to talk about it.
- Goal is not generalization of findings but rich descriptions of phenomenon by those who have experienced it qualitative research methods do not rely as heavily on large sample sizes as quantitative methods, but they can still yield important insights and findings.

Data Collection

After selecting participants the next step of qualitative research process is data collection. The researcher gets close enough to study subjects to observe (with/without participation) usually to understand whether people do what they say they do, and to access tacit knowledge of subjects. Interview the participants involves asking questions, listening to and recording answers from an individual or group on a structured, semistructured or unstructured format in an in-depth manner. Focus group focused (guided by a set of questions) and interactive. Discussion session with a group small enough for everyone to have chance to talk and large enough to provide diversity of opinions. Other methods rapid assessment procedure (RAP), free listing, pile sort, ranking, life history (biography). The form of data collection will depend on the research methodology. For example, case study research usually relies on interviews and documentary materials, whereas ethnography research requires considerable fieldwork.

Data Saturation

Theoretical saturation of data is a term in qualitative research, mostly used in the grounded theory approach. Theoretical saturation of data means that researchers reach a point in their analysis of data that sampling more data will not lead to more information related to their research questions. No additional data can be found to develop new properties of categories and the relationships between the categories are disentangled. Researchers see in their data similar instances over and over again and that make them empirically confident that their categories are saturated, the descriptions of these categories are thick and a theory can emerge. Researchers are allowed to stop sampling data and to round off their analysis.

Analyze Your Data

The analysis of qualitative research notes begins in the field, at the time of observation, interviewing, or both, as the researcher identifies problems and concepts that appear likely to help in understanding the situation. Simply reading the notes or transcripts is an important step in the analytic process. Researchers should make frequent notes in the margins to identify important statements and to propose ways of coding the data. Qualitative data analysis (QDA) is the range of processes and procedures whereby we move from the qualitative data that have been collected into some form of explanation, understanding or interpretation of the people and situations we are investigating. QDA is usually based on an interpretative philosophy. The idea is to examine the meaningful and symbolic content of qualitative data. Approaches in analysis is deductive approach. In data analysis the researcher compare patterns of first case with those of second case and develop a working hypothesis as common patterns emerge across studies. In data analysis the researcher immerses self in data to bring order and meaning to vast narrative which begins with 1st data collection episode. Data analysis started by reading, rereading, intuiting, analyzing, synthesizing and reporting on data. It is a cyclical and recursive process that requires an extensive amount of time for preparing final report. The researcher has to interpret data by looking for concepts and theories in what has been collected so far and formulating additional research questions and modification of questions, based on analysis. Scientific adequacy tested by RIGOR in qualitative research is less about the adherence to rules and more about fidelity to the spirit and standards of qualitative work. At conclusion of study a protracted period of data immersion in which conclusions are reviewed in the context of the whole study. Data similar in meaning are clustered together into preliminary categories.

Literature Review

A cursory review may be done initially to focus the study, otherwise it is generally conducted after the data has been collected and analyzed. Rationale for delaying the literature review is to avoid leading the participants in the direction of what has already been discovered. Purpose of literature review is to show how current findings fit into what is already known the rationale for delaying the literature review is to avoid leading the participants in the direction of what has already been discovered.

Determine the Implication and Draw Conclusion

Once a researcher has developed his over-arching themes, he/she needs to draw out conclusion and think about the implications. A conclusion section refocuses the purpose of the research, revealing a synopsis of what was found and leads into the implications of the findings. A conclusion may also include limitations of the study and future research needs. Why is the research work is important, why should anyone pay attention to it? What are the implications within each community? How are the partners within the communities reacting to the findings? This is where the action comes in from participatory action research. The findings from the research should help us not only in identifying strategies to bring about change, or to be more responsive to a community's needs, but also help us find realistic ways of implementing those strategies.

Write final report and dissemination the results: After completion of any research it needs to write the final report. There is not all that much difference between reporting quantitative and qualitative data the main issue is to present the findings of a study in such a way that those who wish to use them can understand what has been done and what the results are. The common questions which readers want qualitative reports to cover include the following:

- **Design:** How were subjects selected?
- **Research situation:** What information was given to the participants beforehand for example?
- **Transcription:** How thorough was the transcription and what instructions were given to the transcribers?
- **Analysis:** How was the analysis constructed, was it based on a personal intuitive interpretation or were some formal procedures applied?
- **Verification:** Which measures were taken to ensure the validity of the findings?

Dissemination the Results

Dissemination the results should be done carefully, sensitively and in conjunction with those affected. It is important to remember that some study results are sensitive to some people and communities. So we ask ourselves, 'what is the most appropriate way to let people know of the results of the study'? There are many options to disseminate the result, e.g., newspaper, mail, radio or video council meeting, focus groups and community workshops/seminars.

TERMINOLOGY

Applied Research

It is a methodology used to find a solution to an immediate specific practical problem of an individual or group.

Basic Research

It is systematic study directed toward greater knowledge or understanding of the fundamental aspects of phenomena and of observable facts without specific applications towards processes or products in mind. The research that is conducted to generate knowledge rather than to solve immediate problems.

Clinical Nursing Research

Nursing research studies involving clients or that have the potential for affecting clients.

Empirical Data

This data, also known as sense experience, is a collective term for the knowledge or source of knowledge acquired by means of the senses, particularly by observation and experimentation.

Nursing Research

A systematic, objective, process of analyzing phenomena of importance to nursing and provides evidence used to support nursing practices.

Outcomes Research

It is a branch of public health research, which studies the end results of the structure and processes of the healthcare system on the health and well-being of patients and populations. It also includes health services research that focuses on identifying variations in medical procedures and associated health outcomes.

Qualitative Research

Research that is concerned with the subjective meaning of an experience to an individual. It is used to gain an understanding of underlying reasons, opinions, and motivations. It provides insights into the problem or helps to develop ideas or hypotheses for potential quantitative research.

Quantitative Research

Research that is concerned with formal, objective, tight controls over the research situation systematic process to describe, examine the cause-effect interaction among variables, and the ability to generalize findings.

Accessible Population

This population is a subset of the target population which is available to the researcher for a particular study.

Assumptions

Beliefs that are held to be true but have not necessarily been proven; assumptions may be explicit or implicit.

Data

The term data refers to any kind of information researchers obtain on the subjects, respondents or participants of the study during a research.

Dependent Variable

The 'effect' a response or behavior that is influenced by the independent variable; sometimes called the criterion variable.

Hypothesis

A tentative statement of the predicted relationship between two or more variables and the validity of which is usually unknown.

Independent Variable

The 'cause' or the variable that is thought to influence the dependent variable; in experimental research it is the variable that is manipulated by the researcher.

Limitations

Limitations of a dissertation are potential weaknesses in the research study that are mostly out of researcher's control, given limited funding, choice of research design, statistical model constraints, or other factors.

Operational Definition

The definition of a variable that identifies how the variable will be observed or measured. An operational definition in research is how we (the researcher) decide to measure the variables in study.

Pilot Study

Pilot study is a small-scale, trial run of an actual research study.

Population

A complete set of persons or objects that possess some common characteristic that is of interest to the researcher.

Research Design

The design of a study is the end result of a series of decisions made by the researcher concerning how the study will be conducted. It is the overall plan for gathering data in a research study.

Sample

A subset of the population that is selected to represent the population.

Target Population

The entire group of people or objects to which the researcher wishes to generalize the findings of a study.

Variable

A characteristic or attribute of a person or object that differs among the persons or objects that are being studied (e.g., age, blood type).

Anonymity

Anonymity is the condition of being anonymous means the identity of research subjects is unknown, even to the study investigator.

Confidentiality

The identity of the research subjects is known only to the study investigator(s).

Informed Consent

A subject voluntarily agrees to participate in a research study in which he or she has full understanding of the study before the study begins.

Bivariate Study

A research study in which the relationship between two variables is examined.

Multivariate Study

A research study in which more than two variables are examined.

Replication Study

A research study that repeats or duplicates an earlier research study, with all of the essential elements of the original study held intact. A different sample or setting may be used.

Univariate Study

A research study in which only one variable is examined.

Abstract (Research Abstracts)

Brief summaries of research studies, generally contain the purpose, methods, and major findings of the study.

Indexes

Indexes are special lookup tables that the database search engine can use to speed up data retrieval. Indexes are the compilation of reference materials that provide information on books and periodicals.

Primary Source

In the research literature, it is an account of a research study that has been written by the original researcher(s); in historical studies, primary sources consist of firsthand information or direct evidence of an event.

Secondary Source

In the research literature, it is an account of a research study that has been written by someone other than the study investigators; in historical studies, secondary sources are secondhand information or data provided by someone who did not observe the event.

Concept

A word picture or mental idea of a phenomenon.

Conceptual Framework

A background or foundation for a study; a less well-developed structure than a theoretical framework; concepts are related in a logical manner by the researcher.

Conceptual Model

Symbolic presentation of concepts and the relationships between these concepts.

Construct

A highly abstract phenomenon that cannot be directly observed but must be inferred by certain concrete or less abstract indicators of the phenomenon.

Deductive Reasoning

A reasoning process that proceeds from the general to the specific, from theory to empirical data.

Empirical Generalization

A summary statement about the occurrence of phenomena that is based on empirical data from a number of different research studies.

Grand Theories

Theories that are concerned with a broad range of phenomena in the environment or in the experiences of humans which require further specification through research before they can be fully tested.

Inductive Reasoning

A reasoning process that proceeds from the specific to the general from empirical data to theory.

Middle-range Theories

Theories that have a narrow focus; they are concerned with only a small area of the environment or of human experiences.

Model

A symbolic representation of some phenomenon or phenomena.

Proposition

A proposition (a structural element of a theory) is a statement or assertion of the relationship between concepts.

Theoretical Framework

A theoretical framework is the application of a theory, or a set of concepts drawn from one and the same theory, to offer an explanation of an event, or shed some light on a particular phenomenon or research problem. It is a study framework based on propositional statements from a theory.

Theory

A set of related statements that describes or explains phenomena in a systematic way. A theory is like a blueprint, a guide for modeling a structure.

Hypothesis

Complex hypothesis: A hypothesis that concerns a relationship where two or more independent variables, two or more dependent variables, or both are being examined.

Directional Research Hypothesis

A type of hypothesis in which a prediction is made of the type of relationship that exists between variables.

Interaction Effect

The result of two variables acting in conjunction with each other.

Nondirectional Research Hypothesis

A type of research hypothesis in which a prediction is made that a relationship exists between variables, but the type of relationship is not specified.

Null Hypothesis (H_0)

A statistical hypothesis that predicts there is no relationship between variables; the hypothesis that is subjected to statistical analysis.

Research Hypothesis (H_1)

An alternative hypothesis to the statistical null hypothesis; predicts the researcher's actual expectations about the outcome of a study; also called scientific, substantive, and theoretical.

Simple Hypothesis

A hypothesis that predicts the relationship between one independent and one dependent variable.

Comparative Studies

Studies in which intact groups are compared on some dependent variable. The researcher is not able to manipulate the independent variable, which is frequently some inherent characteristic of the subjects, such as age or educational level.

Comparison Group

A group of subjects in an experimental study that does not receive any experimental treatment or receives an alternate treatment such as the 'normal' or routine treatment.

Control Group

A group of subjects in an experimental study that does not receive the experimental treatment (*See* comparison group).

Correlation

The extent to which values of one variable (X) are related to the values of a second variable (Y). Correlations may be either positive or negative.

Correlation Coefficient

A statistic that presents the magnitude and direction of a relationship between two variables. Correlation coefficients range from –1.00 (perfect negative relationship) to +1.00 (perfect positive relationship).

Correlational Studies

Research studies that examine the strength of relationships between variables.

Descriptive Studies

Research studies in which phenomena are described or the relationship between variables is examined; no attempt is made to determine cause-and-effect relationships.

Experimenter Effect

A threat to the external validity of a research study that occurs when the researcher's behavior influences the subjects' behavior in a way that is not intended by the researcher.

Explanatory Studies

Research studies that search for causal explanations; usually experimental in nature.

Exploratory Studies

Research studies that are conducted when little is known about the phenomenon that is being studied.

Ex Post Facto Studies

Studies in which the variation in the independent variable has already occurred in the past, and the researcher, 'after the fact,' is trying to determine if the variation that has occurred in the independent variable has any influence on the dependent variable that is being measured in the present.

External Validity

The degree to which study results can be generalized to other people and other research settings.

Extraneous Variable

A type of variable that is not the variable of interest to a researcher but that may influence the results of a study. Other terms for extraneous variable are intervening variable and confounding variable.

Field Studies

Research studies that are conducted 'in the field' or real-life setting.

Hawthorne Effect

A threat to the external validity of a research study that occurs when study participants respond in a certain manner because they are aware that they are involved in a research study.

History

A threat to the internal validity of an experimental research study; some event besides the experimental treatment occurs between the pretreatment and post-treatment measurement of the dependent variable, and this event influences the dependent variable.

Instrumentation Change

A threat to the internal validity of an experimental research study that involves changes from the pretest measurements to the post-test measurements as a result of inaccuracy of the instrument or the judges' ratings rather than as a result of the experimental treatment.

Validity

Internal validity: The degree to which changes in the dependent variable (effect) can be attributed to the independent or experimental variable (cause) rather than to the effects of extraneous variables.

Laboratory Studies

Research studies in which subjects are studied in a special environment that has been created by the researcher.

Manipulation

The independent or experimental variable is controlled by the researcher to determine its effect on the dependent variable.

Maturation

A threat to the internal validity of an experimental research study that occurs when changes that take place within study subjects as a result of the passage of time (growing older, taller) affect the study results.

Methodological Studies

Research studies that are concerned with the development, testing, and evaluation of research instruments and methods.

Mortality

A threat to the internal validity of an experimental research study that occurs when the subject drop-out rate is different or characteristics are different between those who drop out of the experimental group and those who drop out of the comparison group.

Negative Relationship (Inverse Relationship)

A relationship between two variables in which there is a tendency for the values of one variable to increase as the values of the other variable decrease.

Nonequivalent Control Group Design

A type of quasi experimental design; similar to the pretest-post-test control group experimental design, except that there is no random assignment of subjects to groups.

One-group Pretest-post-test Design

A type of pre-experimental design; compares one group of subjects before and after an experimental treatment.

One-shot Case Study

A type of pre-experimental design; a single group of subjects is observed after a treatment to determine the effects of the treatment. No pretest measurement is made.

Positive Relationship (Direct Relationship)

A relationship between two variables in which the variables tend to vary together; as the values of one variable increase or decrease, the values of the other variable increase or decrease.

Post-test-only Control Group Design

True experimental design in which subjects in the experimental and comparison groups are given a post-test after the experimental group receives the study treatment.

Pre-experimental Design

A type of experimental design in which the researcher has little control over the research situation; includes the one-shot case study and the one-group pretest-post-test design.

Pretest-post-test Control Group Design

True experimental design in which subjects in the experimental and comparison groups are given a pretest before and a post-test after the administration of the study treatment to the experimental group.

Prospective Studies

Studies in which the independent variable or presumed cause (e.g., use of birth control pills) is identified at the present time and then subjects are followed for sometime in the future to observe the dependent variable or effect (e.g., thrombophlebitis or myocardial infarctions).

Quasi Experimental Design

A type of experimental design in which there is either no comparison group or no random assignment of subjects to groups; includes the nonequivalent control group design and time-series design.

Random Assignment

A procedure used in an experimental study to ensure that each study subject has an equal chance of being placed into any one of the study groups.

Reactive Effects of the Pretest

A threat to the external validity of a research study that occurs when subjects are sensitized to the experimental treatment by the pretest.

Retrospective Studies

Studies in which the dependent variable is identified in the present (e.g., a disease condition) and an attempt is made to determine the independent variable (e.g., cause of the disease) that occurred in the past.

Rosenthal Effect

The influence of interviewers on respondents' answers.

Selection Bias

A threat to the internal validity of an experimental research study that occurs when study results are attributed to the experimental treatment when, in fact, the results may be due to pretreatment differences between the subjects in the experimental and comparison groups.

Simulation Studies

Laboratory studies in which subjects are presented with a description of a case study or situation that is intended to represent a real-life situation.

Solomon Four-group Design

True experimental design that minimizes threats to internal and external validity.

Survey Studies

Research studies in which self-report data are collected from a sample to determine the characteristics of a population.

Testing

A threat to the internal validity of a research study that occurs when a pretest is administered to subjects; the effects of taking a pretest on responses on the post-test.

Time-series Design

Quasi-experimental design in which the researcher periodically observes subjects and administers an experimental treatment between two of the observations.

True Experimental Design

An experimental design in which the researcher (a) manipulates the experimental variable, (b) includes at least one experimental and one comparison group in the study, and (c) randomly assigns subjects to either the experimental or comparison group; includes the pretest-post-test control group design, post-test only control group design, and solomon four-group design.

Case Studies

Research studies that involve an in-depth examination of a single person or a group of people. A case study might also examine an institution.

Content Analysis

A data collection method that examines communication messages that are usually in written form.

Ethnographic Studies

Research studies that involve the collection and analysis of data about cultural groups.

External Criticism (External Appraisal, External Examination)

A type of examination of historical data that is concerned with the authenticity or genuineness of the data. External criticism might be used to determine if a letter was actually written by the person whose signature was contained on the letter.

Focus Group
A small group of individuals who meet together and are asked questions by a moderator about a certain topic or topics.

Grounded Theory Studies
Research studies in which data are collected and analyzed and then a theory is developed that is 'grounded' in the data.

Historical Studies
Research studies that are concerned with the identification, location, evaluation and synthesis of data from the past.

Internal Criticism
A type of examination of historical data that is concerned with the accuracy of the data. Internal criticism might be used to determine if a document contained an accurate recording of events as they actually happened.

Phenomenological Studies
Research studies that examine human experiences through the descriptions of the meanings of these experiences provided by the people involved.

Saturation
The researcher is hearing a repetition of themes or ideas as additional participants are interviewed in a qualitative study.

Triangulation
Combining both qualitative and quantitative methods in one study.

Cluster Random Sampling
A random sampling process that involves two or more stages. The population is first listed by clusters or categories (e.g., hospitals) and then the sample elements (e.g., hospital administrators) are randomly selected from these clusters.

Cohort Study
A special type of longitudinal study in which subjects are studied who have been born during one particular period or who have similar backgrounds.

Convenience Sampling (Accidental Sampling)
A nonprobability sampling procedure that involves the selection of the most readily available people or objects for a study.

Cross-sectional Study
A research study that collects data on subjects at one point in time.

Disproportional Stratified Sampling

Random selection of members from population strata where the number of members chosen for each stratum is not in proportion to the size of the stratum in the total population.

Element

A single member of a population.

Longitudinal Study

Subjects are followed during a period in the future; data are collected at two or more different time periods.

Nonprobability Sampling

A sampling process in which a sample is selected from elements or members of a population through nonrandom methods; includes convenience, quota, and purposive.

Power Analysis

A procedure that is used to determine the sample size needed to prevent a Type II error.

Probability Sampling

The use of a random sampling procedure to select a sample from elements or members of a population; includes simple, stratified, cluster, and systematic random sampling techniques.

Proportional Stratified Sampling

Random selection of members from population strata where the number of members chosen from each stratum is in proportion to the size of the stratum in the total population.

Purposive Sampling (Judgmental Sampling)

A nonprobability sampling procedure in which the researcher uses personal judgment to select subjects who are considered to be representative of the population.

Quota Sampling

A nonprobability sampling procedure in which the researcher selects the sample to reflect certain characteristics of the population.

Sampling Bias

- ❖ The difference between sample data and population data that can be attributed to a faulty selection process.
- ❖ A threat to the external validity of a research study that occurs when subjects are not randomly selected from the population.

Sampling Error

Random fluctuations in data that occur when a sample is selected to represent a population.

Sampling Frame

A listing of all the elements of the population from which a sample is to be chosen.

Simple Random Sampling

A method of random sampling in which each element of the population has an equal and independent chance of being chosen for the sample.

Snowball Sampling

A sampling method that involves the assistance of study subjects to help obtain other potential subjects.

Stratified Random Sampling

A random sampling process in which a sample is selected after the population has been divided into subgroups or strata according to some variable of importance to the research study.

Systematic Random Sampling

A random sampling process in which every kth (e.g., every fifth) element or member of the population is selected for the sample.

Table of Random Numbers

A list of numbers that have been generated in such a manner that there is no order or sequencing of the numbers. Each number is equally likely to follow any other number.

Volunteers

Subjects who have asked to participate in a study.

Concurrent Validity

A type of criterion validity in which a determination is made of the instrument's ability to obtain a measurement of subjects' behavior that is comparable to some other criterion used to indicate that behavior.

Construct Validity

The ability of an instrument to measure the construct that it is intended to measure.

Content Validity

The degree to which an instrument covers the scope and range of information that is sought.

Criterion Validity

The extent to which an instrument corresponds or correlates with some criterion measure of the information that is being sought; the ability of an instrument to determine subjects' responses at present or predict subjects' responses in the future.

Equivalence Reliability

The degree to which two forms of an instrument obtain the same results or two or more observers obtain the same results when using a single instrument to measure a variable.

Face Validity

A subjective determination that an instrument is adequate for obtaining the desired information; on the surface or the 'face' of the instrument it appears to be an adequate means of obtaining the desired data.

Factor Analysis

A type of validity used to identify clusters of related items on an instrument or scale.

Internal Consistency Reliability (Scale Homogeneity)

The extent to which all items of an instrument measure the same variable.

Interobserver Reliability

See interrater reliability.

Interrater Reliability (Interobserver Reliability)

The degree to which two or more independent judges are in agreement about ratings or observations of events or behaviors.

Interval Level of Measurement

Data can be categorized and ranked, and the distance between the ranks can be specified; pulse rates and temperature readings are examples of interval data.

Known-groups Procedure

A research technique in which a research instrument is administered to two groups of people whose responses are expected to differ on the variable of interest.

Measurement

A process in scientific research that uses rules to assign numbers to objects.

Nominal Level of Measurement

The lowest level of measurement; data are 'named' or categorized, such as race and marital status.

Ordinal Level of Measurement

Data can be categorized and placed in order; small, medium, and large is an example of a set of ordinal data.

Predictive Validity

A type of criterion validity of an instrument in which a determination is made of the instrument's ability to predict behavior of subjects in the future.

Ratio Level of Measurement

Data can be categorized and ranked, the distance between ranks can be specified, and a 'true' or natural zero point can be identified; the amount of money in a checking account and the number of requests for pain medication are examples of ratio data.

Reliability

The consistency and dependability of a research instrument to measure a variable; types of reliability are stability, equivalence, and internal consistency.

Research Instruments (Research Tools)

Devices used to collect data in research studies.

Stability Reliability

The consistency of a research instrument over time; test-retest procedures and repeated observations are methods to test the stability of an instrument.

Validity

The ability of an instrument to measure the variable that it is intended to measure.

Ambiguous Questions

Questions that contain words that may be interpreted in more than one way.

Attitude Scales

Self-report data collection instruments that ask respondents to report their attitudes or feelings on a continuum.

Attribute Variables

In science and research, **attribute** is a characteristic of an object (person, thing, etc.). Demographic variables only explain the characteristics of a person but attribute variables explain the characteristic of an object (person, thing, etc.).

Close-ended Questions

Questions that require respondents to choose from given alternatives.

Collectively Exhaustive Categories

Categories are provided for every possible answer.

Contingency Questions

Questions that are relevant for some respondents and not for others.

Delphi Technique

A data collection method that uses several rounds of questions to seek a consensus on a particular topic from a group of experts on the topic.

Demographic Questions

Questions that gather data on characteristics of the subjects (*See* demographic variables).

Demographic Variables

Subject characteristics, such as age, educational levels, and marital status.

Double-barreled Questions

Questions that ask two questions in one.

Event Sampling

Observations made throughout the entire course of an event or behavior.

Filler Questions

Questions used to distract respondents from the purpose of other questions that are being asked.

Interview

A method of data collection in which the interviewer obtains responses from a subject in a face-to-face encounter or through a telephone call.

Interview Schedule

An instrument containing a set of questions, directions for asking these questions, and space to record the respondents' answers.

Likert Scale

An attitude scale named after its developer, Rensis Likert. These scales usually contain five or seven responses for each item, ranging from 'strongly agree' to 'strongly disagree.'

Mutually Exclusive Categories

Categories are uniquely distinct; no overlap occurs between categories.

Nonparticipant Observer-covert

Research observer does not identify herself or himself to the subjects who are being observed.

Nonparticipant Observer-overt

Research observer openly identifies that she or he is conducting research and provides subjects with information about the type of data that will be collected.

Observation Research

A data-collection method in which data are collected through visual observations.

Open-ended Questions

Questions that allow respondents to answer in their own words.

Participant Observer-covert

Research observer interacts with subjects and observes their behavior without their knowledge.

Participant Observer-overt

Research observer interacts with subjects openly and with the full awareness of those people who will be observed.

Personality Inventories

Self-report measures used to assess the differences in personality traits, needs, or values of people.

Pre-existing Data

Existing information that has not been collected for research purposes.

Probes

Prompting questions that encourage the respondent to elaborate on the topic that is being discussed.

Projective Technique

Self-report measure in which a subject is asked to respond to stimuli that are designed to be ambiguous or to have no definite meaning. The responses reflect the internal feelings of the subject that are projected on the external stimuli.

Q-sort (Q Methodology)

A data-collection method in which subjects are asked to sort statements into categories according to their attitudes toward, or rating of, the statements.

Questionnaire

A paper-and-pencil, self-report instrument used to gather data from subjects.

Semantic Differential

Attitude scale that asks subjects to indicate their position or attitude about some concept along a continuum between two adjectives or phrases that are presented in relation to the concept that is being measured.

Semistructured Interviews

Interviewers ask a certain number of specific questions, but additional questions or probes are used at the discretion of the interviewer.

Structured Interviews

Interviewers ask the same questions in the same manner of all respondents.

Structured Observations

The researcher makes the determination of behaviors to be observed before data collection. Usually some kind of checklist is used to record behaviors.

Telephone Interviews

Data are collected from subjects through the use of phone calls rather than in face-to-face encounters.

Time Sampling

Observations of events or behaviors that are made during certain specified time periods.

Unstructured Interviews

The interviewer is given a great deal of freedom to direct the course of the interview; the interviewer's main goal is to encourage the respondent to talk freely about the topic that is being explored.

Unstructured Observations

The researcher describes behaviors as they are viewed, with no preconceived ideas of what will be seen.

Visual Analogue Scale

Subjects are presented with a straight line that is anchored on each end with words or phrases that represent the extremes of some phenomenon, such as pain. Subjects are asked to make a mark on the line at the point that corresponds to their experience of the phenomenon.

Bar Graph

A figure used to represent a frequency distribution of nominal or ordinal data.

Bimodal
A frequency distribution that contains two identical high frequency values.

Class Interval
A group of scores in a frequency distribution.

Coefficient of Determination (r^2, r^2)
A statistic obtained by squaring a correlation coefficient and is interpreted as the percentage of variance shared by two variables.

Contingency Table
A table that visually displays the relationship between sets of nominal data.

Descriptive Statistics
That group of statistics that organizes and summarizes numerical data obtained from populations and samples.

Frequency Distribution
A listing of all scores or numerical values from a set of data and the number of times each score or value appears; scores may be listed from highest to lowest or lowest to highest.

Frequency Polygon
A graph that uses dots connected with straight lines to represent the frequency distribution of interval or ratio data. A dot is placed above the midpoint of each class interval.

Histogram
A graph used to represent the frequency distribution of variables measured at the interval or ratio level.

Inferential Statistics
That group of statistics concerned with the characteristics of populations and uses sample data to make an 'inference' about a population.

Interquartile Range
Contains the middle half of the values in a frequency distribution.

Mean (m)
A measure of central tendency; the average of a set of values that is found by adding all values and dividing by the total number of values. The population symbol is μ and the sample symbol is $\bar{x}$.

Measures of Central Tendency
Statistics that describe the average, typical, or most common value for a group of data.

Measures of Relationship
Statistics that present the correlation between variables.

Measures of Variability
Statistics that describe how spread out values are in a distribution of values (e.g., range, standard deviation).

Measures to Condense Data
Statistics that are used to condense and summarize data.

Median (md, mdn)
A measure of central tendency; the middle score or value in a group of data.

Modal Class
The category with the greatest frequency of observations; used with nominal and ordinal data.

Mode (mo)
A measure of central tendency; the category or value that occurs most often in a set of data.

Multimodal
A frequency distribution in which more than two values have the same high frequency.

Negatively Skewed
A frequency distribution in which the tail of the distribution points to the left.

Nonsymmetrical Distribution (Skewed Distribution)
Frequency distribution in which the distribution has an off-center peak. If the tail of the distribution points to the right, the distribution is said to be positively skewed; if the tail of the distribution points to the left, the distribution is said to be negatively skewed.

Normal Curve
A bell-shaped curve that graphically depicts a normally distributed frequency distribution (*See* normal distribution).

Normal Distribution
A symmetrical, bell-shaped theoretical distribution; has one central peak or set of values in the middle of the distribution.

Parameter
A numerical characteristic of a population (e.g., the average educational level of people living in the United States).

Percentage (%)
A statistic that represents the proportion of a subgroup to a total group, expressed as a percent ranging from 0 to 100%.

Percentile
A data point below which lies a certain percentage of the values in a frequency distribution.

Positively Skewed
A frequency distribution in which the tail of the distribution points to the right.

Range
A measure of variability; the distance between the highest and lowest value in a group of values or scores.

Scatter Plot (Scatter Diagram, Scattergram)
A graphic presentation of the relationship between two variables. The graph contains variables plotted on an X-axis and a Y-axis. Pairs of scores are plotted by the placement of dots to indicate where each pair of X's and Y's intersect.

Semiquartile Range
Determined by dividing the interquartile range in half (*See* interquartile range).

Standard Deviation (sd; s)
A measure of variability; the statistic that indicates the average deviation or variation of all the values in a set of data from the mean value of that data.

Statistic
A numerical characteristic of a sample (e.g., the average educational level of a random sample of people living in the united states).

Symmetrical Distributions
Frequency distributions in which both halves of the distribution are the same.

Unimodal
A frequency distribution that contains one value that occurs more frequently than any other.

Variance (sd^2; s^2)
A measure of variability; the standard deviation squared.

Z-score

A standard score that indicates how many standard deviations that a particular value is away from the mean of the set of values.

Analysis of Covariance (ANCOVA)

A statistical test that allows the researcher to statistically control for some variable(s) that may have an influence on the dependent variable.

Analysis of Variance (ANOVA)

A parametric statistical test that is used to compare the difference between the means of two or more groups or sets of values.

Canonical Correlation

Examines the correlation between two or more independent variables and two or more dependent variables.

Central Limit Theorem

The phenomenon in which sample values tend to be normally distributed around the population value.

Chi-square Test

A nonparametric statistical test that is used to compare sets of data that are in the form of frequencies or percentages (nominal level data).

Confidence Interval

A range of values that, with a specified degree of probability, is thought to contain the population value.

Critical Region (Region of Rejection)

An area in a theoretical sampling distribution that contains the critical values, which are values that are considered to be statistically significant.

Critical Value

A scientific cut-off point that denotes the value in a theoretical distribution at which all obtained values from a sample that are equal to or beyond that point are said to be statistically significant.

Degrees of Freedom (DF)

A concept in inferential statistics that concerns the number of values that are free to vary.

Dependent t-test

A form of the t-test that is used when one set of scores or values is associated or dependent on another set of scores or values.

Independent t-test

A form of the t-test that is used when there is no association between the two sets of scores or values that are being compared.

Level of Significance (Probability Level)

The probability of rejecting a null hypothesis when it is true; symbolized by lowercase Greek letter alpha; also symbolized by p.

Meta-analysis

A technique that combines the results of several similar studies on a topic and statistically analyzes the results as if only one study had been conducted.

Multiple Regression

A statistical procedure used to determine the influence of more than one independent variable on the dependent variable.

Multivariate Analysis of Variance (MANOVA)

A statistical test that examines the difference between the mean scores of two or more groups on two or more dependent variables that are measured at the same time.

Nonparametric Tests (Distribution-free Statistics)

Types of inferential statistics that are not concerned with population parameters, and requirements for their use are less stringent; can be used with nominal and ordinal data and small sample sizes.

One-tailed Test of Significance

A test of statistical significance in which the critical values (statistically significant values) are sought in only one tail of the theoretical sampling distribution (either the right or the left tail); used when a directional research hypothesis has been formulated for a study.

Parametric Tests

Types of inferential statistics that are concerned with population parameters. When parametric tests are used assumptions are made that (a) the level of measurement of the data is interval or ratio, (b) data are taken from populations that are normally distributed on the variable that is being measured, and (c) data are taken from populations that have equal variances on the variable that is being measured.

Power of a Statistical Test
The ability of a statistical test to reject a null hypothesis when it is false (and should be rejected).

Sampling Distribution
A theoretical frequency distribution that is based on an infinite number of samples. Sampling distributions are based on mathematical formulas and logic.

Standard Error of the Mean
The standard deviation of the sampling distribution of the mean.

T-test (t)
A parametric statistical test that examines the difference between the means of two groups of values. Types of t-tests are the independent t-test (independent samples t-test) and the dependent t-test (paired t-test).

Two-tailed Test of Significance
A test of statistical significance in which critical values (statistically significant values) are sought in both tails of the sampling distribution; used when the researcher has not predicted the direction of the relationship between variables.

Type I Error
A decision is made to reject the null hypothesis when it is actually true; a decision is made that a relationship exists between variables when it does not.

Type II Error
A decision is made not to reject the null hypothesis when it is false and should be rejected; a decision is made that no relationship exists between variables when, in fact, a relationship does exist. Boxes in a table that are formed by the intersection of rows and columns.

Columns
Vertical entries in a table.

Rows
Horizontal entries in a table.

Blind Review
Manuscript reviewers are not made aware of the author's identity before the manuscript is evaluated.

Call for Abstract

A request for a summary of a study that the researcher wishes to present at a research conference.

Galley Proofs

Sheets of paper that show how an article or book will appear in typeset form.

Nonrefereed Journal

A journal that uses editorial staff members or consultants to review manuscripts.

Peer Review

The review of a research manuscript by professional colleagues who have content or methodological expertise concerning the material that is presented in the manuscript.

Query Letter

A letter of inquiry sent to a journal to determine the editor's interest in publishing a manuscript. The letter usually contains an outline of the manuscript and important information about the content of the manuscript.

Refereed Journal

A journal that uses experts in a given field to review manuscripts.

Research Report

A written or oral summary of a research study.

SUMMARY

- Scientific research involves a systematic process that focuses on being objective and gathering a multitude of information for analysis so that the researcher can come to a conclusion.
- Any research done without documenting the study so that others can review the process and results is not an investigation using the scientific research process.
- There are five major phases in the quantitative research process: (1) The conceptual phase, (2) Phase of construction of research design, (3) Empiric phase, (4) Analytic phase, (5) Disseminative phase.
- A basic distinction in quantitative studies is between experimental and nonexperimental research.
- In experimental research, researchers actively intervene or introduce a treatment, whereas in nonexperimental research, researchers make observations of existing situations and characteristics without intervening.
- Qualitative research often is strongly rooted in research traditions that originate in the disciplines of anthropology, sociology, and psychology. Three such traditions have had strong influence on qualitative nursing research: grounded theory, phenomenology, and ethnography.

- There is difference in steps of qualitative and quantitative research process. In qualitative research process a cursory review may be done initially to focus the study, otherwise it is generally conducted after the data has been collected and analyzed.
- In qualitative research process after data collection data saturation was done. Theoretical saturation of data is a term in qualitative research, mostly used in the grounded theory approach. Theoretical saturation of data means that researchers reach a point in their analysis of data that sampling more data will not lead to more information related to their research questions.

QUESTIONS TO TEST YOUR KNOWLEDGE

Q1. Enumerate the major phases of quantitative research process. (15)

Q2. Explain how the steps of qualitative research process is differ from quantitative research process. (10)

Q3. Describe the steps under construction phase of quantitative research process. (10)

Q4. Multiple choice questions: (10 × 1 = 10)

   I. A condition or characteristic that can take on different values or categories is called:
   - a. Constant
   - b. Variable
   - c. Cause-and-effect relationship
   - d. Descriptive relationship

   II. A good qualitative problem statement,
   - a. Defines the independent and dependent variables
   - b. Conveys a sense of emerging design
   - c. Specifies a research hypothesis to be tested
   - d. Specifies the relationship between variables that the researcher expects to find

   III. In qualitative research process, the researcher has to explicate researcher's own belief which may affect the study process. A method by which it is done is called is:
   - a. Confidentiality
   - b. Anonymity
   - c. Triangulation
   - d. Bracketing

   IV. A complete set of persons or objects that possess some common characteristic that is of interest to the researcher is termed as:
   - a. Population
   - b. Assessable population
   - c. Target population
   - d. Sample

   V. The variable which is going to change by manipulation is:
   - a. Independent variable
   - b. Dependent variable
   - c. Discrete variable
   - d. Continuous variable

   VI. To test the feasibility of study a small scale study was conducted named:
   - a. Small scale study
   - b. Pilot study
   - c. Main study
   - d. Smaller study

   VII. Predictions of the outcome of the research are stated as:
   - a. Methodology
   - b. Samples
   - c. Hypothesis
   - d. Chi square

   VIII. The analyzing of time, money, materials and prior to beginning the study is called:
   - a. Validity
   - b. Feasibility
   - c. Reliability
   - d. Researchability

   IX. The researcher expects to achieve after completion of study is called as:
   - a. General objectives
   - b. Specific objectives
   - c. Intermediate objectives
   - d. Hypothesis

X. The abstractions or mental representations inferred from behavior or characteristics is known as:
   a. Conceptual framework
   b. Variables
   c. Phenomenon
   d. Theory

ANSWERS

| I. b | II. b | III. d | IV. a | V. b |
| VI. b | VII. c | VIII. b | IX. a | X. c |

Q5. State True or False (T/F): (1 × 10)
   a. Bivariate study is a research study in which the relationship between two or more variables is examined.
   b. Indexes are brief summaries of research studies.
   c. A word picture or mental idea of a phenomenon is called contruct.
   d. A reasoning process that proceeds from the general to the specific, from theory to empirical data is called deductive reasoning.
   e. A numerical characteristic of a population is Parameter.
   f. When researchers reach a point in their analysis of data that sampling more data will not lead to more information related to their research questions this is called data saturation.
   g. The entire group of people or objects to which the researcher wishes to generalize the findingis of a study is assessable population.
   h. The analysis of quantitative research notes begins in the field.
   i. Ethnography is the study of the subjective experiences of others.
   j. Ideally in qualitative studies the in-depth review of literature should be done after analyzing the data.

Ans. a. False b. False c. False d. True e. True f. True g. False h. False i. False j. True.

Chapter 3
Research Problems, Objectives, Variables Hypothesis, Delimitation, and Assumptions

Learning Objectives

After completion of this chapter, the students will be able to:
- Describe the concept of research problem.
- Explain the sources of research problems.
- Identify the characteristics of a good research problem.
- List down the qualities of a good research questions.
- Describe the steps in developing a research problem.
- Enumerate the concept, characteristics, importance and types of research objectives.
- Explain the concept and different types of variables.
- State the purposes and types of hypothesis and identify the importance of hypothesis in quantitative studies.
- Describe the characteristics and functions of hypothesis.
- Enumerate the concept, types and uses of delimitations.
- Identify the limitations for the study and how it will be differ from delimitation.
- Describe the concept, types and uses of assumptions.
- Differentiate between assumption and hypothesis.

INTRODUCTION

In order to begin to identify research problems is it first necessary to understand what is meant by the term research and to have an understanding of how the research problem fits into the whole research process. A number of different definitions for research exist however common to all of them is an agreement that research is systematic, disciplined and focused on gathering information to understand a phenomena, answer questions or solve research problems. The systematic nature of the research process means that research is undertaken in a methodological fashion using a rigorous approach to collect information (data) about a phenomena or research problem and to analyze and interpret that information in order to begin to answer questions or solve problems. Since research is directed at ultimately helping us to answer a question or address a problem, it is critical that we are as clear as possible about the research problem, we are interested in. Thus, developing a problem statement is a critical first step in the research process. In research process, the first and foremost step is selecting and properly defining a research problem. A researcher must find the problem and formulate it when he/she is interested to make a research study and a research problem is one which requires a researcher to find out the best solution for the given problem, i.e., to find out by which course of action the objective can be attained optimally in the context of a given environment. It is an enigmatic, perplexing, or troubling condition for the researcher. Both qualitative and quantitative researchers identify a research problem within a broad topic area of interest. The purpose of study for them is to "solve" the problem or to contribute to its solution by accumulating relevant information.

DEFINITIONS OF RESEARCH PROBLEM

❖ A research problem, in general refer to some difficulty which a researcher experience in the contest of either a theoretical or practical situation and wants to obtained a solution for the same.
❖ A research problem is a situation involving enigmatic, perplexing, or troubling condition and the purpose of it to solve the problem to be solved.

MEANING OF RESEARCH PROBLEM

❖ Research problem is a situation in need of a solution, improvement, or alteration.

or

❖ A discrepancy between the way things are and the way they ought to be. Research questions are the specific queries researchers want to answer in addressing the research problem.

SOURCES OF RESEARCH PROBLEMS

When a reviewer or consumer critiquing, reviewing or utilizing research questions being puzzled about the origins of research problems. Generally before starting research project their doubt should be cleared regarding development how to select research problem and formulate problem statement. As research is a time consuming enterprise, curiosity about and interest in a topic are essential to a project's success. There are a variety of sources for searching research problem. At the most basic level, research topics originate with researchers' interests. Explicit sources that might fuel researchers' curiosity include experience, the nursing literature, social issues, theories, and ideas from others. The sources of research problems are enlisted as follows (Fig. 3.1):

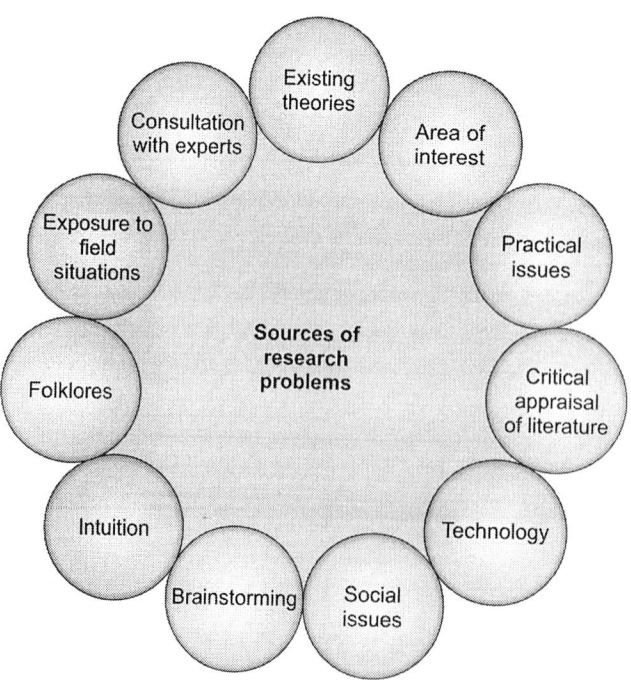

Fig 3.1: Sources of research problems.

Personal Experience

The first credible source of information is what a person comes to know by direct personal experience. In the course of professional training and experiences at work, a nurse feel uncomfortable with some certain things or facing problems in day to day activities which can be changed or improved on. This allows the nurse to embark on solving the problems by which they will conduct research. Sometime personal practical experiences can pursue a nurse to make some changes by carrying out research where they are getting problems. Personal experience, such as gripe, professional wishes, curiosity, new person/experience are also provocative factors for research.

Existing Theories

One good source for completing the research is deducting from the existing theories and hence finding its discrepancies and conclusions. There is good relationship between theories and research. Research is a process of theory development and theory testing because theories are proved by research. Nurses use many theories from other disciplines in their practices. If an existing theory is used in developing a researchable problem, that specific statement from the theory must be isolated. Generally, parts of the theory are subjected to testing in the clinical situation.

Area of Interest

Research is all about exploring and probing new areas that have not been worked upon. A researcher can choose any field or area that interests him and then gather all the existing knowledge about it. This would help to strengthen the grip of the researcher over the topic. Once you know the existing areas, it can observe where there is need for further work. The discrepancies in the research can serve as the basis of the new research where it can try to explore new dimensions and avenues and update the existing knowledge. This would serve as a source for research problem.

Practical Issues

Practical issues can be a source of research ideas. Some current problems facing in nursing education (new learning strategy) nursing practice (new intervention or quality care), nursing administration (e.g., problem facing administrators) can be taken as research problem. Nurses gets plenty of ideas to formulate research problems from their clinical experiences. Every curious nurse has several questions to be answered which are encountered during clinical experience. For example, a nurse finds that unrestricted visiting hours in surgical wards reduced the analgesic demand among postoperative patients. Such clinical experiences could be rich sources of ideas to identify a significant research problem.

Critical Appraisal of Literature

When we critically study books and articles relating to the subject of our interest, including research report, opinion articles, and summaries of clinical issues, pertinent questions may arise in our mind. These may strike reader's mind indirectly by stimulating imagination and directly by stating what additional research is needed. For example, a nurse reads an article on the prevalence of the pin site infection among patients with external fixators while reading this article nurse learns that there is lack of consensus about pin site care. This information may serve as a basis to formulate a research problem. There may be areas, as revealed by a dearth of available literature on the topic that remain unexplored that can be identified through the review, discovering the areas how much has been explored and what is remaining can helps to get a research problem.

Past research can be an excellent source of research ideas. It is probably the most important source of research ideas. That's because a great deal of research that has already been conducted on a multitude of topics and, importantly, research usually generates more questions than it answers. This is also the best way to come up with a specific idea that will fit into and extend the research literature. For students planning on writing a thesis or dissertation, the use of past research is extremely helpful, and remember to not just look at the variables and the results, but also carefully examine how they conducted the study. In research every research report suggests areas for continued study which can be referred as source. No study can stand by itself, must be replicated for confidence in the results which can be referred as source.

Technology

Advance technology may have different type of influence on human life. There are many adverse effects of advance technology also which can be considered as research problem. For example, effect of continuous improper uses mobile phone on the health of the individual or the effect of continuous use of computer on the health of the official workers (using computer at least 8 hours in a day). In medical science also different drugs are banned due to such types of adverse effects.

Social Issues

Sometimes, topics are suggested by more global contemporary social or political issues of relevance to the healthcare community. For example, HIV/AIDS, female feticide, sexual harassment, domestic violence, and gender equality in healthcare and in research are some of the current social and political issues of concern for healthcare professionals.

Brainstorming

Brainstorming sessions are good techniques to find new questions, where an intensified discussion among interested people of the profession is conducted to find more ideas to formulate a good research problem. For example, ideas for studies may emerge from reviewing research priorities by having brainstorming session with other nurses, researchers, or nursing faculties.

Intuition

Traditionally institutions are considered good sources of knowledge as well as sources to find new research problems. It is believed that reflective mind is good sources of ideas, which may be used to formulate a good research problem.

Folklores

Common beliefs could be right or wrong. Peoples have a variety of believe and practice which may affects the health conditions can be tested for right or wrong. Let's take a small example, it is generally believed that studying just before the test decrease the score. We believe we should not study just before test to relax our mind. Researchers can conduct a research study on whether one should study before the test or no. In this way the common myths can also be tested.

Exposure to Field Situations

During field exposure, researchers get variety of experiences, which may provide plenty of ideas to formulate research problems. For example, while working in field a researcher observed a specific traditional practice for cure of disease condition, which can be used as research problem to investigate its efficacy.

Consultation with Experts

Experts are believed to have sound experience of their respective field, which may suggest a significance problem to be studied. In addition, expert may help in finding a current problem of discipline to be solve, which may serve as basis for formulation of research problem.

RESEARCH PROBLEMS TO BE AVOIDED (FIG. 3.2)

The research problem undertaken for study must be carefully selected. Generally the less expert person or the students casually select any topic for research without knowing the consequences. Researcher use to conduct a research either for the partial fulfillment of her/his studies or publishing any index journal or presenting any national or international seminar. Even though it is for the partial fulfillment of her/his studies of publication purpose. It should be carefully selected because conducting study is not an easy or small thing. During selection the research has to avoid some of the problem statements which are described below. Otherwise he/she will face problems later during conducting studies.

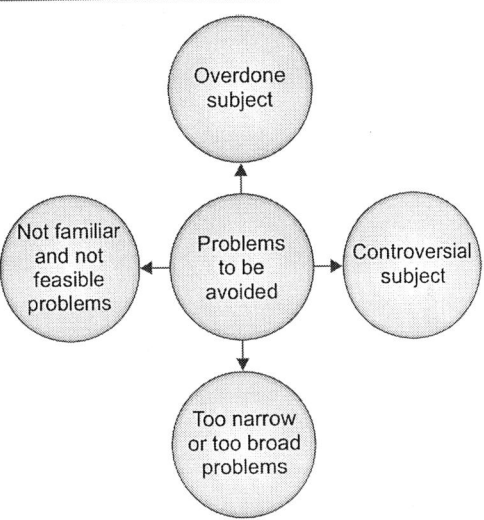

Fig 3.2: Research problems to be avoided.

Overdone Subject

Subject which is overdone should not be normally chosen because people are already aware about that and its results then what's the new in selecting such topic. For example, effectiveness of warm compress and back massage in reducing labor pain. If it is already proved by so many researcher that warm compress and back massage is helpful in reducing labor pain then no need to repeat again and again. In such types of studies the result said something new also it will create controversy.

Controversial Subject

So many subjects/problems having controversy on the result or the research or in the research methodology it is wise not to select such type of problem because there may be many issues that can arises due to controversy. So this type of research problems should be avoided.

Too Narrow or Too Broad Problems

Too narrow or too vague problems should be avoided. If a researcher select a too narrow research problem there will be difficult to get the reviews on that. It will be difficult in constructing tools on that and the generalization will be a limited group with limited area. Vague problem should be avoided because it is necessary that problem statement should be clear. Too broad problems should be avoided because it will be difficult to conduct due to too broad problem. For example a study on methods of family planning is too broad than only conventional contraceptive and it is also broad than only the emergency contraceptive pills. Similarly study to assess nutritional deficiency disorder is too broad which is difficult to conduct whereas a study to assess vitamin A deficiency disorders is narrower than it. Similarly a study to assess bitot spots due to vitamin A disorder is more narrower than the above two problem statements.

Not Familiar and Not Feasible Problems

The subject selected for research should be familiar and feasible so that the related research material or sources of research are within one's reach. Not familiar and not feasible problems should be avoided. The feasibility of research problem in reference to time, availability to subjects, facilities, equipment and money, and ethical considerations should be checked. The time needed for a research study is depend upon what type of the study that is based on which a problem statement may be select. The maximum allotment of time for an undergraduate (UG) or a postgraduate (PG) student will be one to two week. So a cross-sectional and quantitative studies should be selected by them. Similarly the researcher must consider realistically the financial resources available for research projects and the cost for conducting the study. Based on the capacity of the researcher to spend money or funding agency contracts the problem statement must be selected. Similarly availability to subjects, facilities, equipment and money, and ethical considerations and the qualification and expertise of the researcher must be taken into consideration.

CHARACTERISTICS OF A GOOD RESEARCH PROBLEM

The major characteristics of good research problem statement are (**Fig. 3.3**):

Interesting

This is a subjective criteria, the study must be interesting to the person who is conducting the study. It depends upon the individual's choice. Generally new study will be arouse interest of the researcher and others also. A research problem can only be considered good fit is an accordance with researcher's field of interest. A research problem must be as per the motivation of the researcher and it should be fascinating. It is one that grows as it is exercised and that provides the intensity of effort needed for overcoming the many hurdles and frustrations of the research process.

Solvable/Researchable

Problem selected is considered good only if it is solvable so that chances of insolvability of problem should be minimized. It will enhance relevant results. For example, a researcher selects a research problem to know the existence of God in this universe. These sorts of problems are ambiguous and impossible to solve. Therefore, the researcher must ensure that a research in the variables should be precisely defined and measured and lead to an answer to the question.

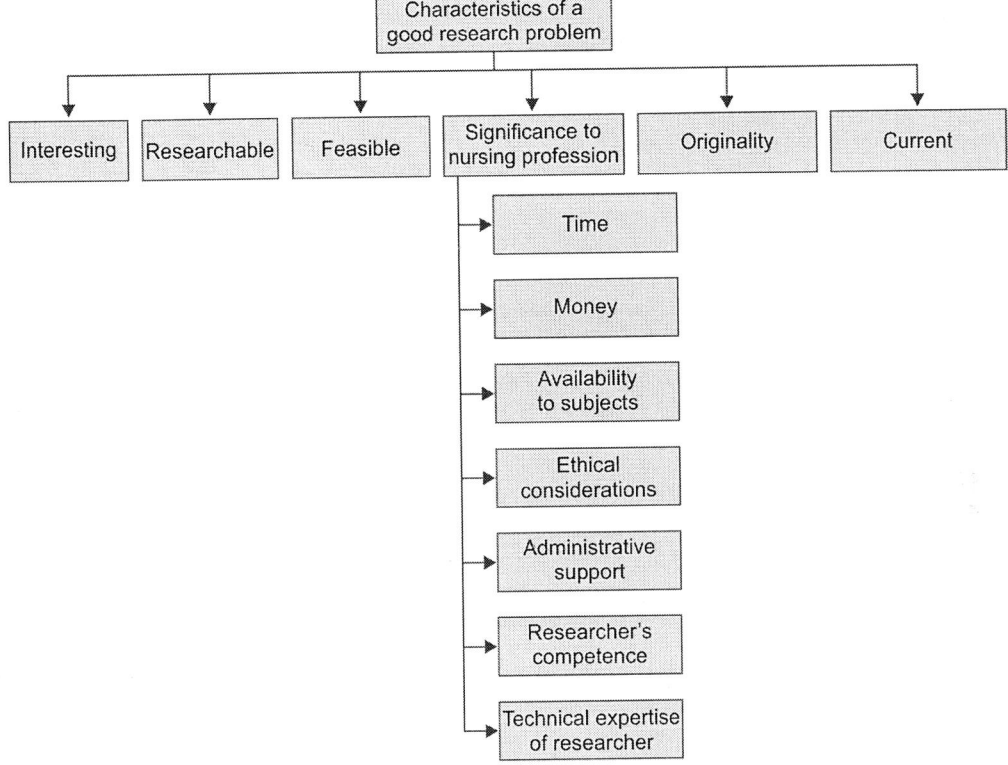

Fig. 3.3: Characteristics of a good research problem.

Feasible/Practicable

Before deciding to carry out the research project, or to select any research problem it must be observed whether it would be feasible to conduct? Can the study be conducted by the researcher? Feasibility is an essential consideration of any research project. Regardless of how significant or researchable a problem may be, the feasibility of research problem in reference to time, availability to subjects, facilities, equipment and money, and ethical considerations should be checked. It will help the researcher to decide whether selected problem is appropriate or inappropriate and study can be.

Significance to Nursing Profession

A problem which a researcher is selecting should have significance to nursing profession or it will not serve any purpose. A research problem is significant for nursing profession when it is directed to develop or refine, the body of professional knowledge. A research problem could be considered significant for nursing profession if it fulfills the following criteria: Patients, nurses, and generate information to get practical implications for nursing profession.
    Will the results make a difference that matters to the profession?
- Make a difference in patient care
- Add to professional practice knowledge
- Related to more general conceptual issues
- An instance of a larger class of events

- ❖ Provides solutions of current nursing practice needs
- ❖ Promotes nursing theory development or testing
- ❖ The results will improve clinical nursing practices
- ❖ Healthcare fraternity will benefit from the study

Time

The time needed for a research study is depend upon what type of the study that is. A longitudinal survey a correlational research study that involves repeated observations of the same variables over long periods of time—often many decade but a cross-sectional study is not like this. A qualitative generally takes more time than a quantitative study. Sufficient time should be allowed for a researcher for conducting a study. During selection of problem statement this factor must be considered otherwise the study cannot be completed.

Money

The researcher must consider realistically the financial resources available for research projects and the cost for conducting the study; some studies are much more expensive than others. Therefore, before making the final decision to conduct a study, an accurate determination of the needed equipment is essential. All research projects require some type of resources supplies. Supplies should be ensured and supplies in the early phases of a research project, ensure there are less chances of the project to be revised or discarded later because of equipment or supply. The feasibility of the study must be tested by assessing the ability to pay by the investigator or any funding agencies.

Availability to Subjects

Sometimes after selection of statement it is difficult to carry out the study due to unavailability of participant or participant in sufficient number. For example, the researcher selected a study on the effect of consanguineous marriage on their offspring's. For conducting such type of study such type couple is essential who had undergone consanguineous marriage which is very uncommon in Odisha. Only in south side of Odisha or in the state Andhra Pradesh these type of couple may available. Similarly if a researcher wants to conduct a study on assessing the cause of sickle cell anemia, she has to search the patient suffering with such disorders. So the availability to subjects can determine the feasibility of the study.

Ethical Considerations

A researcher must ensure that the research problem can be considered by the ethical committee without undue hurdles and unless it is in accordance with ethical guideline. If the study poses unacceptable physical risks or invasion of privacy the investigator must seek other ways to answer the question. If there is uncertainty about whether the study is ethical, it is helpful to discuss it at an early stage with a representative of the institutional review board.

Administrative Support

Financial as well as psychological support from administrative is very helpful. The nurse researcher may find it very difficult to conduct research independently. Many research projects require administrative support knowing that the superiors support the research efforts can be very powerful motivating force.

Researcher's Competence

A research problem can only be feasible if it is in accordance with researcher's competence. Researcher competence is essential in selection of problem statement selection of study subject and research design everything. During selection of problem statement the competence of researcher will also be obtained because all studies are not alike. Some studies can be carried out by less expertise person whereas for some other studies expert person is essential.

Technical Expertise of Researcher

The investigators must have the skills, equipment, and experience needed for designing the study, recruiting the subjects, measuring the variables, and managing and analyzing the data. Consultants can help to shore up technical aspects that are unfamiliar to the investigators, but for major areas of the study it is better to have an experienced colleague steadily involved as a coinvestigator.

Originality

It is fundamentally considered that every research problem should be new and unique in itself. Therefore, it is the key responsibility of a researcher that an innovative knowledge is used for selecting a research problem, so as to extend the growth of existing body of knowledge on a profession.

Current

A good research problem must be based on the current problems and needs of a profession, so that results generated will be of more use. Furthermore, more number of the professionals will be interested in the research conducted on the current issues of their profession.

QUALITIES OF A GOOD RESEARCH QUESTIONS

- It is grounded in a theoretical framework.
- It is builds on, but also offers something new to, previous research.
- It has the potential to suggest directions for future research.
- It is a purpose or question that the researcher is sincerely interested and/or invested in.
- It addresses directly or indirectly some real problem in the world.
- It takes ethical issues into consideration.
- It clearly states the variables or constructs to be examined.
- It is not biased in terminology or position.
- It has multiple possible answers.
- It is simple, or at least manageable.

STEPS IN DEVELOPING A RESEARCH PROBLEM (FIG. 3.4)

Decide on the General Area of Study or Investigation

The researcher will formulate of a research problem begins with selection of a broad research topic from personal experience, literature, previous research, and theories in which researcher

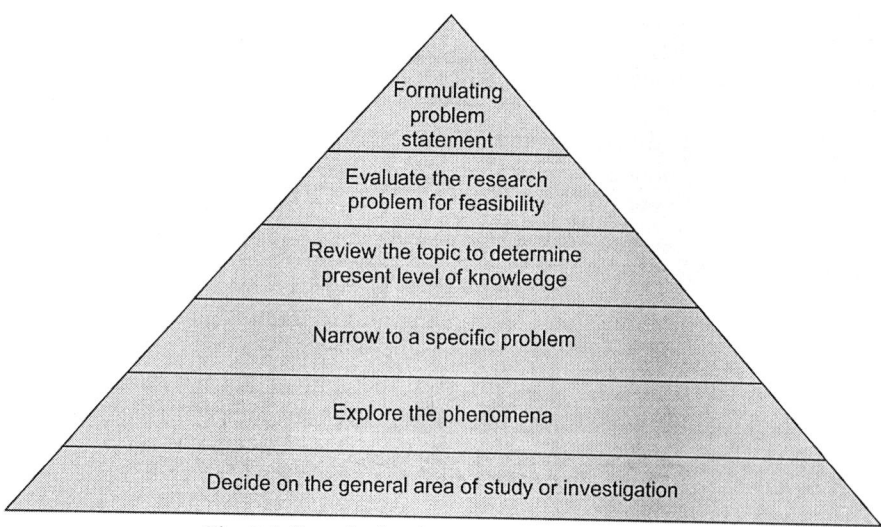

Fig. 3.4: Steps in developing a research problem.

is interested and has significance for nursing profession. Some broad general ideas about things that makes wonder the researcher in practice can be selected. It depends upon the researcher's interest. Choosing a topic in a familiar area will help to make decisions about the need for further research in the area, as well as the feasibility of particular research approaches but here the researcher will select abroad topic. For example, a researcher will select a topic on nutritional deficiencies. Therefore, he or she initially begins with such broad research.

Explore the Phenomena

Phenomena mean a fact or situation that is observed to exist or happen, especially one whose cause or explanation is in question. The researcher will explores the different specific area on which the study can be conducted on this. He/she will identify different specific areas under that broad areas. For example, in the area of nutritional deficiencies what are the specific areas, such as under nutrition, vitamin A deficiencies disorders, iodine deficiencies disorders and nutritional anemia's and so on which is more prevalent. In this stage, the investigator will undergo the review also.

Narrow the Topic to a Specific Problem

In this step, researcher proceeds from a general area of interest to more specific topic of research to conduct a study. For example, from the area of nutritional deficiencies the researcher will select any specific problem like vitamin A deficiencies disorders and formulate the statement 'A study to assess the vitamin A deficiencies disorders among school going children'.

Review the Topic to Determine Present Level of Knowledge

After getting a problem for research, he or she needs to review the nursing literature and theories. Literature is reviewed to know what has already been done in this selected area of research. Review of nursing theories provides an opportunity for nurses researcher to plan a research problem to contribute towards either testing or development of a theory/conceptual model. What different studies are already done on this weather select problem is appropriate or not.

Evaluate the Research Problem for Feasibility

Once researcher is clear about the specific research problem, next the research problem must be carefully evaluated for its significance, research ability, and feasibility. Feasibility of the research problem should be evaluated for time, cost, availability of subjects and resources, administrative and peer support, ethical consideration, researcher's competence and interest.

Formulating Final Statement of Research Problem

After establishing the significance, research ability, and feasibility, then researcher finally formulates a final statement of a research problem. A statement of research problem could be in declarative or interrogative format. Example of declarative or statement form of problem statement, a study to assess the effectiveness of video assisted teaching module (VATM) regarding prevention of malnutrition among under-fives on knowledge of the mothers in a selected rural community, Odisha and the same problem statement in question form is, what is the effectiveness of VATM regarding prevention of malnutrition among under-fives on knowledge of the mothers in Odisha?

CRITERIA FOR DEVELOPING PROBLEM STATEMENT

Clear and Unambiguous

The problem statement should be stated clearly and unambiguously, between 10 and 15 words long and should clearly identify for the reader the purpose of the study. The problem statements that are too long or too short can be confusing or misleading. The researcher has to find out whether the title clear, accurate and unambiguous or not.

Relationship between Variables

The problem statement in quantitative studies should depict the relationship between two or more variables. Generally, a problem statement consist at least two variables named dependent and independent variable but sometime more than two variables, for example, effectiveness of warm compress and back massage on 1st stage of labor pain. In this problem statement the relationship between two independent variables and one dependent variable exist. Sometime in descriptive or qualitative studies there is only one variable known as research variable.

Possibility of Empirical Testing

The problem statement should imply the possibility of empirical testing which means practical applicability. During selecting the researcher will judge the significances of research problem statement which is planned to be done.

RESEARCH OBJECTIVES

Concept and Definitions

Research is an organized investigation of a problem in which there is an attempt to gain solution to a problem. Clearly defined objectives enlighten the way in which the researcher has to proceed to get right solution of a right problem. Sometime objectives are directed towards identifying the relationship or difference between two variables. Generally research objective focus on the ways to measure the variables, such as to identify or describe them objective should be closely related to the statement of the problem. A research objective is a clear, concise, declarative statement, which provides direction to investigate the variables. That are the results sought by the researcher at the end of the research process, i.e., what the researcher will be able to achieve at the end of the research study. The objectives of a research project summarize what is to be achieved by the study research objectives is a concrete statement describing what the research is trying to achieve.

Definitions of Objectives

- Objectives can be broadly defined as a general statement which attempts to give both shape and direction to set off more detailed intention for the future. —*Davis, 1999*
- It is also defined as a broad general statement of goal direction which contains reference to the worth whileness of achieving it. —*Sankaranarayanan, 2000*

Definition of Research Objectives

- Research objectives are clear concise declarative statement expressed in the present tense and measure through statistical method.
- Research objective is the specific accomplishment of the researcher that hopes to achieve by conducting the study. The objectives include obtaining answer to research questions or testing research hypothesis.

Characteristics of Research Objectives (Fig. 3.5)

A well-worded objective will be SMART, (i.e., specific, measurable, attainable, realistic, and time-bounded). It should be relevant, feasible, logical, observable, and unequivocal.

Other than this it should be logical, unequivocal, feasible, and observable.

The overall objectives of research project characteristics summarizes below:

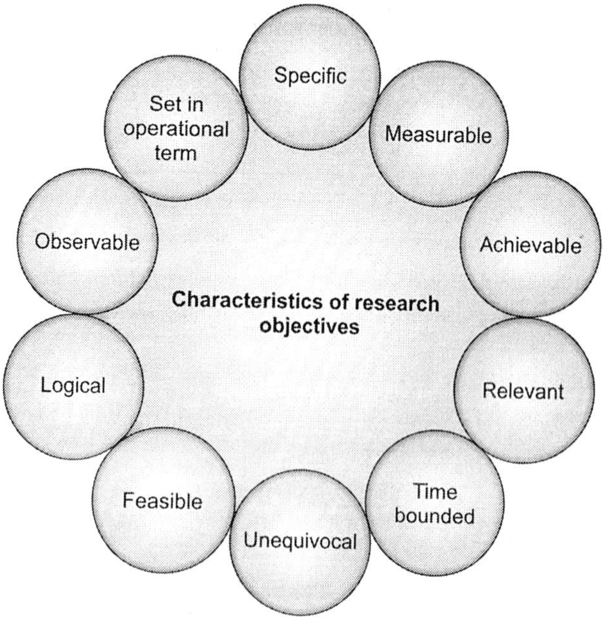

Specific

The objectives should be simple indicating what to achieve, sensible which means it should be practicable and significant not trivial.

Measurable

Fig. 3.5: Characteristics of research objectives.

The existence of a criterion for measurement will make it easier to choose or in construct a valid evaluation mechanism. The objectives can be measurable means it can be evaluated how much fully objectives achieved, partially achieved or not achieved. It should be meaningful and motivating.

Achievable

Achievable means it should not be beyond our capacities and can be attainable within our limited resources.

Relevant

Relevancy means reasonable, realistic or applicable. It should be free of any superfluous material but cover every point relating to the aim in view. In case of nursing research the objectives should be relevant to nursing research only.

Time bounded

Time-based, time limited, time/cost limited, timely, time-sensitive.
Other than this it should be logical, unequivocal, feasible, observable.

Unequivocal

Equivocal means allowing the possibility of several different meanings which create biases. The objectives should be unequivocal means free from biases. The research objectives should be clearly stated what the researcher will be achieved at last.

Feasible

The objectives is feasible means achievable. It should be achievable within specific period of time, with limited planned budget, with the limited sample sizes and with the target setup and so on. Finally if it is possible to achieve that objectives than we can tell the objective is feasible.

Logical

The objective must be logical means rational. We cannot write research objectives by our own. The objective must be internally consistent. We cannot change research objectives by our own.

Observable

Unless there is some means of observing progress towards 'an objective, it will be impossible to tell whether the objective has been achieved.

Importance of Research Objective

- The formulation of research objectives will help researcher for solving problem that he or she has defined.
- The formulation of research objectives helps the researcher avoid the collection of data which are not strictly necessary for understanding.
- With clearly defined objectives, the researchers can focus on the study.
- Properly formulated, specific objectives will facilitate the development of research methodology. The formulation of objectives organize the study in clearly defined parts or phases and will help to orient the collection, analysis, interpretation, and utilization of data.

Types of Research Objective

Generally research objectives are classified as two types:

General Objectives

The general objectives of the study state what the researcher expects to achieve by the study in general terms. General objectives are broad goals to be achieved. It is corresponding to the function of researcher/learner after completion of study. That means according to the problem what achievement was gain by researcher?

Specific Objectives

General objectives can break into small logically connected parts to form specific objectives. Specific objectives are narrow goals. They systematically address various aspects of problem as defined under 'the statement of problem' and they should specify what the researcher will do in the study, where, key factor that is assumed to influence or causes the problem and for what purpose? The specific objectives corresponding or desired from precise professional task whose result are observable and measurable against given criteria.

Objectives of Research According to Different Types of Study

The objective of research is different according to different types of study. The main purpose of research is to find out truth which is hidden and which has not been discovered as yet.

Through each research study has its own specific purpose, we may think of research objectives as following into a number of following broad group headings.

- To gain familiarity with a phenomenon or to achieve new insight into it (studies with this object in view are termed as exploratory or formulative research studies).
- To portray accurately the characteristics of a particular individual situation or group (studies with this object in view are known as descriptive research studies).
- To determine the frequency with which something occurs or with which it is associated with something else (studies with this object in view are known as diagnostic research studies).
- To test a hypothesis of a casual relationship between variables (hypothesis testing, research studies).

Objectives	Uses
To identify	For identification of variables under the study: A study to identify the factors associated with malnutrition among urban slum under-five children. For the problem statement the overall objective is to identify the factors associated with malnutrition among urban slum under-five children
To describe	For description of the variables under the study: Describing the characteristics or variables generally followed in descriptive research or qualitative research. To descriptive the perception of patients towards health care
To determine	To find out the difference between the variables: To determine means to evaluate. A study to assess effectiveness of music therapy on reducing pain among postoperative patients in selected hospitals, Odisha. Here the objective is to determine the effectiveness of music therapy on reducing pain among postoperative patients
To compare or to associate	To find rational between the variables: A study to compare the effectiveness of drumstick leaves powder and homo nutria ladu in reduction of anemia. The objective may be to compare the effectiveness of drumstick leaves powder and homo nutria ladu in reduction of anemia Other examples are "to find out the association between postoperative knowledge scores of adolescence girls with their selected demographic variables"

Chapter 3: Research Problems, Objectives, Variables Hypothesis, Delimitation, and Assumptions

For a problem statement 'A study to assess the effectiveness of VATM regarding prevention of malnutrition among under-fives on knowledge of the mothers in a selected rural community'. The general objectives will be: to assess the effectiveness of video-assisted teaching module regarding prevention of malnutrition on knowledge of the mother among under-five children

- To assess the knowledge of mothers regarding prevention of malnutrition among under-five children before implementation of VATM.
- To develop a video-assisted teaching module on knowledge of mothers regarding prevention of malnutrition among under-five children.
- To assess the knowledge of mothers regarding prevention of malnutrition among under-five children after implementation of VATM.
- To differentiate pre and post-test knowledge score
- To compare knowledge of mothers regarding prevention of malnutrition among under-five children with their selected demographic variables.
- To find out association between the post-test KS of mothers with their selected demographic variables.

Similarly for a study effectiveness of self-instructional module (SAM) on knowledge of adolescent girls regarding breast self-examination to prevent breast cancer in selected girls high schools (Cuttack). In this study, the general objective is:

- To assess the effectiveness of self-instructional module on knowledge of adolescent girls regarding breast self-examination to prevent breast cancer
- To assess the knowledge of adolescent girls regarding breast self-examination to prevent breast cancer before implementation of self-instructional module
- To develop a self-instructional module on knowledge of adolescent girls regarding breast self-examination to prevent breast cancer
- To assess the knowledge of adolescent girls regarding breast self-examination to prevent breast cancer after implementation of self-instructional module
- To compare knowledge of adolescent girls regarding breast self-examination to prevent breast cancer with their selected demographic variables
- To find out association between the post-test KS of adolescent girls regarding breast self-examination to prevent breast cancer with their selected demographic variables

For a research study to identify the associated risk factors of malnutrition among under-five children in a selected urban slum area, Berhampur, Ganjam, Odisha. In this problem statement, the general objective for this study is, to identify the associated risk factors among under-five children in a selected urban slum area.

- The specific objectives for this study is:
  - To assess the prevalence of malnutrition among under-five children
  - To assess the risk factors of malnutrition among under-five children
  - To determine the relationship of prevalence of malnutrition with its risk factors.

Similarly for a research study, "Effectiveness of curry leaf powder on reduction of blood sugar among diabetes patient in a selected community."

- The general objective is to assess the effectiveness of curry leaf powder on reduction of blood sugar among diabetes clients.
- Specific objectives are:
  - To assess blood sugar level among diabetic clients before administration of curry leaf powder in experimental group.
  - To assess blood sugar level among diabetic clients before administration of curry leaf powder in control group

- To prepare curry leave powder and prepares pouches with adequate amount of curry leave powder for single administration and administer in experimental group
- To assess blood sugar level among diabetic clients after administration of curry leaf powder in experimental group.
- To assess blood sugar level among diabetic clients after administration of curry leaf powder in control group
- To compare the changes in sugar level within the experimental and control groups.

Table 3.1: Action verbs used for objectives in cognitive domain.

Remember	Understand	Apply	Analyze	Evaluate	Create
• Define	• Choose	• Apply	• Analyze	• Appraise	• Arrange
• Identify	• Cite examples of	• Demonstrate	• Appraise	• Assess	• Assemble
• List	• Demonstrate use of	• Dramatize	• Calculate	• Choose	• Collect
• Name	• Describe	• Employ	• Categorize	• Compare	• Compose
• Recall	• Determine	• Generalize	• Compare	• Critique	• Construct
• Recognize	• Differentiate between	• Illustrate	• Conclude	• Estimate	• Create
• Record	• Discriminate	• Interpret	• Contrast	• Evaluate	• Design
• Relate	• Discuss	• Operate	• Correlate	• Judge	• Develop
• Repeat	• Explain	• Operationalize	• Criticize	• Measure	• Formulate
• Underline selects, States	• Express	• Practice	• Deduce	• Rate	• Manage
	• Give in own words	• Relate	• Debate	• Revise	• Modify
	• Identify	• Schedule	• Detect	• Score	• Organize
	• Interpret	• Shop	• Determine	• Select	• Plan
	• Locate	• Use	• Develop	• Validate	• Prepare
	• Pick	• Utilize	• Diagram	• Value	• Produce
	• Report	• Initiate	• Differentiate	• Test	• Propose
	• Restate		• Distinguish		• Predict
	• Review		• Draw conclusions		• Reconstruct
	• Recognize		• Estimate		• Set-up
	• Select		• Evaluate		• Synthesize
	• Tell		• Examine		• Systematize
	• Translate		• Experiment		• Devise
	• Respond		• Identify		
	• Practice		• Infer		
	• Simulates		• Inspect		
			• Inventory		
			• Predict		
			• Question		
			• Relate		
			• Solve		
			• Test		
			• Diagnose		

VARIABLES CONCEPT

In Layman statement variables is something that can change and or can have more than one value. 'A variable, as the name implies, is something that varies'. It may be weight, height, anxiety levels, income, body temperature and so on. Each of these properties varies from one person to another and also has different values along a continuum. It could be demographic, physical or social and include religion, income, occupation, temperature, humidity, language, food, fashion, etc. Some variables can be quite concrete and clear, such as gender, birth order, types of blood group, etc., while others can be considerably more abstract and vague. Thus the variables are quality property or characteristics of person things or situation that changes or vary.

Types of Variables

There are three types of classification of variables:
1. Independent and dependent variables
2. Extraneous and confounding variables
3. Continuous and categorical variables

Dependent Variables

Dependent variables act as the effect in that they change as a result of being influenced by an independent variable. The dependent variable is the variable a researcher is interested in. The changes to the dependent variable are what the researcher is trying to measure with all their fancy techniques. For example, a nurse researcher had undergone study on effectiveness of back massage and warm compress on reducing labor pain in 1st stage of labor among prime gravida mothers in labor room of selected hospital, here the dependent variable is labor pain of prime gravid mothers which will be going to reduce.

Independent Variable

Independent variables act as the 'cause' in that they precede, influence, and predict the dependent variable. An independent variable is a variable believed to affect the dependent variable. This is the variable that the researcher, will manipulate to see if it makes the dependent variable change. In above example, back massage and warm compress are the dependent variable. To reiterate, the independent variable is the thing over which the researcher is manipulating. In this study, the researcher is manipulating the labor pain of prime gravid women by back massage and warm compress which are the independent variable. The dependent variable is believed to be dependent on the independent variable.

Active and Attribute Variables

Variables are often characteristics of research subjects, such as their age, health beliefs, or weight, etc., which cannot be manipulated are attribute variables and the variables that the researcher creates are the active variables. Active variables can also be called as independent variables, e.g., effectiveness of self-instructional module on knowledge of staff nurses regarding infection control in labor room. Here active variable is self-instructional module which is also called independent variables.

Discrete Variables

Discrete variables also called categorical variables belongs to a kind of measurement called nominal. In nominal measurements there are two or more subsets of the set objects being measured. 'They have a simple requirement that all the members of the subset are considered the same and all are assigned the same name (nominal) and the same numeral.' That is, they can be measured only in terms of whether the individual items belong to certain distinct categories, but we cannot quantify or even rank order the categories. These variables has restricted category. Gender has two categories, male and female and socioeconomic status has three categories—low, middle and high. These variables take on only a handful of discrete nonquantitative values are categorical variables.

Continuous Variables

Sometimes variables take on a wide range of values on a continuum. 'A continuous variable can assume an infinite number of values between two points.' If we consider the continuous variable weight between 1 and 2 kg, the number of values is limitless: 1.005, 1.7, 1.33333, and so on. Continuous measures in actual use are contained in a range continuous variables are measured on a scale that theoretically can take on an infinite number of values test scores range from a low of 0 to a high of 100, attitude scales, students' age score are the example of continuous variables. Continuous variables can be converted to categorical or discrete variables, but categorical variables cannot be converted to continuous variables, i.e., IQ is a continuous variable, but the researcher can choose to group students into three levels based on IQ scores—low is below a score of 84, middle is between 85 and 115, and high is above 116 test scores are continuous, but teachers typically assign letter grades on a ten point scale (i.e., at or below 59 is an F, 60 to 69 is a D, 70 to 79 is a C, 80–89 is a B, and 90 to 100 is an A).

Extraneous Variables

Extraneous variables are those that affect the dependent variable but are not controlled adequately by the researcher. Sometimes after completion of the study we wonder that the actual result is different than what we expected. In spite of taking all the possible measures the outcome is unexpected. It is because of extraneous variables. Variables that may affect research outcomes but have not been adequately considered in the study are termed as extraneous variables. Extraneous variables exist in all studies and can affect the measurement of study variables and the relationship among these variables. 'Extraneous variables that are not recognized until the study is in process.' It is known as the issue of contaminating factors means it will contaminate the study and change the study results. For example, in a problem statement effects of drumstick leave powder on increasing hemoglobin's level among anemic adolescent girls the extraneous variables are diet iron tablets and so on. Even though we will try to control the extraneous variable sometime it's difficult to control in natural situation. We cannot control the diet of girl even we try a lot also. If we can control on extraneous variables then only our study will be fruitful.

Confounding Variables

Confounding variables are those that vary systematically with the independent variable and exert influence of the dependent variable. Confounding variables recognized before the study is initiated but cannot be controlled, are referred to as confounding variables. They can influence the outcome of a study in a ways that are not intended by the investigator. These variables are not a part of primary investigation but exist as a part of the investigation. Since the majority of nursing studies take place in the real world with human subjects, it is impossible to eliminate confounding variables are used interchangeable.

For example, effect of a planned exercise and training program on weight reduction and blood pressure control among hypertensive patients. In given experimental study age, gender, in other sociodemographic variables are considered as demographic variables are considered as confounding variable and could affect study results.

❖ **Intervening variables:** Certain external variables may influence the relationship between the research variables, even though researcher cannot see it. These variables are called *intervening variables*. For example, girl's knowledge and practices helps in maintaining menstrual hygiene. Here, motivation, mother and friends, mass media, are some intervening

variables which may also help in maintaining menstrual hygiene. Thus, if these two factors are not controlled it would be impossible to know what the underlying cause really is.
* **Demographic variables:** Demographic variables are characteristics or attributes of subjects that are collected to describe the sample. They are also called sample characteristics. It means these variables describe study sample and determine if samples are representative of the population of interest. Although demographic variables cannot be manipulated, researchers can explain relationships between demographic variables and dependent variables. Some common demographic variables are age, gender, occupation, marital status, income, etc.

Research Variables

In descriptive, exploratory, comparative and qualitative research studies, variables are observed or measured in natural setting as they exist without manipulating or imposing the effect of intervention or treatment. Here no independent variable is manipulated and no cause effect relationship is examined. These variables are considered as research variable. Therefore research variables can be defined as qualities, attributes, properties, or characteristics which are observed or measured in a natural setting without manipulating and establishing cause effect relationship.

For example, an exploratory study on factors responsible for upper respiratory tract infection (URTI) among women on reproductive age group is a research variable, which is observed in natural setting without manipulating it.

In nonexperimental research (descriptive, exploratory, comparative, correlational) and qualitative studies variables are observed in natural setting without undue manipulation or change. These variable are observed to describe or explore a particular phenomenon, called research variables.

For example, a descriptive study on burden and coping strategies among caregiver of mentally ill patients. In this study, 'burden' and 'coping strategies' are research variables.

According to variables the studies are classified into three types, they are:

1. **Univariate study:** When there is only one variable in the study all, that can be termed as univariate study, e.g., 'a study to assess the knowledge of adolescent girls regarding reproductive health care' or 'a study to assess the prevalence of malnutrition among school going children in urban slum area'. These studies are having only one variable hence called as univariate study.
2. **Bivariate study:** These studies are having two variables one dependent and one independent variables. These studies are generally experimental studies. The example of these types of studies are 'effectiveness of planned teaching program on knowledge of staff nurses regarding infection control in labor room'. Here there are two variables one dependent, i.e., knowledge of staff nurses regarding infection control and another independent planned teaching program. These types of studies are bivariate study.
3. **Multivariate study:** When the studies are having more than two variables they are called multivariate studies. The studies may have more than one dependent and/or more than one independent variables, e.g., effectiveness of planned teaching program on knowledge and practice of staff nurses regarding infection control in labor room. Here one independent variable planned teaching program but two dependent variable knowledge and practice. Another example is 'effectiveness of warm compress and back massage on reducing labor pain in 1st stage of labor among prime gravid mothers admitted in labor room of a selected hospital'. Here two independent variables warm compress and back massage and one dependent variable is reducing labor pain in 1st stage of labor. These type of studies are called multivariate study.

HYPOTHESIS CONCEPT

The word hypothesis is derived from the Greek words 'hypo' means under 'tithemi' means place. Hypothesis explain the known facts (variables) of the problem to explain relationship between these. It is a tentative prediction or explanation about the relationship between variables. A hypothesis is not a question, but rather it is a statement about the relationship between two or more variables. It helps to translate the research problem and objectives into a clear explanation or prediction of the expected results or outcomes of the research study. A hypothesis is the tool of quantitative studies usually only found in experimental quantitative research studies. A hypothesis thus translates a quantitative research question into a precise prediction of expected outcomes. In qualitative studies, researchers do not begin with a hypothesis, in part because there is usually too little known about the topic to justify a hypothesis, and in part because qualitative researchers want the inquiry to be guided by participants' viewpoints rather than by their own to be complete a hypothesis must include three components:
1. The variables
2. The population
3. The relationship between the variables

Definitions

- Hypothesis is proposition, condition or principle which is assumed, perhaps without belief, in order to draw its logical consequences and by this method to test its accord with facts which are known or may be determined (Webster's New International Dictionary of English).
- A tentative statement about something, the validity of which is usually unknown (Black JA, Champion DJ. Method and Issues in Social Research, New York: John Wiley and Sons, Inc, 1976).
- Hypothesis is proposition that is stated is a testable form and that predicts a particular relationship between two or more variable. In other words, if we think that a relationship exists, we first state it is hypothesis and then test hypothesis in the field (Baily KD. Methods of Social Research, 3rd edition. New York: The Free Press, 1978).
- A hypothesis is a formal statement of the expected relationship or relationship between two variables in a specified population (Nanci Burn, 2005).
- Hypothesis is written in such a way that it can be proven or disproven by valid and reliable data—in order to obtain these data that we perform our study (Grinnell R Jr. Social Work Research and Evaluation, 3rd edition, Itasca, Illinois, FE Peacock Publishers, 1988).
- A hypothesis may be defined as a tentative theory or supposition set up and adopted provisionally as a basis of explaining certain facts or relationships and as a guide in the further investigation of other facts or relationships (Crisp RD. Marketing Research, New York: McGraw Hill Book Co., 1957).

Purposes of Hypothesis

- It provides bridge between theory and reality and in this sense unifying of two domains.
- It provides powerful tool, for the advancement of knowledge since they enable the researcher to objectively enter new areas of discovery.
- It provides direction for any research endeavor by tentatively identifying the anticipated outcome.
- It is guide to the thinking process and the process of discovery.
- It serves as a framework for drawing conclusions.

Importance of Hypothesis in Quantitative Studies (Fig. 3.6)

Hypotheses Provide Objectivity to the Research Activity

Hypotheses enable the researcher to objectively investigate new areas of discovery. Thus, it provides a powerful tool for the advancement of knowledge and hypotheses provides clear relevance of data and specific goals to the researchers. These clear and specific goals provide the investigator with a basis for selecting sample and research procedures to meet these goals. Hypotheses facilitates objectivity in data collection.

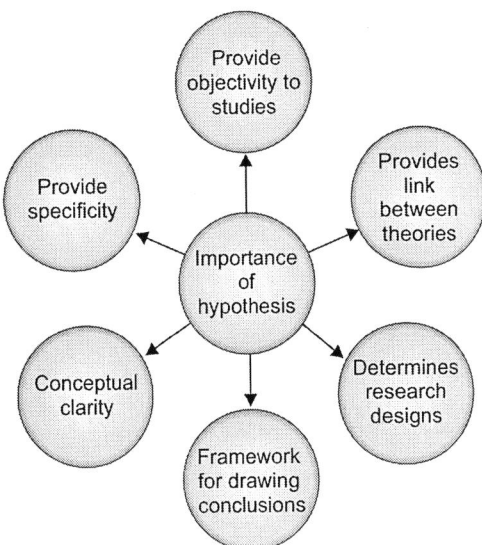

Fig. 3.6: Importance of hypothesis.

Hypotheses Provides Link Between Theories

It provides a bridge between theory and actual practical researches, and it stimulates the thinking process of researcher as the researcher forms the hypothesis by anticipating the outcome.

Determines Research Designs

As it is a tentative statement of anticipated results, it guides the researcher towards the direction in which the research should proceed. A hypothesis suggests which type of research designs is likely to be most appropriate. So it determines the most appropriate research designs without hypotheses, research would be like aimless.

It Serves as Framework for Drawing Conclusions of a Research Study

Hypotheses provide understanding to the researchers about what expect from the results of the research study. During hypothesis testing the result of the study weather sign, there is significant relationship or not is obtained. So hypothesis itself is a framework for drawing conclusions of a research study.

Conceptual Clarity

Hypothesis should consist of clearly defined and understandable concepts which should be stated in very terms, the meaning and empirical referents. Research must have an ultimate empirical referent. No usable hypothesis can embody moral judgments. A good hypothesis must have empirical basis from the area of enquiry implication of which cannot be doubted. To facilitate the conceptual clarity, hypothesis can be stated in declarative statement, in present tense.

Provide Specificity

Hypothesis should be specific, not general, keeps the research activity free from researcher value—judgment and should explain the expected relations between variables. For example, regular yoga reduces stress.

Characteristics of Hypothesis

- Unknown validity
- Specifies relation between two or more variables
- Researchable
- Stated in declarative form
- State, in definite terms, the relationship between variables
- Testable
- Follow the findings of previous studies
- Be related to a body of theory
- Tentative proposition

Functions of Hypothesis

- Bringing clarity to the research problem
- Provides a study with focus
- Signifies what specific aspects of a research problem is to investigate
- What data to be collected and what not to be collected
- Enhancement of objectivity of the study
- Formulate the theory
- Enable to conclude with what is true or what is false

Types of Hypothesis

- Null and alternative hypothesis
- Simple and complex hypothesis
- Directional and nondirectional hypothesis
- Casual and associative hypothesis

Null and Alternative Hypothesis

Null Hypothesis

A null hypothesis is designated as Ho which shows there is no relationship between variables.

It is contrary to the positive statement made in the alternate hypothesis formulated to disprove the contrary of an alternate hypothesis. When a researcher rejects a null hypothesis, he/she actually proves alternate hypothesis. In statistics, to mean a null hypothesis usually Ho is used. Typically will imply no association between explanatory and response variables in our applications, e.g., $H0_1$; There is no significant difference between the pre and post-test KS of mothers with under-five children regarding prevention of malnutrition.

Alternate Hypothesis

The alternative hypothesis states that the population parameter is different than the value of the population parameter in the null hypothesis. The alternative hypothesis is what you might believe to be true or hope to prove true. An alternate hypothesis is formulated when a researcher totally rejects null hypothesis. He/she develops such hypothesis with adequate reasons. Alternate hypothesis statement contradictory to the null hypothesis, e.g., H1; There is significant difference between the pre and post-test KS of mothers with under-five children regarding prevention of malnutrition.

Simple and Complex Hypothesis

Simple Hypothesis

Simple hypothesis express relationship between one dependent and one independent variable. It may be null or may be alternative but when there is one dependent and one independent variables we can called that as simple hypothesis.

For example, there is no significant association between the pre and post-test knowledge score of adolescent girls regarding reproductive health care after implementation of video-assisted teaching module.

Another example is two hourly positions—changing of a fully bedridden patient will prevent bedsore. In the example 2 hourly positions changing is independent variable and bedsore prevention is dependent variable. The statement shows that there exists a relationship between 2 hourly positioning and bedsore prevention.

Complex Hypothesis

When the hypothesis express relationship between more than one dependent and/or more than one independent variable we can called it as complex hypothesis. Example—for a fully bed ridden patent 2 hourly position changing, 2 hourly back care and a high protein diet will build up body resistance, will promote blood circulation and will prevent bedsore. In the above example, three independent variable are: (1) 2 hourly position changing, (2) 2 hourly back care, (3) high protein diet and three dependent variable are: (1) promotion of blood circulation, (2) building up of body resistance, (3) prevention of bedsore. Another example of complex hypothesis is 'The post-test mean knowledge and practice score of staff nurses regarding infection control in labor room will be high then the pretest mean knowledge and practice score after implementation of planned teaching program'. Here one independent variable planned teaching program but two dependent variable knowledge and practice score. Another example is warm compress and back massage will be reduce labor pain in 1st stage of labor'. Here two independent variables warm compress and back massage and one dependent variable is labor pain in 1st stage of labor. In all of the above example there is either more than one dependent or independent variables so these are consider as complex hypothesis.

Directional and Nondirectional Hypothesis

Directional Hypothesis

Directional hypothesis specifies not only the existence, but also the expected direction of the relationship between variables when direction of relationship exist it specify some direction, e.g., mean pretest knowledge score will be more than mean post-test knowledge score. Directional hypothesis express the direction of relationship between variables by using some directional terms that are positive, negative, less, more, increased, decreased, greater, higher, lower, etc. It is directional because it predicts that there will be a difference between the two groups and it specifies how the two groups will differ example high quality of nursing education will lead to high quality of nursing practice skills.

Nondirectional Hypothesis

When direction of relationship does not exist, if past research providing conflicting result and the researcher is confused regarding the result in that case a researcher can adopt non-directional hypothesis. Here nature of the relationship between two or more variables, such as positive, negative, or no relationship has not specified and the hypothesis simply predicts that there will be a difference between the two groups, then it is a nondirectional hypothesis. It is nondirectional because it predicts that there will be a difference but does not specify how the groups will differ. Example, teacher student relationship influence student's learning here the direction of relation does not exist.

Casual and Associative Hypothesis

Casual Hypothesis

Casual hypothesis predicts a cause and effects relationship or interaction between the independent variable and dependent variable. This hypothesis predicts the effect of the independent variable on the dependent variable. In this the independent variable is the experimental or treatment variable. The dependent variable is the outcome variable identify cause effect interaction when there is treatment, e.g., early postoperative ambulation will lead to prompt recovery. Or another example is 'planned teaching module will be enhancing the knowledge of adolescent girls regarding reproductive health care'.

Associative Hypothesis

Associative hypothesis predicts an associative relationship between the independent variable and the dependent variable. When there is a change in any one of the variables, changes also occurs in the other variable. Relationships is associative when there is no treatment variables occur or exist together. The associative relationship between the independent and dependent variables may have either positive association or negative association.

DELIMITATIONS

Concept

Delimitations are boundaries that are set by the researcher in order to control the range of a study. They are created before any investigations are carried out, in order to reduce the amount of time spent in certain areas that may be seen to be unnecessary, and perhaps even unrelated, to the overall study. The delimitations are those characteristics that limit the scope and define the boundaries of the study which are in the control of researcher. Delimiting factors include the choice of objectives, the research questions, variables of interest, theoretical perspectives that was adopted (as opposed to what could have been adopted), and the population chosen for investigation. The first delimitation was the choice of problem itself implying there are other related problems that could have been chosen but were rejected or screened off from view. The purpose statement explains the intent that clearly sets out the intended accomplishments, and also includes an implicit or explicit understanding of what the study will not cover. This section of the study will explicate the criteria of participants to enroll in the study, the geographic region covered in the study, and the profession or organizations involved. It will also explicate the criteria of participants to enroll in the research study.

The researcher makes conscious exclusionary and inclusionary decisions regarding the geographical location of the study, study setting, sample size, the variables studies the theoretical perspectives, the instrument, the generality, etc.

In delimitations following parameters are identified and addressed to clearly define the scope of study and to make the study more feasible.

- Confinement of a particular geographical area or study setting/study center, e.g., this study was limited to the single health care center of the city because of limited time and funds for study.
- The population, which the researcher is not studying, e.g., this study will be restricted to nurses with diploma qualification.
- Defining the restriction about sampling technique/sampling size, e.g., in the present study, samples was not drawn using random sampling technique, because of nonavailability of sampling frame.
- The literature will not review, e.g., in the present study only locally published studies were considered for literature review and for the discussion of the study findings, because of the inability to access international literature.
- The methodological procedures will not use, e.g., in the present study, randomized control trial design was not used because of quasi nature of independent variable.
- The particular tools was not used for the study, e.g., researcher was limited to data collected through telephonic method because of limited time for the present study.
- The things that researcher are not doing, e.g., the researcher limited the follow-up of patients for only five days because as per hospital protocol, patients who underwent laparotomy are discharged on the fifth postoperative day.

Overall delimitation are the choices made by the researcher that should be mentioned in the research study. They describe the boundaries' that researcher has set for the study. The parameters used are:

- The study does not cover.
- The researcher limited this research.

Let us take an example, if a study was selected 'to assess the knowledge of mothers of under-five children regarding prevention of malnutrition in a rural community' the delimitations in selection of samples are, the mothers who were:

- Living in selected rural community
- Having one or more under-five children
- Able to understand and speak the language developed in tool
- Willing to participate in the study
- Present during the period of data collection

The delimitation is fully depends upon the researcher. The researcher for his conveniences can makes the delimitation as which characteristics he will accept for his/her study. In above study the researcher had developed a tool in a local language but some migrant people may not be understood it and the researcher does not have enough resource to develop another tool which can be understood by migrant people or can provide a translator who can translate it in that language.

Uses of Delimitation

- The delimitation of the study is delimiting a study by geographical location, age, sex, population traits, population size and other similar consideration. It is used to make study better and more feasible and practicable and not just for the interest of the researcher.
- It is also identifies the constraints or weakness of the study which are not control by the researcher, so that strengthening of evidence.
- The delimitations generated through study may be determined.
- It helps to clearly define the scope of the study to avoid the parametric ambiguities in the research study.

- Define the boundaries of the selected study parameters, such as geographic location, age, gender, population traits, population size, sample size, study instrument or other similar considerations.
- Researcher usually mention delimitation of their study. So that the readers can have an idea about the creditability and generalizability of the research findings.
- Researchers usually mention delimitations of their study, so that the readers can have an idea about the creditability and generalizability of the research findings.

Types of Delimitation

Delimitations are restriction of the study because of theoretical or methodological reasons, which may decrease the creditability generalizability of the findings. Usually two types of delimitation in research study are as follows:

Theoretical Delimitation

Theoretical delimitation limiting the study within specific theory. They defined the study variables through specific operational definitions and restricts the ability of research findings to generalize because of the use of specific theoretical concepts in the study or limiting the study of variables through operational definitions.

Methodological Delimitation

Methodological delimitation usually result from some of the methodological factors, such as unrepresentative sample, weak design, single settings, and limited control over extraneous variables, poor implementations of treatment protocol, research tools with limited reliability and validity, poor data collection procedure, ineffective use of statistical analysis, etc.

Points to Remember while Writing Delimitation

When discussing the delimitations of a research study researcher must ensure:
- Describe each delimitation in detailed but concise term.
- Explain reasons for not considering certain parameters of the study.
- Mention why a particular delimitation is considered for a research study.
- Identify and mention the intended impact of each delimitation in relation to the overall findings and conclusions of a study.

LIMITATIONS

Limitations of a dissertation are potential weaknesses in the research study that are mostly out of researcher's control, given limited funding, choice of research design, statistical model constraints, or other factors. In addition, a limitation is a restriction on your study that cannot be reasonably dismissed and can affect researcher's design and results, e.g., if a researcher using a sample of convenience, as opposed to a random sample, then the results of researcher's study cannot be generally applied to a larger population, another limitation is time. A study conducted over a certain interval of time is a snapshot dependent on conditions occurring during that time. Due to limitation it is always possible that the future research may cast doubt on the validity of any hypothesis or conclusion from a study.

There are different types of limitations in different research study. In qualitative research study there is limitations in their validity and reliability as it is carried out in natural setting, and it is extreme difficult to replicate the study. In a case study we cannot make casual inference because it is always unclear about the generality of the findings. A case study involves the behavior of one person group or organization. The behavior of a person, group or organization may not reflect the behavior of similar entities. In correlational research also the correlational findings always not generalize to all situation due to present of different confounding factors for different populations. Similarly the experimental studies are influencing by extraneous variables which are difficult to control.

ASSUMPTIONS

An assumption is a realistic expectation which is something that we believe to be true. However, no adequate evidence exists to support this belief. In other words, an assumption is an act of faith which does not have empirical evidence to support. Assumption provide a basis to develop theories and research instrument and therefore, influence the development and implement of research process. Assumptions are those things we take for granted in the study, the statements by the researcher that certain elements of the research are understood to be true. While assumed, they should still be explicitly stated in the body of the dissertation.

Definition

- ❖ Assumptions are statements that are taken for granted or are considered true, even though they have not been scientifically tested.
- ❖ Assumption are principles those are accepted as being true based on logic or reasons, but without proof or verification.

Uses of Assumption in Research

- ❖ Research is built upon assumptions since a foundation is needed to move forward on must assume something to discover something.
- ❖ Assumptions listed in research paper may be good sources of the research topics.
- ❖ Assumptions provide basis to conduct of the research study.
- ❖ Tested assumptions through research studies expand the professional body of knowledge.

Types of Assumptions

Assumptions are basically classified into three board categories, these are (**Fig. 3.7**):

Universal Assumptions

Universal assumptions are the beliefs that are assumed to be true by large part of society. Universally accepted assumptions are known

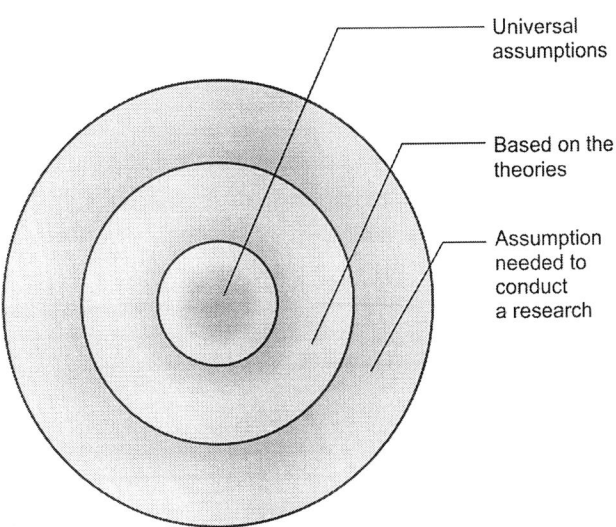

Fig. 3.7: Types of assumptions.

as universal assumptions, but testing such assumptions are not always possible examples of universal assumptions are 'there is a supernatural power which governs this universe' or, 'all human being needs love and affection' or crow is black. The testing of such assumptions are not possible.

Assumptions Based on Theories

Assumptions may also be drawn from theories. If a research is based on theory, the assumption of particular theory may become assumption of that particular research study. In addition the result of previous study can forms the basis of assumption in the present research investigation.

Example: Ray's adaptation model will use assumption of this particular theoretical model.

Assumption Needed to Conduct a Research

Some of the common sense assumptions may be developed to conduct a particular study. This assumptions are based on the needs of the research. Let us take an example, a nurse researcher is conducting a study on the attitude of the father on parenting the children. Here the father consider by the family can accepted as real father. Sometimes the researcher in his/her study take assumption to his/her data source. The data collected from the antenatal mothers are the true data.

Another classification of assumptions is warranted assumptions and unwarranted assumptions.

- **Warranted assumptions:** Warranted assumptions are the assumptions that stated along with evidenced to support. Assumptions that developed from theories are also warranted assumptions, e.g., regular exercises can maintain your health.
- **Unwarranted assumptions:** These unwarranted assumptions are stated without any supportive evidence. It is mainly based on believes, e.g., almighty god exists everywhere in this universe.

Examples of Assumption

Williams (1980) reviewed published nursing studies and other health care literature where following common assumptions were found.
- People are aware of the experiences that most effect their life choices.
- People in underserved areas feel underserved.
- People want to assume control of their own health problems.
- Stress should be avoid.
- Health is the priority for most of the people.
- Most measurable attitudes are held strongly enough to direct behavior.
- Health professionals view health care in a different manner than laypersons.
- Human biological and chemical factors show less variation than cultural and social factors.
- The nursing process is the best way of conceptualizing nursing practices.
- Statistically significant differences relate to the variables under consideration.
- Receiving health care at home is preferred to receiving health care in an institution.
- People operate on the basis of cognitive information.
- Increased knowledge about an event lowers anxiety about the event.

Difference between Assumption and Hypothesis

Assumption	Hypothesis
Assumption are basically beliefs and ideas that we hold to be true	Hypothesis is a prediction often with little or no evidence and are not statistically tested in research
Beliefs about the variables may be tested previously or not	Hypothesis can be statistically tested and may be accepted or rejected
In assumption there is no need of argument	Hypothesis is an argument put forward to explain a phenomenon or sets of phenomena
Anything taken for granted is an assumption. When a hypothesis has been proved by repeated verification, the assumption can be drawn from it	Hypothesis is not a theory until it has been proved and verified under different circumstances

SUMMARY

- In research process, the first and foremost step is selecting and properly defining a research problem. A researcher must find the problem and formulate it when he/she is interested to make a research study.
- A research problem, in general refer to some difficulty which a researcher experience in the contest of either a theoretical or practical situation and wants to obtained a solution for the same.
- Researchers usually identify a broad topic, narrow the scope of the problem, and then identify questions consistent with a paradigm of choice.
- The most common sources of ideas for nursing research problems are experience, critical appraisal of literature, social issues, practical issues, theory, brainstorming, technology, and external sources.
- Various criteria should be considered in assessing the value of a research problem. The problem should be clinically significant, relevant, researchable, feasible, and of researcher's personal interest.
- Feasibility involves the issues of time, cooperation of study participants and other people, availability of facilities and equipment, researcher experience, and ethical considerations.
- Research objective is the specific accomplishment of the researcher that hopes to achieve by conducting the study. The objectives include obtaining answer to research questions or testing research hypothesis. These are clear concise declarative statement expressed in the present tense and measure through statistical method.
- A well-worded objective will be SMART, (i.e., specific, measurable, attainable, realistic, and time-bounded). It should be relevant, feasible, logical, observable, and unequivocal. Other than this it should be logical, unequivocal, feasible, and observable.
- In research studies the variables have been used. A variable is something that can change and or can have more than one value. There are three types of classification of variables, such as independent versus dependent variables, extraneous versus confounding variables, and continuous and categorical variables.
- In quantitative studies, a hypothesis is a statement of predicted relationships between two or more variables. A testable hypothesis states the anticipated association between one or more independent and one or more dependent variables. The hypothesis can be classified as null and alternative hypothesis, simple and complex hypothesis, directional and non-directional hypothesis, casual and associative hypothesis.

QUESTIONS TO TEST YOUR KNOWLEDGE

Q1. What do you research problem? Explain the sources and characteristics of good research problem.
(3 + 6 + 6)

Q2. Describe the steps in developing a research problem statement. Explain these steps with help of examples.
(7 + 3)

Q3. Define objective and research objective. Explain the types research objectives with examples. Write down the characteristics of research objectives.
(4 + 6 + 5)

Q4. Explain different types of variables with examples. Enumerate the classifications of studies based on the variables.
(10 + 5)

Q5. Explain the concept and classification of hypothesis.

Q6. Write short notes on the following:
(5 × 5 = 25)
- a. Criteria problem statement
- b. Delimitations
- c. Importance of hypothesis
- d. Types of assumptions
- e. Limitations

Q7. Multiple choice questions:
(1 × 11)

I. The beliefs that are assumed to be true by large part of society is termed as:
- a. Assumptions
- b. Universal assumptions
- c. Warranted assumptions
- d. Assumptions based on theories

II. Potential weaknesses in the research study that are mostly out of researcher's control is_____.
- a. Delimitations
- b. Limitations
- c. Extraneous variables
- d. Assumptions

III. _____is a quality of good hypothesis.
- a. Small in size
- b. Durability
- c. Applicability
- d. Conceptual clarity

IV. Things we take for granted in the study is called as:
- a. Objectives
- b. Delimitations
- c. Assumptions
- d. Sampling

V. _____hypothesis express relationship between one dependent and one independent variable.
- a. Simple hypothesis
- b. Complex hypothesis
- c. Alternate hypothesis
- d. Null hypothesis

VI. _____ from theory leads to hypothesis.
- a. Deduction
- b. Induction
- c. Logical deduction
- d. Observation

VII. A variable that is presumed to cause a change in another variable is called a(n):
- a. Categorical variable
- b. Dependent variable
- c. Independent variable
- d. Intervening variable

VIII. Function of a hypothesis is to:
- a. Guide the researcher to meet the objective
- b. Support statement
- c. Formulate problem statement
- d. None of the above

IX. _____are boundaries that are set by the researcher in order to control the range of a study.
- a. Delimitations
- b. Hypothesis
- c. Variables
- d. Objectives

X. _____ is a quality of good hypothesis.
- a. Small in size
- b. Durability
- c. Applicability
- d. Conceptual clarity

Chapter 3: Research Problems, Objectives, Variables Hypothesis, Delimitation, and Assumptions

XI. Which of the following is not selected by the interest of a researcher but automatically that may influence the study results?
   a. Delimitations
   b. Limitations
   c. Extraneous variables
   d. Assumptions

ANSWERS

I. b	II. b	III. d	IV. c	V. a
VI. c	VII. c	VIII. a	IX. a	X. d
XI. c				

Q8. Fill in the blanks
   a. Things we take for granted in the study is called as_____.
   b. When the studies are having more than two variables they are called as _____.
   c. Potential weaknesses in the research study that are mostly out of researcher's control is_____.
   d. Certain external variables may influence the relationship between the research variables, even though researcher cannot see it. These variables are called as _____.
   e. _____ variables that affect the dependent variable but are not controlled adequately by the researcher.
   f. _____ variables take on a wide range of values on a continuum.

Ans. a. Assumptions b. Multivariate studies c. Limitations d. Intervening variables e. extraneous variables f. Continuous variables

Chapter 4

Review of Literature

Learning Objectives

After completion of this chapter, the students will be able to:
- Enumerate the concept and purposes of literature review.
- Recognize the importance of literature review.
- Identify the sources of literature review.
- Perform literature review by following necessary steps.

INTRODUCTION

Review of literature is one of the most important steps in the research process. Review usually means an overview summarizing major parts and bringing them together to build a picture of what's out there. Different fields of study will have different standards on whether a review is supposed to be more of a straightforward summary or if it is supposed to have a deep analysis and discussion literature 'means the major writings—especially scholarly writings—on the topic. Depending on your field 'the literature' can include all sorts of things like journal articles, books, published essays, government reports and so on. The main thing is that 'the literature' is the body of scholarly, professional information that is used by professionals and scholars working on that topic area. It is an account of what is already known about a particular phenomenon. The main purpose of literature review is to convey to the reader about the work already done and knowledge and ideas have been already established on a particular topic of research. Review' usually means an overview summarizing major parts and bringing them together to build a picture of what's out there.

A literature review discusses published information in a particular subject area, and sometimes information in a particular subject area within a certain time period. It can be just a simple summary of the sources, but it usually has an organizational pattern and combines both summary and synthesis and recap of the important information of the source, but a *synthesis* is a re-organization, or a reshuffling, of that information. It might give a new interpretation of old material or combine new with old interpretations. Or it might trace the intellectual progression of the field, including major debates and depending on the situation, the literature review may evaluate the sources and advise the reader on the most pertinent or relevant.

A literature review is the effective evaluation of selected documents on a research topic. It may form an essential part of the research process or may constitute a research project in itself. In the context of a research paper or thesis the literature review is a critical synthesis of previous research. The evaluation of the literature leads logically to the research question. A literature review is an account of the previous efforts and achievement of scholars and researchers on a phenomenon. Actually, it is a piece of discursive another.

It is a laborious task, but it is essential if the research process is successful research studies are usually undertaken within the context of an existing knowledge base, because research cannot be conducted in an intellectual vacuum.

- Before starting any research, a literature review of previous studies and experience related to the proposed investigations has to be done.
- One of the most satisfying aspects of the literature review is the contribution it makes to the new knowledge, insight and general scholarship of the researches.

Nursing research may be considered as a continuing process in which knowledge gained from earlier studies is an integral part of research in general.

MEANING OF LITERATURE REVIEW

A review of literature is a description and analysis of the literature relevant to a particular field or topic. It provides an overview of what work already has been carried out, who are the key researchers who did that work, which of the questions are already answered regarding a particular area of research interest, what methods and methodologies were used to answer the particular questions and what are the prevailing theories and hypotheses.

A literature review discusses published information in a particular subject area, and sometimes information in a particular subject area within a certain time period. It may be just a simple summary of the related studies or documents, but it usually has an organizational pattern and combines both summary and synthesis. Generally, a summary is a recap of the important information of the document, but a synthesis is a reorganization, or a reshuffling, of that information. It might give a new interpretation of old material or combine new with old interpretations. Or it might trace the intellectual progression of the field, including major debates. And depending on the situation, the literature review may evaluate the sources and advise the reader on the most pertinent or relevant. The format of a review of literature may vary from discipline to discipline and from studies to studies. A review may be a self-contained unit—an end in itself—or a preface to and rationale for engaging in primary research. A review is a required part of grant and research proposals and often a chapter in theses and dissertations. Generally, the purpose of a review is to analyze critically a segment of a published body of knowledge through summary, classification, and comparison of prior research studies, reviews of literature, and theoretical articles.

Overall a literature review is the effective evaluation of selected documents on a research topic. It may form an essential part of the research process or may constitute a research project in itself. In the context of a research paper or thesis the literature review is also a critical synthesis of previous research. The evaluation of the literature leads logically to the research question.

DEFINITIONS

- Literature review may be defined as selection of available document, both published and unpublished on the topic of research interest, which contain information, ideas, data and evidence written from a particular stand point to fulfil certain aims or express certain views on the nature of the topic and how it is to be investigated and the effective evaluation of these document in relation to the research being proposed.
- A literature review uses as is database reports of primary or original scholarship and does not report new primary scholarship itself. The primary reports used in the literature may be verbal, but in the vast majority of cases, reports are written documents. The types of scholarship may be empirical, theoretical, critical/analytic methodological in nature. Second

a literature review seeks to describe, summarize, evaluate, clarify and/or integrate the content of primary reports.
—*HM Cooper, 1988*
- A literature review is an evaluative report of information found in the literature related to selected area of study. The review describes, summarizes, evaluates and clarifies this literature. It gives a theoretical base for the research and helps to determine the nature of research.
—*Queensland University, 1999*
- A literature review is a body of text that aims to review the critical points of knowledge on a particular topic of research.
—*ANA, 2000*
- A literature review is an account of what has been already established or published on a particular research topic by accredited scholars and researches.
—*University of Toronto, 2001*
- Literature review is defined as a broad, comprehensive, in depth, systematic and critical review of scholarly publication, unpublished printed or audio visual material and personal communications.
—*SK Sharma, 2005*

PURPOSES OF LITERATURE REVIEW

The purpose of a literature review is to convey to the reader previous knowledge and facts established on a topic and their strengths and weakness. The literature review allows the reader to be updated the state of research in a field and any contradictions that may exist which challenges finding of other research studies. Furthermore, literature review enhances researcher knowledge. It helps to developed research investigative tools and to improve research methodologies. It also provides the knowledge about the problem faced by the previous researchers' while studying the same topic. Besides enhancing researchers' about the topic, writing a literature review helps to:
- Place each in the context of its contribution to the understanding of subject under review.
- Describe the relationship of each study to other research studies under consideration.
- Identify new ways to interpret and shed light on any gaps in previous research.
- Resolve conflicts amongst seemingly contradictory previous studies.
- Identify areas of prior scholarship to prevent duplication of effort.
- Point a way forward for further research.
- See what has and has not been investigated.
- Develop general explanation for observed variations in a behavior or phenomenon.
- Identify potential relationship between conflicts and to identify researchable hypothesis.
- Learn how others have defined and measured key concept.
- Identify data sources that other researchers have used.
- Develop alternative research project.
- Discover how a research project is related the work of others.
- Place one's original work (in case of thesis or dissertation) in context of the existing literature.
- Placing the research in a historical context to show familiarity with state-of-the-art developments.

IMPORTANCE OF LITERATURE REVIEW

Literature review provides a practical guide to a particular topic. For healthcare professionals they are useful reports that keep them updated with what is present in the field. For scholars, the depth and breadth of the literature review highlights the credibility of the writers in their respective fields. Literature reviews also provide a solid background for a research study.

Comprehensive knowledge of the literature of the field is essential to most research studies. Review of relevant literature can help in fulfillment of the following objectives:
- Identification of a research problem and development or refinement of research question.
- Generation of useful research questions or projects/activities for the discipline.
- Orientation to what is known and not known about an area of inquiry to ascertain what research can best contribution to knowledge.
- Determination of any gaps or inconsistencies in a body of knowledge.
- Provides evidence that a selected research problem is of importance.
- Discovery of unanswered questions about subjects, concepts or problems.
- Determination of a need a replicate a prior study in different study setting or different samples or sizes or different study populations.
- Identification of relevant theoretical or conceptual framework for research problem.
- Identification or development of new or refined clinical interventions to test through empirical research.
- Description of the strengths and weakness of designs/methods of inquiry and instruments used in earlier research work.
- Development of hypothesis to be tested in a research study.
- Helps in planning the methodologies of the present research study.
- Helps in the development of research instruments.
- Identification of suitable design and data collection method for a research study.
- Assistance in interpreting study finding and in developing implications and recommendation.

SOURCES OF LITERATURE REVIEW

The types of information sources for a review of literature are conceptual and data-based literature. The common sources of literature are books, chapters of books, journal articles; abstracts critique reviews, abstract published in conference proceeding, professional and governmental reports and unpublished doctoral dissertations.

The kinds of information available in written documents can be categories into five broad classes.
1. Facts, findings or results
2. Theory
3. Researcher procedure or methods
4. Opinions, points of view or personal, commentaries
5. Anecdotes or impression on a particular events or situation

Literature can be reviewed from two main sources, i.e., primary sources and secondary sources.

Primary Sources

Primary sources provides direct or firsthand evidence about an event, object, person, or work of art and also provide the original materials on which other research is based and enable students and other researchers to get as close as possible to what actually happened during a particular event or time period. Primary sources are generally original, peer-reviewed and published research journal articles reported by original researchers. In other words, primary sources are the research reports, which are description of studies written by researchers who conducted it. It is written by a person who developed the theory or conducted the research or is the description of an investigation written by the person who conducted it. Most of the primary sources are found in published literature, for ex-nursing research article. A credible literature review reflects the use of mainly primary sources. For example, an original qualitative study on patient.

Secondary Sources

Secondary sources describe, discuss, interpret, comment upon, analyze, evaluate, summarize, and process primary sources. It is generally one or more steps removed from the event or time period and are written or produced after the fact with the benefit of hindsight. Secondary source research documents are description of studies prepared by someone other than the original researcher. They are written by people other than the individuals who developed the theory or conducted the research. The secondary sources include the comments and summaries of multiple research studies on one topic, e.g., systemic reviews, meta-analysis, meta-synthesis. Secondary sources are usually paraphrased and may be based on the secondary author's interpretation of the primary work. It is necessary then to review primary source whenever possible to ensure accuracy. However, the secondary sources may be used when primary sources are not available or if researchers want external opinions on an issue or problem or even the results of their own research.

The main sources from where literature can be searched are as follows:

Electronic Sources

Computer-assisted literature search has revolutionized the review of literature. These searches however, for a variety of literature of reasons may not provide the desired references.

Electronic literature search through web may be very useful, but sometimes it web pages that can lead to information overload and confusion. However, currently it is one of the most important sources of literature searches.

The most useful and relevant database are as follows:
- CINAHL-cumulative index to nursing and allied health literature.
- Other online database: Other online database can be searched for free by nurses from the following websites.
   - http://www.aidsinfo.nih.gov (HIV/AIDS information)
   - http://www.hazmap.nim.nih.gov (information on hazardous agents)
   - http://www.child.nih.gov (combined health information database)
   - http://www.toxinet.nlm.nih.gov (toxicology database network).
- Cancer lit (cancer literature)
- EMBASE (excerpt medical database)
- ETOH (alcohol and alcohol problems science database)
- HEALTH STAR (health services technology administration and research)
- RADIX (nursing and managed care database)
- CD-ROM (compact disc-read only memory) with research database

Printed Sources

Printed sources are also used for literature review. Printed research summary may be located from published abstracts, such as nursing research abstract, psychological abstracts, dissertation abstract international, masters abstracts international, etc.

References of the other printed sources may be located through indices, such as cumulative index to nursing and allied health literature, nursing studies index and index medicus.

Following are the main printed sources that can be used to review the relevant literature.

Journals

There are several national and international journals that can be used to review the research-related literature. Some of the main national and international nursing journals are as follows:

Names of national nursing journals
- Nursing and Midwifery Research Journal
- Indian Journal of Nursing and Midwifery
- The Nursing Journal of India
- Nightingale Nursing Times
- Community Health Nursing Spectrum
- Nurses of India
- Journal of Nursing Research Association India
- **MEDLINE:** Medical literature analysis and retrieved system online.
- **Pubmed:** Used to search research abstracts. Available at http://www.pubmed.com
- **British nursing index:** It is a leading UK nursing database providing bibliographic reference to journal articles from all the major British nursing and midwifery journals, as well as a selection of English-language internationals journals.
- **Medline plus:** It is the national library of medicine's websites for consumer health information.
- **Registry of nursing research:** Sigma theta tau international honor society of nursing makes this database available through its Virginia Henderson International Nursing Library.
- **Cochrane database of system reviews:** Health care related literature can be searched from this source.
- **ERIC:** The ERIC database is the largest source of education information.
- **PSYCINFO:** This database belongs to American Psychological Association and covers literature from psychological or related discipline.
- **Dissertations abstracts online:** Abstract of masters and doctoral these are available on this electronic database.
- **Online journals:** Following are the website addresses for journals and magazines that are available online:
  - http://www.nsna.org
  - http://www.health web.org
  - http://www.medbioworid.com
  - http://www.nursingweek.com
  - http://www.juns.nursing.arizona.edu
  - International Journal of Nursing Education
  - Indian Journal of Nursing Studies

Names of international journals
- Nursing Research
- Research in Nursing and Health
- Nursing Sciences Quarterly
- Western Journal of Nursing Research
- Applied Nursing Research

- ❖ Biological Research for Nursing
- ❖ Advances in Nursing Sciences
- ❖ Clinical Nursing Research
- ❖ World views on Evidence-based Nursing
- ❖ Journal of Qualitative Research
- ❖ American Journal of Nursing
- ❖ International Journal of Nursing Studies
- ❖ Canadian Journal of Nursing Research
- ❖ Evidence-based Nursing
- ❖ Journal of Nursing Measurement
- ❖ Journal of Nursing Scholarship
- ❖ Oncology Nursing Forum
- ❖ Scholarly Inquiry of Nursing Practice
- ❖ Research Reports
- ❖ Unpublished Dissertations and Theses
- ❖ Magazines and Newspapers
- ❖ Conference Papers and Proceedings
- ❖ Encyclopedias and Dictionaries
- ❖ Books

Following steps should be followed for good literature review.

STEPS FOLLOWED FOR GOOD LITERATURE REVIEW (FIG. 4.1)

Step 1: Formulating Questions for a Review

This is the first step of the review of literature. After selecting problem statement a researcher should have understood the concept and identify its components. The broad problem questions will be divided into small narrow parts. The problems to be addressed by the review should be specified in the form of clear, unambiguous and structured questions before beginning the review work. Once the review questions have been set, modifications to the protocol should be allowed only if alternative ways of defining the populations, interventions,

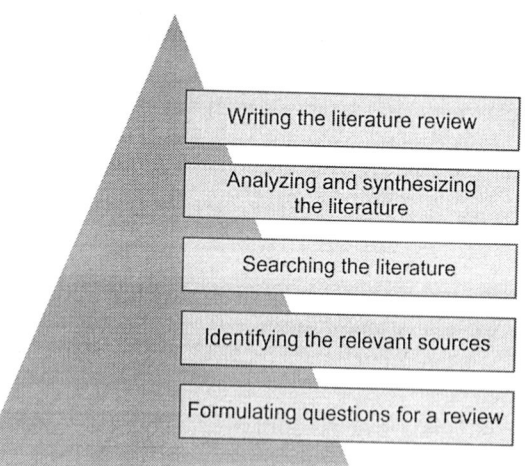

Fig. 4.1: Steps followed for good literature review.

outcomes or study designs become apparent. The researcher wants to know what is the current state of knowledge on the questions that will be addressing the study. The researcher has to formulate two types of questions—primary questions and secondary questions. In primary questions the researcher can address directly the questions the study want but in secondary questions the researcher kept supportive questions, e.g., a researcher selected a problem statement to find out the effectiveness of diet therapy in preventing malnutrition, here primary question is what is the effectiveness of that diet in preventing malnutrition and secondary questions are prevalence of malnutrition, what other factors affecting nutritional status of the group.

Step 2: Identifying the Relevant Sources

By deciding what to include and what to exclude, the researcher prepare herself to search more effectively and efficiently. Here the researcher will think where she will get all the related studies. Here are a lot of books and journals that can be followed by the researcher. Nowadays, literature searches are undertaken most commonly using computers and electronic databases. Computer databases offer access to vast quantities of information, which can be retrieved more easily and quickly than using a manual search. There are numerous electronic databases, many of which deal with specific fields of information. It is important therefore to identify which databases are relevant to the topic. University and hospital libraries often subscribe to a number of databases and access can be gained using student or staff. Generally, journals are regarded as being more up-to-date than books as sources of information. Books can be dated due to the length of time it takes for publication. However, this does not mean they should be excluded as they are an acceptable and valuable source of information, before undergoing review the researcher should identify the relevant sources. The questions determine the areas of literature review what the research wants.

Step 3: Searching the Literature

When undertaking a literature search an important question in determining whether a publication should be included in your review is defining the type of source. A systematic approach is considered most likely to generate a review that will be beneficial in informing practice. Keyword searches are the most common method of identifying literature. However, keywords need carefully consideration in order to select terms that will generate the data being sought. For American databases, such as CINAHL, the keywords used to identify terms may differ from the British in spelling and meaning (for example, tumour/tumor, paediatric/pediatric, transcultural/multicultural). It is a good idea to consider alternative keywords with similar meanings that might elicit further information (for example, if you are undertaking a review in an aspect of pressure ulcers, you would need to include terms, such as 'pressure sores' and 'decubitus ulcers'. The search include answer to all primary and secondary question. The researcher will gather studies and different data as her study want. When searching the book and journal the researcher can search the content or index of the book but during assessing the internet directly the researcher can visit to the specific site or can type the keywords selected for literature review.

Step 4: Analyzing and Synthesizing the Literature

At this point of the process, what has been determined as appropriate literature will have been gathered. While the focus of the literature may vary depending on the overall purpose, there are several useful strategies for the analysis and synthesis stages that will help the construction and writing of the review. Initially, it is advisable to undertake a first read of the articles that have been collected to get a sense of what they are about. Most published articles contain a summary or abstract at the beginning of the paper, which will assist with this process and enable the decision as to whether it is worthy of further reading or inclusion. At this point, it may also be of benefit to undertake an initial classification and grouping of the articles by type of source. Once the initial overview has been completed, it is necessary to return to the articles to undertake a more systematic and critical review of the content. Focused on the criteria of quality, credibility and accuracy when appraising this type of literature. Quality and credibility encompassed issues related to the journal, the processes of peer review, the standing of the author(s) and the claims being made. In addition, content is judged for its accuracy and its coherence with what is already known on the subject. The final stage of appraisal is to write a short summary of each article and may include key thoughts, comments, strengths and weaknesses of the publication. It should be written in your own words to facilitate your understanding of the material. It also forms a good basis for the writing of the review.

Step 5: Writing the Literature Review

This is the final stage. Finally the researcher writes the literature review based on research questions. Literature review can done for each and every chapter, or otherwise we can mention that the review can be organized into three distinct headings that are introduction, body and summary with conclusion.

Introduction

The introduction should include definitions of general topics, issues under study and a brief overview of the 'problem'. It is important that the literature sources and the key search terms are outlined.

Any limits, boundaries or inclusion/exclusion criteria should be clearly described. Some comment on what was found in the literature should be offered, i.e., whether there was a dearth or wealth of literature on the topic. This gives the reader some insight into the breadth and depth of the literature This introduction part include just concepts, classifications and general facts about the topic.

Main Body

The main body of the report presents and discusses the findings from the literature. There are several ways in which this can be done regardless of the manner in which the main body of the review is framed, there are key points that must be considered. Literature that is central to the topic should be analyzed in-depth here. When discussing empirical or research literature a critical review of the methodologies used should be included. Care must be taken, however, that the review does not end up just as a description of a series of studies. In addition, it is best to avoid broad sweeping statements about the conclusiveness of research studies. It suggest that when describing a study's findings, it is best to use language that indicates the tentativeness of the results rather than making definite statements about the research. The body of the review should contain all the areas in an analytic and synthetic form and in each aspect the reference should be given.

Similarly, it is necessary for the reviewer to remain objective about the literature and personal opinions about the quality of research studies should not be included. Neither should it be a series of quotes or descriptions but needs to be written succinctly in the writer's own words.

The reader should know that the reviewer has understood and synthesized the relevant information, rather than merely describing what other authors have found. In review the body of the text summarizes and synthesizes the literature. The summarization and synthesization material in a way that allows the researcher not only to report, but also to compare, contrast, critically review and comment on what has been said in the literature. In each work, the similarities, differences, strengths and weaknesses need to be identified.

Conclusion

The review should conclude with a concise summary of the findings that describes current knowledge and offer a rationale for conducting future research. In a review, which forms part of a study, any gaps in knowledge that have been identified should lead logically to the purpose of the proposed study. In some cases, it may also be possible to use the developed themes to construct a conceptual framework that will inform the study. In all reviews, some recommendations or implications for practice, education and research should be included. In conclusion mention the main contribution of important studies. Specify the gaps of study findings and in consistencies in methodologies. Mention the most significant findings when concluding.

Step 6: Referencing and Reviewing the Final Draft of Literature

In this last step of literature review the final draft of literature is reviewed for completeness, accuracy and relevance of the content. Furthermore the reference citation and the list of reference in bibliography should be checked.

Bibliography

The literature review should conclude with a full bibliographical list of all the books, journal articles, reports and other media, which were referred to in the work. Regardless of whether the review is part of a course of study or for publication, it is an essential part of the process that all sourced material is acknowledged. This means that every citation in the text must appear in the reference/bibliography and vice versa. Omissions or errors in referencing are very common and students often lose vital marks in assignment because of it. A useful strategy is to create a separate file for references and each time a publication is cited, it can be added to this list immediately.

A literature review is central to the research process and can help refine a research question through determining inconsistencies in a body of knowledge. Similarly, it can help inspire new research innovations and ideas while creating greater understanding about a topic. It can enable a novice researcher to gain insight into suitable designs for a future study, as well as providing information on data collection and analysis tools. Whether the approach is qualitative or quantitative will often dictate when and how it is carried out. Various types of literature reviews may be used depending on the reasons for carrying out the review and the overall aims and objectives of the research. Writing a review of the literature is a skill that needs to be learned. By conducting them, nurses can be involved in increasing the body of nursing knowledge and ultimately enhancing patient care through evidence-based practice.

TIPS TO REMEMBER WHEN DOING LITERATURE REVIEW

1. Identify the points on what you have to search for.
2. Be specific and avoid long description.
3. Take the material from a study which is appropriate to meet your research questions.
4. Always search for recent studies
5. The statistics should not be more than 5 years
6. Give importance to primary sources.
7. Ensure evidence for claims (mention the name of the author who is proving that)
8. Follow any one style of writing bibliography.
9. Collect review (statistical data) from more source and write it concisely rather than a long description from only a few source.
10. Each and every review must followed with citation and for each citation there will be a bibliography.
11. Write the review in your own language without changing it's meaning.

12. The sentence structure must be simple and accurate.
13. Group the sentence that express one aspect of a particular topic.
14. All similar aspects will be written together.
15. Effective use of transition ward which link the paragraph should be a contrast ward to development the argument (e.g., hence, therefore, whereas, etc.)
16. A literature should be organized beads on the subheading not by the references.
17. The writer may cite several reference on same paragraph or same reference in different paragraph.
18. Avoid technical terms and abbreviations.

SUMMARY

❖ A review of literature is a description and analysis of the literature relevant to a particular field or topic. It provides an overview of what work already has been carried out, who are the key researchers who did that work, which of the questions are already answered regarding a particular area of research interest, what methods and methodologies were used to answer the particular questions and what are the prevailing theories and hypotheses.

❖ Literature review may be defined as selection of available document, both published and unpublished on the topic of research interest, which contain information, ideas, data and evidence written from a particular stand point to fulfil certain aims or express certain views on the nature of the topic and how it is to be investigated and the effective evaluation of these document in relation to the research being proposed.

❖ The purpose of a literature review is to convey to the reader previous knowledge and facts established on a topic and their strengths and weakness. The literature review allows the reader to be updated the state of research in a field and any contradictions that may exist which challenges finding of other research studies.

❖ The importance of literature review is it provides a practical guide to a particular topic. For healthcare professionals they are useful reports that keep them updated with what is present in the field. For scholars, the depth and breadth of the literature review highlights the credibility of the writers in their respective fields. Literature reviews also provide a solid background for a research study.

❖ The sources of literature review is classified as primary and secondary sources. Primary sources provides direct or firsthand evidence about an event, object, person, or work of art and also provide the original materials where as secondary sources describe, discuss, interpret, comment upon, analyze, evaluate, summarize, and process primary sources.

❖ There are six steps in literature review. Those are formulating questions for a review, identifying the relevant sources, searching the literature, analyzing and synthesizing the literature, writing the literature review and referencing and reviewing the final draft of literature.

QUESTIONS TO TEST YOUR KNOWLEDGE

Q1. Describe the concept of literature review. Enumerate the purposes and importance of literature review.
(5 + 5 + 5)

Q2. Explain different sources of literature review.
(15)

Q3. Enumerate the steps of conducting literature review. Write the points to remember when doing literature review. (10 + 5)

Q4. Multiple choice questions: (1 × 10)

I. What do you mean by literature review?
  a. Analysis of the literature relevant to a particular field or topic
  b. Analysis of research findings
  c. Analysis of all published and nonpublished research articles
  d. Analysis of the significant studies which support the findings

II. The full form of CINAHL is:
  a. Cumulative index to nursing and allied health literature
  b. Cumulative international to nursing and allied health literature
  c. Cumulative index to nursing and assisted health literature
  d. Cumulative index to nutrition and allied health literature

III. When a researcher conducting reviews he/she should considered:
  a. Only research articles from published journal
  b. Research articles from published journal and books
  c. Published and nonpublished research articles
  d. Published and nonpublished research articles along with books

IV. When the literature review should be done.
  a. Early in research process
  b. After writing of first chapter
  c. Near the end of the research process
  d. Throughout the research process

V. Database differ from search engine in the following manner:
  a. A database stores the information
  b. A search engine takes you to the information
  c. Database are specialized by area of knowledge
  d. All of the above

VI. Which of the following is most appropriate way to organize the review?
  a. Thematic organization
  b. Year wise organization
  c. Alphabetical organization
  d. None of the above

VII. Published research journal articles reported by original researcher is an example of _____ source of review.
  a. Primary sources
  b. Secondary sources
  c. Printed sources
  d. Online sources

VIII. MEDLINE stands for:
  a. Medical electronic data online
  b. Medical literature analysis and retrieved system online
  c. Medical electronic data system online
  d. Medical literature data analysis system online

IX. Published meta-analysis is an example of:
  a. Primary sources
  b. Secondary sources
  c. Printed sources
  d. Online sources

X. Plagiarism is appropriately use for:
  a. Coping any material from internet without cite the real author's name
  b. Coping any material from internet with cite the real author's name
  c. Coping any material from any source without cite the real author's name
  d. Coping any material from journals without cite the real author's name

ANSWERS				
I. a	II. a	III. d	IV. d	V. d
VI. a	VII. a	VIII. b	IX. b	X. c

Chapter 5

Theoretical and Conceptual Frameworks

Learning Objectives

After completion of this chapter, the students will be able to:
- Explain of concepts of theories and nursing theories.
- Describe historical evolution and types of nursing theories.
- Identify the characteristics and enumerate the uses of nursing theories.
- Formulate and use the theoretical and conceptual framework in research work.
- Describe the role of theoretical and conceptual framework in nursing research.
- Differentiate between conceptual and theoretical framework.

INTRODUCTION

Good research generally integrates research findings into an orderly, coherent system. Such integration typically involves linking new research and existing knowledge by performing a thorough review of the prior research on a topic and by identifying or developing an appropriate conceptual framework. These activities are important because they provide a rich context for a research project and because they help to be studied. A framework provides an explicit explanation why the problem under study exists by showing how the variables are related to each other.

When the researcher plans to conduct a research project the primary need is a framework based on which the research project can be developed. That framework will act as a guide for the researcher during his/her research work. The framework may be a theoretical or conceptual framework, but can act as the overall conceptual underpinnings of a study.

SOME COMMON TERMS

Theory

Theories are constructed in order to explain, predict and master phenomena (e.g., relationships, events, or the behavior). A theory makes generalizations about observations and consists of an interrelated, coherent set of ideas and models.

The basic elements that structure a theory are concepts and propositions. In a theory, propositions represent how concepts affect each other. A concept is the basic building block of a theory.

Concept

Concept is a vehicle of thought and a 'complex mental formulation of our perceptions of the world.' It is an image or symbolic representation of an abstract idea and it labels or names a phenomenon, an observable fact that can be perceived through the senses and explained. A concept assists us in formulating a mental image about an object or situation. Concepts help us to name things and occurrences in the world around us and assist us in communicating with each other about the world. Independence, self-care, and caring are just a few examples of concepts frequently encountered in health care. Theories are formulated by linking concepts together.

It is the complex mental formulation of an object, property or event that is derived from individual perceptual experience. It is an idea, a mental image or generalization formed and developed in the mind.

Proposition

A proposition (another structural element of a theory) is a statement that proposes a relationship between concepts. An example of a non-nursing proposition might be the statement 'people seem to be happier in the springtime.' This proposition establishes a relationship between the concept of happiness and the time of the year.

Conceptual Model

A conceptual framework or model is a structure that links global concepts together and represents the unified whole of a larger reality. The specifics about phenomena within the global whole are better explained by theory. A set of relatively abstract and general concepts and the propositions that describe or link those concepts.

Philosophy

Concerned with the values and beliefs of a discipline and with the values and beliefs held by members of the discipline.

Assumptions

Assumptions are the statements that describe concepts or connect two concepts. They are the 'taken for granted' statements that determine the nature of the concepts, definitions, purpose, relationships and structure of the theory.

Phenomenon

Phenomenon are an aspect of reality that can be consciously sensed or experience generally nursing theories focus on the phenomena of nursing and phenomena reflect the domain of nursing practice.

CONCEPTS OF THEORIES AND NURSING THEORIES

A theory is a set of interrelated concepts, which structure a systematic view of phenomena for the purpose of explaining or predicting. A theory is like a blueprint, a guide for modeling a structure. A blueprint depicts the elements of a structure and the relation of each element to the other, just as a theory depicts the concepts, which compose it and the relation of concepts with each other. Chinn and Kramer (1999) define a theory as an 'expression of knowledge....a creative and rigorous structuring of ideas that project a tentative, purposeful, and systematic view of phenomena.'

DEFINITIONS

- ❖ A theory is a group of related concepts that propose action that guide practice.
- ❖ Theory refers to 'a coherent group of general propositions used as principles of explanation.'

- Theories as a set of interrelated concepts that give a systematic view of a phenomenon (an observable fact or event) that is explanatory and predictive in nature.
- Theories are composed of concepts, definitions, models, propositions and are based on assumptions.
- A set of concepts, definitions and propositions that projects a systematic view of phenomena by designating specific interrelationships among concepts for purposes of describing, explaining, predicting and controlling phenomena.

PURPOSE OF A THEORY

In scientific disciplines a theory guides the research and enhances the science by supporting existing knowledge or generating new knowledge. A theory not only helps us to organize our thoughts and ideas, but it may also help direct us in what to do and when and how to do it.

CHARACTERISTICS OF A THEORY

A theorist can get the following characteristics in theories:
- Interrelate concepts in such a way as to create a different way of looking at a particular phenomenon.
- Must be logical in nature.
- Should be relatively simple yet generalizable.
- The bases for hypothesis that can be tested or for theory to be expanded.
- Contribute to and assist in increasing the general body of knowledge within the discipline through the research implemented to validate them.
- Used by practitioners to guide and improve their practice.
- Consistent with other validated theories, laws, and principles but will leave open unanswered questions that need to be investigated.

NURSING THEORY

A nursing theory is a set of concepts, definitions, relationships, and assumptions or propositions derived from nursing models or from other disciplines and project a purposive, systematic view of phenomena by designing specific inter-relationships among concepts for the purposes of describing, explaining, predicting, and/or prescribing.

Nursing theory is conceptualization of some aspect of nursing communicated for the purpose of describing phenomena explaining relationships between phenomena predicting consequences or prescribing nursing care.

Nursing theory provides a perspective from which to define the *what* of nursing, to describe the *who* of nursing (who is the client) and *when* nursing is needed, and to identify the boundaries and goals of nursing's therapeutic activities. Theory is fundamental to effective nursing practice and research. The professionalization of nursing has been and is being brought about through the development and use of nursing theory.

Nursing theory defines and enriches the practice of nursing. It focuses attention on issues essential to providing care. It implies criteria with which to evaluate what nurses do. It presents concepts capable of supporting research most useful to nurses. Thereby it helps create knowledge unique to nursing, thus augmenting the status of nursing as a profession. In fostering research, nursing theory upholds nursing education, maintaining it on a par with other academic disciplines.

History and Evolution of Nursing Theory

The work of early nursing theorists in the 1950s focused on the tasks of nursing practice from a somewhat mechanistic viewpoint. Because of this emphasis, much of the art of nursing—the value of caring, the relationship aspects of nursing, and the esthetics of practice—was diminished. During the decades of the 1960s, 1970s, and 1980s, many nursing theorists struggled with making nursing practice, theory, and research fit into the prevailing view of science.

Reflecting changes in global awareness of health care needs, several contemporary nursing theorists have projected a new perspective for nursing that truly unifies the notion of nursing as both an art and a science. Noted nursing theorists, such as Leininger, Watson, Rogers, Parse, and Newman have been urging the discipline of nursing to embrace this new emerging view that is seen as more holistic, humanistic, client focused, and grounded in the notion of caring as the core of nursing. Since the early 1950s, many nursing theories have been systematically developed to help describe, explain, and predict the phenomena of concern to nursing. Each of these established theories provides a unique perspective and each is distinct and separate from other nursing theories in its particular view of nursing phenomena.

- **Nightingale (1860):** To facilitate 'the body's reparative processes' by manipulating client's environment.
- **Paplau (1952):** Nursing is therapeutic interpersonal process.
- **Henderson (1955):** The needs often called Henderson's 14 basic needs.
- **Abdellah (1960):** This theory focus on delivering nursing care for the whole person to meet the physical, emotional, intellectual, social, and spiritual needs of the client and family.
- **Orlando (1962):** To Ida Orlando (1960), the client is an individual; with a need; that, when met, diminishes distress, increases adequacy, or enhances well-being.
- **Johnson's theory (1968):** Dorothy Johnson's theory of nursing 1968 focuses on how the client adapts to illness and how actual or potential stress can affect the ability to adapt. The goal of nursing to reduce stress so that; the client can move more easily through recovery.
- **Rogers (1970):** To maintain and promote health, prevent illness, and care for and rehabilitate ill and disabled client through 'humanistic science of nursing'.
- **Orem (1971):** This is self-care deficit theory. Nursing care becomes necessary when client is unable to fulfill biological, psychological, developmental, or social needs.
- **King (1971):** To use communication to help client reestablish positive adaptation to environment.
- **Neuman (1972):** Stress reduction is goal of system model of nursing practice.
- **Roy (1979):** This adaptation model is based on the physiological, psychological, sociological and dependence-independence adaptive modes.
- **Watson's theory (1979):** Watson's philosophy of caring 1979 attempts to define the outcome of nursing activity in regard to the humanistic aspects of life.

TYPES OF THEORY

Theories are located on the ladder of abstraction relative to their scope. Based on the level of abstraction the theories can be classified as grand theory, middle-range theories and situation specific theories. Classification of theories is shown in **Figure 5.1**.

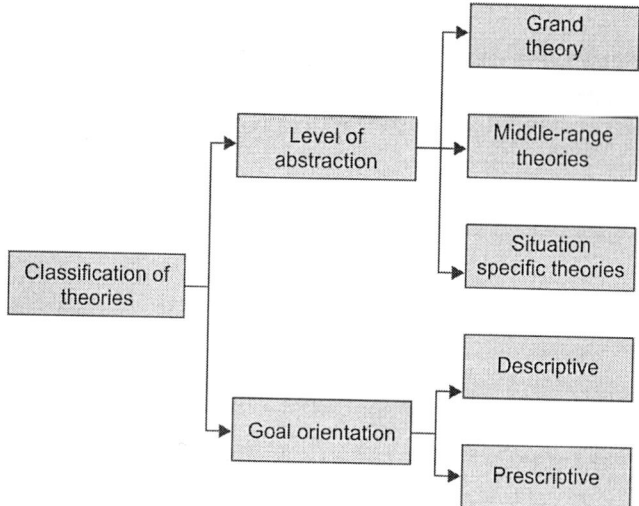

Fig. 5.1: Classification of theories.

Grand Theories

A grand theory is composed of concepts representing global and extremely complex phenomena. It is the broadest in scope, represents the most abstract level of development, and addresses the broad phenomena of concern within the discipline. Typically, a grand theory is not intended to provide guidance for the formation of specific nursing interventions, but rather provides an overall framework for structuring broad, abstract ideas. Grand theories are unique to nursing profession which help the discipline to define how it is different from other disciplines and reflect particular views of person, health, environment and other concepts that contribute to the development of a body of knowledge specific to nursing's concerns. Grand theories are all-inclusive conceptual structures, which tend to include views on person, health and environment to create a perspective of nursing. This most abstract level of theory has established a knowledge base for the discipline and is critical for further knowledge development in the discipline.

Name of grand theories with the name of theorists is listed in **Table 5.1**.

Table 5.1: Name of grand theories with the name of theorists.

Theorist	Theory
Imogene King	Theory of goal attainment
Leininger	Theory of culture care and universality
Margaret A Newman	Health as expanding consciousness
Dorothea Orem	Self-care deficit theory
Parse	Theory of human becoming
Ida Jean Orlando	Nursing process theory
Hildegard E Peplau	Interpersonal relationship theory

Characteristics of Grand Theories

- Systematic constructions of the nature of nursing, the mission of nursing and the goals of nursing care.
- Broad in scope and complex.
- Require further specification through research before they can be fully tested.
- Concepts are abstract.
- Not easily empirically tested.

Middle-range Theories

A theory that addresses more concrete and more narrowly defined phenomena than a grand theory is known as a middle-range theory. Descriptions, explanations, and predictions put forth in a middle-range theory are intended to answer questions about nursing phenomena, yet they do not cover the full range of phenomena of concern to the discipline. A middle-range theory provides a perspective from which to view complex situations and a direction for interventions. Middle-range theory is a focused conceptual structure, which synthesizes practice-research into ideas central to the discipline. Merton (1968), who has been the original source for much of Nursing's description of middle-range theory, says that middle-range theory lie between everyday working hypotheses and all-inclusive grand theories. Middle-range theories address the experiences of particular patient populations or a cohort of people who are dealing with a particular health or illness issue......Because middle-range theories are more specific in what they explain, practitioners often find them more directly applicable.

Characteristics of Middle-range Theory

The middle-range theories are having:
- Limited scope.
- Less abstract concepts.
- Address specific phenomena or concepts.
- Reflect practice (administration, clinical or teaching).
- Increased theory-based research and nursing practice strategies.

Situation Specific Theories

Situation specific theories are the most concrete and narrow in scope. These micro-range theories explains a specific phenomenon of concern to the discipline such as the effect of social supports on grieving and would establish nursing care guidelines to address the problem. There are two levels of micro-range theory, one of higher level abstraction than the other. Micro-range theory at the higher level of abstraction suggest is closely related to middle-range theory, comprised of a limited number of concepts and applicable to a narrow issue or event. In the low-middle theory hypotheses are an example of low abstraction micro-range theories. The critiquer will recall that a hypothesis is a best guess or prediction about what one expects to find the value of micro-range theory, noting that the 'particularistic approach is invaluable for scientists and practitioners as they work to describe, organize and test their ideas'.

Characteristics of Situation Specific Theories

- ❖ Focus on specific nursing phenomena that reflect clinical practice.
- ❖ Limited to specific populations or to a particular field of practice.
- ❖ Limited scope.
- ❖ More direct impact on nursing practice.
- ❖ Predict outcomes and the impact of nursing practice.
- ❖ Called as prescriptive theory.
- ❖ Day-to-day experience of nurses is a major source to situation specific theory.

Based on the goal orientation, theories can be classified as descriptive **theories** and prescriptive theories.

Descriptive Theories

The major characteristics of descriptive theories are to describe a phenomenon, an event, a situation or a relationship needed when very little is known about a phenomena. These theory explore the phenomenon and speculate on why phenomena occur and what are the consequences of a phenomena. Descriptive theories describe all these. These theories have explanatory, relating and predicting utility. They are consider as complete and have the potential for guiding research.

Prescriptive Theories

Generally, prescriptive theory designates the prescription (intervention), the conditions under which the prescription should occur, and the consequences. They are action-oriented which tests the validity and predictability of a nursing intervention. Guide nursing research to develop and test specific nursing interventions.

Table 5.2 shows classification of theories and Table 5.3 enlists name of grand theorist and name of model.

Table 5.2: Classification of theories.

Types of theory	Level of abstraction
Conceptual model	Most abstract
Grand theory	
Middle-range theory	
Situation specific theory	Most concrete

Table 5.3: Name of grand theorist and name of model.

Theorist	Model
Dorothy Johnson	Behavior system model
Myra Levin	Conservation model
Martha Rogers	Science of human beings
Betty Neuman	Systems model
Sister Callista Roy	Adaptation model

CHARACTERISTICS OF A THEORY

- Interrelate concepts in such a way as to create a different way of looking at a particular phenomenon.
- Must be logical in nature.
- Should be relatively simple yet generalizable.
- The bases for hypothesis that can be tested or for theory to be expanded.
- Contribute to and assist in increasing the general body of knowledge within the discipline through the research implemented to validate them.
- Used by practitioners to guide and improve their practice.
- Consistent with other validated theories, laws, and principles but will leave open unanswered questions that need to be investigated.

USES OF THEORIES

The nursing theories provide direction and guidance for structuring professional nursing practice, education, and research. It also differentiates the focus of nursing from other professions. They serve to guide assessment, intervention, and evaluation of nursing care. They provide a rationale for collecting reliable and valid data about the health status of clients, which are essential for effective decision making and implementation. They help to establish criteria to measure the quality of nursing care. They help build a common nursing terminology to use in communicating with other health professionals. Finally, nursing theories enhance the autonomy of nursing by defining its own independent functions.

Nursing research plays a dual and continuing role in theory building and testing. Theories guides and generates ideas for research; research assesses the worth of the theories and provides a foundation for new theories. In nursing education, nursing theories provide a general focus for curriculum design. They guide the curricular decision-making.

In nursing research, nursing theories offer a framework for generating knowledge and new ideas. They assist in discovering knowledge gaps in the specific field of study. Finally, they offer a systematic approach to identify questions for study, select variables, interpret findings, and validate nursing interventions. The relationship between theory and research is reciprocal and mutually beneficial. Theories and models have been built by inductive method from observations, and an excellent source for those observations is prior research, including in-depth qualitative studies which have been conducted before. Concepts and relationships that are validated empirically through research become the foundation for theory development.

Nursing theories provide a framework for thought in which to examine situations. As new situations are encountered, this framework provides a structure for organization, analysis, and decision making. In addition, nursing theories provide a structure for communicating with other nurses and with other members of the healthcare team. **Figure 5.2** shows role of theories in research.

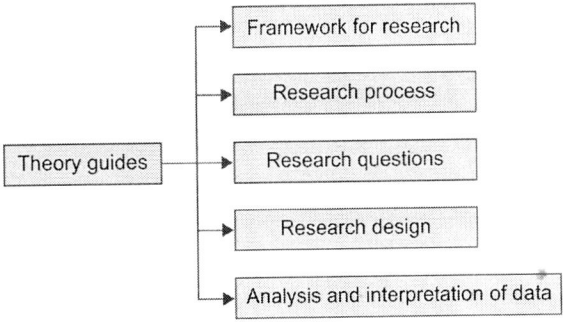

Fig. 5.2: Role of theories in research.

RESEARCH FRAMEWORK

First, it is important to understand what a 'framework' is, within the context of research. A framework for research as a structure that provides 'guidance for the researcher as study questions are fine tuned, methods for measuring variables are selected and analyses are planned.' Once data are collected and analyzed, the framework is used as a mirror to check whether the findings agree with the framework or whether there are some discrepancies; where discrepancies exist, a question is asked as to whether or not the framework can be used to explain them.

- ❖ Frameworks described as the abstract, logical structure of meaning that guides the development of the study.
- ❖ Frameworks are based on the identification of key concepts and the relationships among those concepts.
- ❖ The Oxford Dictionary defines 'Framework' as frame structure, upon or in to which casing or contents be put in and underpin as 'Support from below with masonry strengthen.'

—'O' Toole (2003)

Theoretical Framework

A theoretical framework consists of concepts and, together with their definitions and reference to relevant scholarly literature, existing theory that is used for your particular study. It refers to the theory that a researcher chooses to guide him or her in his or her research. Thus, a theoretical framework is the application of a theory, or a set of concepts drawn from one and the same theory, to offer an explanation of an event, or shed some light on a particular phenomenon or research problem. Theoretical framework present a broad general of relationship of research study by based on an existing theory. It provides a general representation of relationships between things in a given phenomenon. The 'theoretical framework' of an experiment or paper refers to the larger assumptions in which the researcher is working. It provides a large, overarching structure of ideas that the researcher can then draw from in beginning to analyze a phenomenon or a text.

Theoretical framework present a broad general of relationship of research study by based on an existing theory.

When selecting theoretical framework the investigator must understand different theories and models that are relevant to the research topics which is going to be conducted by the researcher.

Importance of Using Theoretical Framework

- ❖ An explicit statement of theoretical assumptions permits the reader to evaluate the research study critically.
- ❖ The theoretical framework connects the researcher to existing knowledge which is known and provides a framework to conduct the study.
- ❖ Guided by a relevant theory means you (the researchers) are given a basis for your hypotheses and choice of research methods.
- ❖ Articulating the theoretical assumptions of a research study forces the researcher to address questions of why and how the methodology chosen and study conducted.
- ❖ The theoretical framework permits researcher to intellectually transition from simply describing a phenomenon you have observed to generalizing about various aspects of that phenomenon.

❖ Having a theory helps the researcher identify the limits to those whom the study will be generalized.
❖ A theoretical framework specifies which key variables influence a phenomenon of interest and highlights the need to examine how those key variables might differ and under what circumstances.

How should the Theoretical Framework Formulated (Fig. 5.3)

❖ Specifies the theory used as basis for your study
❖ Mentions the proponents of the theory.
❖ Cites the main points emphasized in the theory.
❖ Supports his exposition of the theory by ideas from other experts to apply on your study.
❖ Illustrates his theoretical framework by means of a diagram to fit your study.
❖ Reiterates his theoretical proposition in your study

To construct a theoretical framework an existing theory is used to establish relationship between study concepts.

Let us take an example of a study that 'effectiveness of video-assisted teaching module (VATM) regarding prevention of malnutrition among under-fives on knowledge of the mothers in a selected rural community'.

Theoretical framework for this study was based on general system's theory of Bertalanffy (1968).

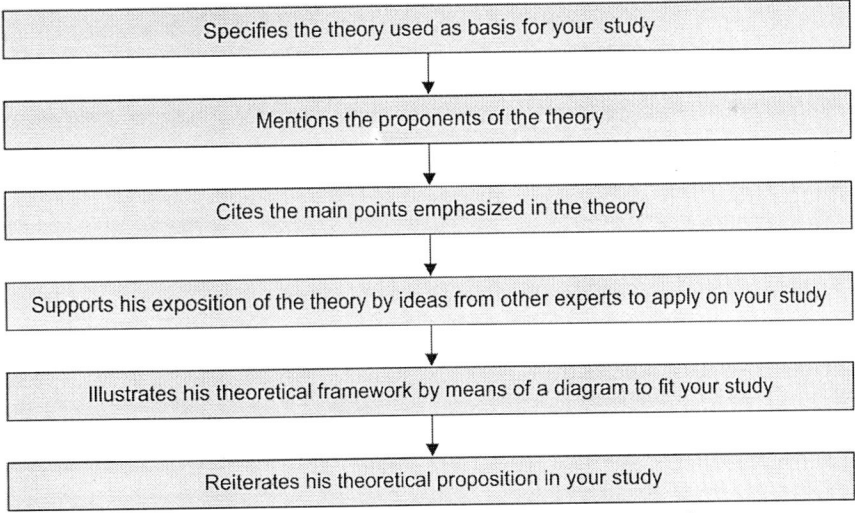

Fig. 5.3: Steps of constructing of theoretical framework.

General System's Theory of Bertalanffy

In this theory main focus was on the part and their inter-relationship which make-up and describes the whole. He defines system, 'as a complex interaction which means that system consists of two or more converted elements which form an organized whole and which interact with each other.' For the present study the knowledge of mother on child nutrition was considered as the whole and various components of the nutrition education are the part of the system **(Fig. 5.4)**.

Input

According to theorist 'input' refers to energy, matter and information. All systems must receive varying type and amount from the environment. In the present study input refers to information on prevention of malnutrition in the form of structured interview schedule and VATM for the mothers. It includes importance of nutrition among under fives, meaning, cause and effect of malnutrition, prevention of malnutrition and consequence of long-term malnutrition. Prevention of malnutrition considered as proper antenatal care, exclusive breastfeeding, weaning, food hygiene, weight monitoring and prevention of common communicable diseases.

Throughput

According to the theory 'throughput' refers to a process by which the system processes input and release output. In the present study throughput is processing of information. It includes pretest, presentation of VATM followed by post-test.

Output

According to the theory, the 'output' refers to the information, energy and matter that leave a system. For the present study the expected outcome considered as the post-test knowledge score obtained through application of structured interview schedule which shows significantly increased which was graded as very poor, poor, average, good, very good and excellent depending on the percentage of knowledge score.

Let us take an example of another problem statement '*Effectiveness of structured teaching on knowledge on prevention of anemia among primi gravida mothers attending outpatient department of selected hospitals.*' Theoretical framework for this study was based on King's theory of goal attainment.

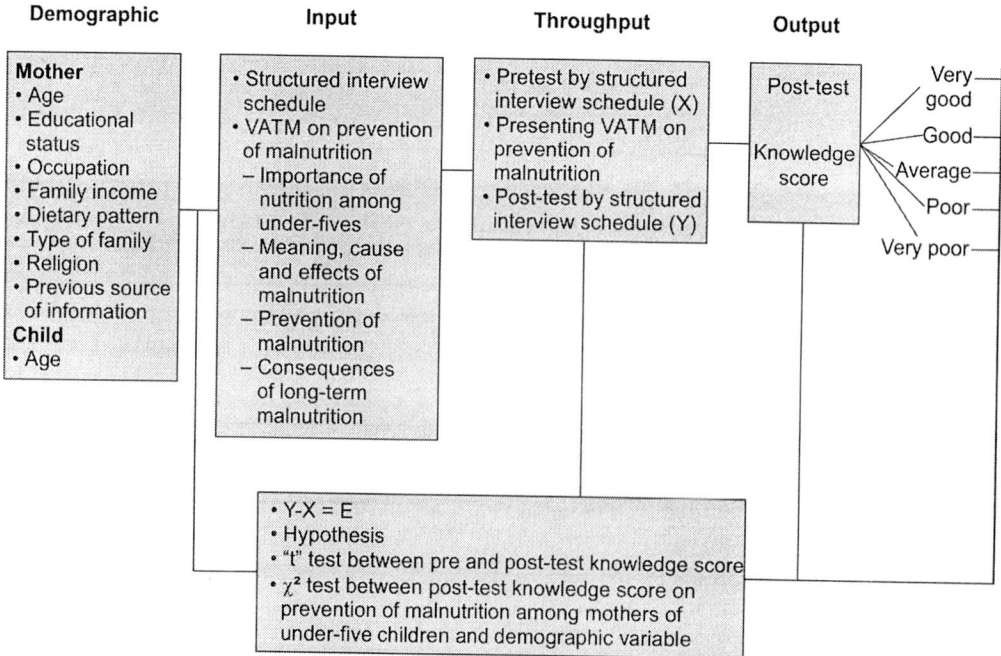

Fig. 5.4: Theoretical framework based on general system theory of Bertanlanffy (1968).

King's Theory of Goal Attainment

According to this theory, human being as patients have rights to obtain information, to participate in decisions that may influence their life, health, and community services, and to accept or reject care. It is the responsibility of health care members to inform individuals of all aspects of health care to help them in making informed decision. This goal attainment can be possible by the perception judgment and action of both nurse and patient (**Fig. 5.5**).

Perception

King explains perception as a process in which data is obtained through the senses and from memory are organized, interpreted and transformed. Here antenatal mother perceived the need of gain knowledge and the nurse by doing duty daily in antenatal OPD perceived that they have lack of knowledge regarding prevention of anemia.

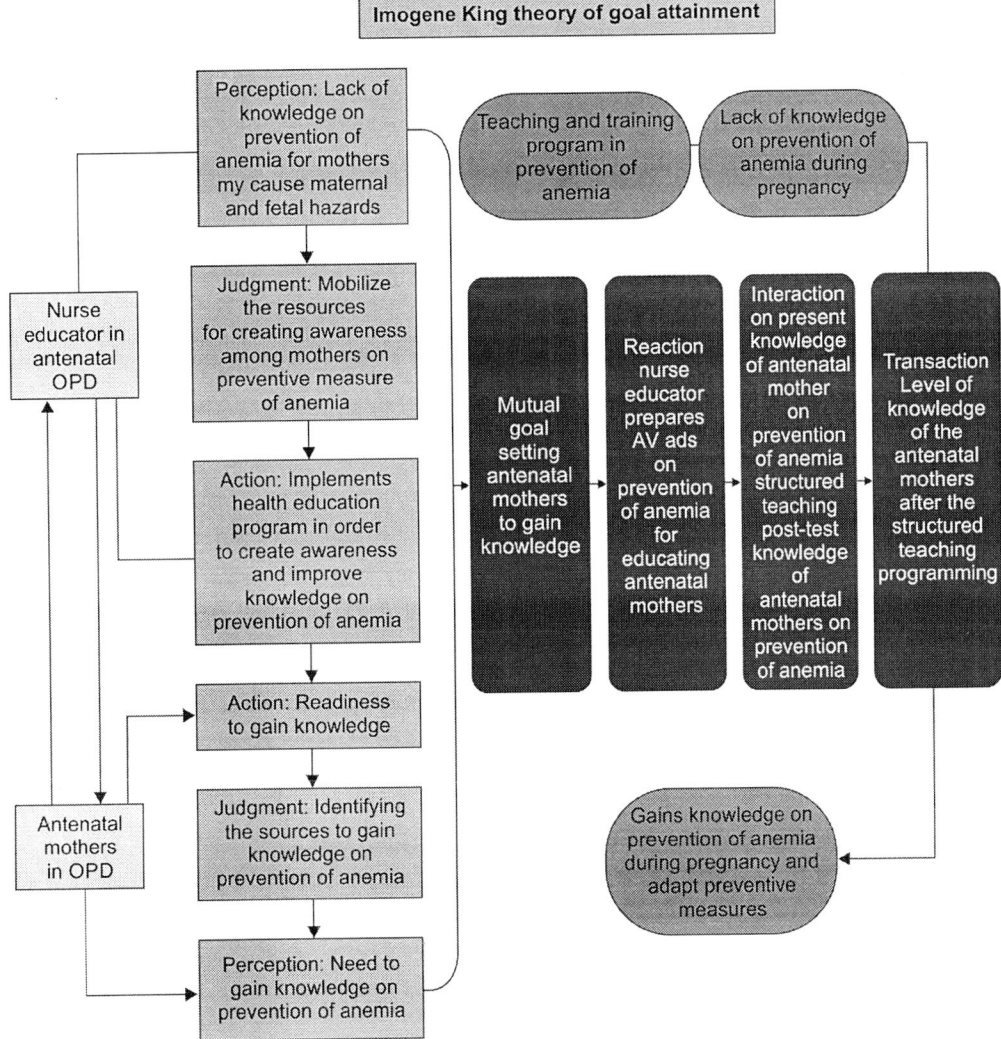

Fig. 5.5: Theoretical framework based on Imogene King's theory of goal attainment.

Judgment

Judgment means decision making. The mothers identified the sources to gain knowledge on prevention of anemia and the nurse taking mobilize the resources for creating awareness among mothers on preventive measures of anemia.

Action

Here action denotes for the nurse researcher is the implements of health education program in order to create awareness and improve their knowledge on prevention of anemia and for antenatal mothers is readiness to gain knowledge and there is mutual goal setting between antenatal mothers and nurse researcher to gain knowledge among the antenatal mothers regarding prevention of anemia.

Reaction

On reaction nurse educator prepares ads on prevention of anemia for educating antenatal mothers.

Interaction

It is defined as the observable behaviors of two or more persons in mutual presence here interaction consists assessment of present knowledge of antenatal mothers on prevention of anemia, then presentation of structured teaching and post-test knowledge of antenatal mothers on prevention of anemia if the level of knowledge of the antenatal mothers after the structured teaching programming increase, they gains knowledge on prevention of anemia during pregnancy and adapt preventive measure then goal achieved. If still there is lack of knowledge on prevention of anemia during pregnancy again every step will continue. This is in transaction phase.

A descriptive study on prevalence of pin-site infection and practices of pin-site care for patients with external skeletal fixation, in orthopedic ward, MKCG Medical College and Hospital, Berhampur, Odisha.

This theoretical framework was based on a single middle-range theory 'epidemiological triad'.

This model explains the factors responsible for any illness that may be classified as agent, host and environment, and is referred to as 'epidemiological triad' (**Fig. 5.6**).

Interaction of these three factors—agent, host and environment initiates the process of variation if any of these factors bringing significant difference in occurrence of an illness in an individual.

Conceptual Framework

Generally, researcher may opine that his or her research problem cannot meaningfully be researched in reference to only one theory, or concepts resident within one theory. In such cases, the researcher may have to 'synthesize' the existing views in the literature concerning a given situation—both theoretical and from empirical findings. The synthesis may be called a *model* or *conceptual framework*, which essentially represents an 'integrated' way of looking at the problem. Such a model could then be used in place of a theoretical framework. Thus, a conceptual framework may be defined as an end result of bringing together a number of related concepts to explain or predict a given event, or give a broader understanding of the phenomenon of interest—or simply, of a research problem. The process of arriving at a conceptual framework is akin to an inductive process whereby small individual pieces

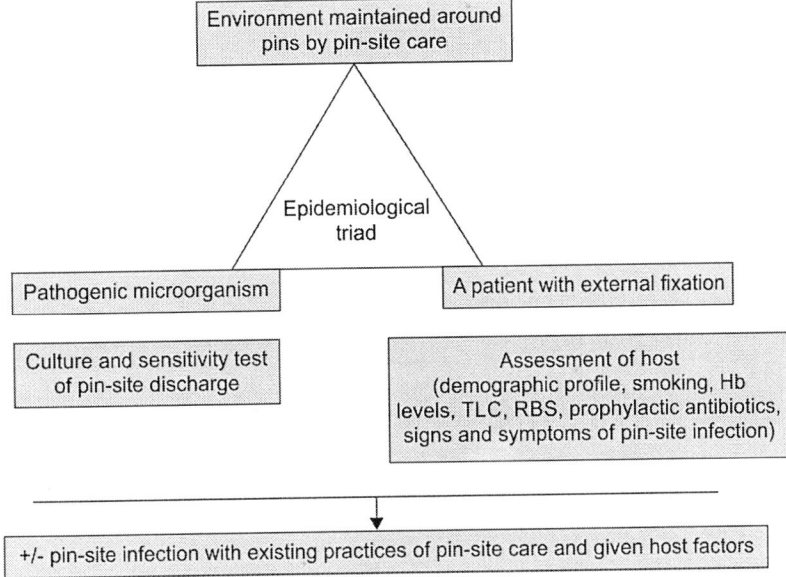

Fig. 5.6: Theoretical framework based on the epidemiological triad model of disease causation.

(in this case, concepts) are joined together to tell a bigger map of possible relationships. Thus, a conceptual framework is derived from concepts, in-so-far as a theoretical framework is derived from a theory, which is a model of systematic representation of some phenomenon. A conceptual framework explains the main things to be studied—the key factors, constructs or variables—and the presumed relationships among them. Frameworks can be rudimentary or elaborate, theory-driven or commonsensical, descriptive or causal. Conceptual framework represent ways of thinking about a problem. It deals with abstractions (concepts) that are assembled by virtue of relevance to a common theme. It is an explanation of how a researcher sees the different concepts and outcomes of study and its relations with each other and can be developed from the researcher's personal experience, previous studies, or from more than one theory or models. It broadly presents understanding of the phenomenon of interest and reflects the assumptions and philosophic view of the designer. It is researcher's own position on the problem—the way the researcher shapes it together.

Definition of Conceptual Framework

Conceptual framework logically constructed concepts to provide general relationship between the concepts of research study without using a single theory.

The most important thing to understand about conceptual framework is that it is primarily a conception or model of what is out there that a researcher plan to study, and of what is going on with these things and why—a tentative *theory* of the phenomena that a researcher is investigating.

Conceptual framework is a written or visual presentation that explains either graphically or in a narrative form, the main things to be studied such as the key factors, concepts, or variables and the presumed relationship among them.

Purposes of Conceptual Framework

- Keeps research on track.
- Provides clear links from the literature to the research goals and questions.
- Helps the researcher to see clearly the variables of the study.
- Clarifies concepts and propose relationships among concepts.
- Provides an organizing structure for the research design and methods.
- Useful to prepare research proposal using experimental or descriptive methods.
- Guides the development and testing of interventions and hypotheses.
- Provides general framework for data analysis.
- The interpretation of findings flows from the conceptualization represented by the framework.
- Makes research findings meaningful and generalizable.
- Provides reference points for discussion of the methodology and analysis of the data.
- Contributes to the trustworthiness of the study.
- Encourages theory development that is useful to practice.
- An abstract, logical structure of meaning that guides the development of the study.
- Enables the researcher to link the findings to the body of nursing knowledge.
- Shows the relationship of the different constructs or concepts that the researcher wants to investigate.

Metaphor in Development of Conceptual Framework

Conceptual Metaphor

Metaphor is an expression, often found in literature, that describes a person or object by referring to something that is considered to have similar characteristics to that person or object. Conceptual metaphor refers to the understanding of one idea, or conceptual domain, in terms of another. These are very often used to understand theories and models. Conceptual metaphor uses one idea and links it to another to better understand something.

Definition

Metaphors are an essential part of scientific creativity, because they provide a means of seeking literal descriptions of the world about us. The literal descriptions are scientific theories.

Metaphor is use of an object or action to represent another. Because theories are literal statements, on these construal metaphor in research is useful only in the pretheoretical stages of emergent disciplines.

In the more established scientific disciplines metaphor is seen as useful in terms of only in pretheoretical stages of emergent disciplines.

Uses of Metaphor

In the more established scientific disciplines, metaphor is seen as useful in terms of only **Exegesis**, e.g., white cells are soldiers in the war against cancer (Bonner and Greenland, 2005).

As a heuristic device to facilitate new discoveries, e.g., styles of thinking are conceptual spaces that can be mapped, explored and transformed (Borden, 1994).

As a pedagogical tool, e.g., to breathe life into dry subjects (Cook and Gordon, 2004).

Theory, Concept-Constructive Metaphor

Theory-constructive metaphors are introduced into scientific theorizing when there seems good reason to believe that there are theoretically important points of similarity between primary and secondary subjects.

When there is no adequate literal expression with which to express the same theoretical claims, metaphorical expressions and statements are theory constructive.

Theoretically constitutive metaphorical expressions allow the introduction, at a relatively early stage of theory construction, of theoretical terms which refer to various plausibility postulated similarities and dissimilarities between target source.

There are entities in the world the essential nature of which renders them referentially imprecise. These are what Boyd (1993) terms homeostatic property cluster phenomena.

Homeostatic cluster phenomena are characterized by a range of cases. Their co-occurrence is typical the result of what may be described either literally or metaphorically as a form of homeostasis.

The homeostasis is appropriate because either the presence of some properties favors the presence of others (under the appropriate conditions) or there are underlying mechanisms or processes which tend to maintain the presence of both (sets of) properties.

Ingredients of Conceptual Framework

A conceptual framework is composed of concepts and the rational linkages between them (called propositional statements).

A concept abstractly describes and names an object or phenomenon, thus providing it with separate identity or meaning.

It is actually the intellectual representation of some aspect of reality, derived from observations made from phenomenon, e.g., anxiety, stress and pain.

Prerequisites to Develop a Conceptual Framework

- Construction of the framework requires researcher's knowledge of theories, findings of the previous similar research studies and related field experience.
- Development of a framework depends on the power of observation, understanding of a problem, imagination and conceptualization about abstract ideas and ability of linking the abstract ideas with logical scheme to generate the facts.
- Frameworks are usually developed through inductive reasoning, where the researcher have the ability to observe and conceptualize to generate the facts.

Components

Miles and Hubermann (1994) gives following components of a conceptual framework.
- Concept or variable
- Relationship
- Statement hierarchy

Concept or Variable
Based on the degree of abstractness of a term, they may be termed as construct, concept or variable. A construct is something which has general meaning.

Relationship

This declares some kind of connection between and among two or more than two concepts. It is center part of a conceptual framework.

The statement of relationship in conceptual framework may be made of objectives, hypothesis, research question, study design, statistical analysis and the findings.

Statement Hierarchy

Statement hierarchy deals with abstractions of conceptual ideas. The level of abstractness are as follows:

* **General proposition:** Highest level of abstractness (conceptual model).
* **Specific proposition:** Moderate level of abstractness (theories).
* **Hypothesis:** It is very specific and lowest level of abstractness.

Steps of Developing Conceptual Framework

Conceptual or theoretical framework of the study may be developed by using following steps (**Fig. 5.7**):

* Identify the general concepts
* Gathering relevant information
* Formulate general scheme of relevant concepts
* Develop a logical construct
* Evaluation and revision
* Establishing the congruity
* Development of conceptual model

Identify the General Concepts

In this step, the researcher identifies the general concepts of the study; these concepts may be used on study variables, previous research findings, or existing theories and models.

Some concepts may be identified from a real-life observation or experience.

For example, a research is planned to develop a conceptual framework for his or her research study titled 'a correlational study on the effect of institutional and home environment on overall development of the students, in selected school, Berhampur.

Here the researcher identifies the general concepts of the study based on study variables, i.e., home environment, institute environment and student development.

Gathering Relevant Information

It involves gathering information about the concepts from the relevant existing theories, previous research findings.

This information helps the researcher to understand the concepts more empirically for establishing a relationship between concepts for development of framework.

A framework is based on a scientific theory or theoretical model; researcher must read about them from primary sources.

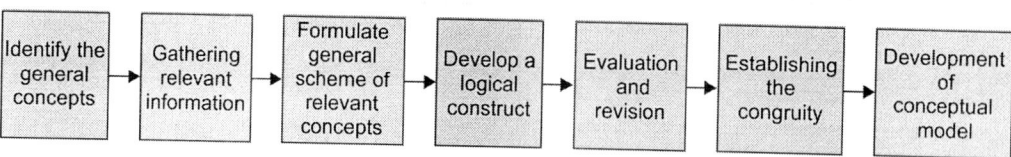

Fig. 5.7: Steps of developing conceptual framework.

Gathering relevant information about concepts enables the researcher to judge the amount of empirical support the theory has received and the way the theory must be adopted in framework.

Once the theory is identified to borrow the concepts to develop the conceptual framework, read this theory in detail and understand each concept and preposition so that you can appropriately adopt and integrate the theoretical concepts in your study concept.

Formulate General Scheme of Relevant Concepts

After learning in-depth about the concepts, the researcher starts establishing the general relationship between the different related and relevant concepts.

The schematic relationship is established through brainstorming and logical reasoning.

If a researcher has identified the problem statement and later develops a conceptual framework, it requires an interactive approach.

Development of Logical Construct

After establishing the logical relationship between two or more variables, the researcher develops a final construct.

Construct is a highly abstract and complex description of a phenomenon (concept) and denoted by a made-up or constructed term.

Construct term is used to indicate a phenomenon that cannot be directly observed but must be inferred by certain concrete or less abstract indicators of the phenomenon.

For example, wellness, mental health and self-esteem are constructs, but are only measures through indefinable and measurable concepts, e.g., wellness can only be assessed with laboratory data.

Evaluation and Revision

Concepts and constructs act as a building block for the framework, which are later evaluated for their relevance and relationship to conclude or generate the facts.

After the evaluation, revisions may be made before development of a framework. A theoretical framework may be evaluated through following:

- Is the theoretical framework consistent with the research question, design, variables and interpretation of the study?
- Are major concepts of the models identified and defined?
- Are the relationships among concepts within the models described?
- Is the conceptual framework based on nursing theory or theory from other related discipline?
- Are the concepts in conceptual framework clearly, adequately and logically defined and articulated in the way that they help either in testing or generation of a theory?

Establishment of Congruity

Congruity means a point of agreement once the researcher develops a framework, it is important to establish the congruity between conceptual framework and its components, the research problem, hypothesis, the description of the operationalization of concepts, and the selection of the research design.

In the real sense, congruity of framework may only be established if most of the research decisions and interpretations of the study findings is based on the framework.

Development of Conceptual Model

Finally, the researcher develop the model which can be validated there after with the experts and then applied in research study.

Conceptual framework is the researcher's own position on the problem and gives direction to the study. It may be an adaptation of a model used in a previous study, with modifications to suit the inquiry. Aside from showing the direction of the study, through the conceptual framework, the researcher can be able to show the relationships of the different constructs that he wants to investigate, etc. Let us take an example of a conceptual framework developed based on a study.

'A study to compare quality of life among tuberculosis new cases tuberculosis retreatment and TB with HIV patients at MKCG Medical College and Hospital, Berhampur with a view to develop counseling guideline.'

Conceptual framework of the present study is developed by taking the concepts from *Wilson and Cleary (1995)* and *Felce and Perry (1995)* (**Fig. 5.8**).

Wilson and Cleary developed a model in 1995 for planning health care intervention to improve health-related quality of life (QOL). This theory focuses to identify determinant of QOL and relationship among them. This model presents five ordered domains of patient outcomes, from biological function (e.g., presence of disease) via symptoms, functional status, and general health perceptions to overall quality of life, implicating a one-way main causal relation. The characteristics of the individual (demographic, biological, e.g., genetics, and psychological factors) as well as characteristics of the environment (social and physical factors), are affect the QOL in one-way direction.

Felce and Perry (1995) expressed that QOL is well-being. According to them QOL is based on multidimensional concept. Objective quality of life is the condition in which individual lives, individual subjective satisfaction in which individual lives that influence QOL which can be weighted by his values, perception and expectations. In this model QOL encompasses five domain namely material, physical, social, emotional and productive well-being.

In this present study the conceptual framework consists of components that are:
- ❖ **Controlling factor:** These are the factor present in external and internal environment of individual (including natural, political, social and economic environments) that have constant interaction with him. It includes individual characteristics, functional status, disease's symptom, individual satisfaction and environmental interaction.
- ❖ **Category of patient:** In these present study three categories of patient has included, e.g., TB new case, TB retreatment and HIV TB coinfection.

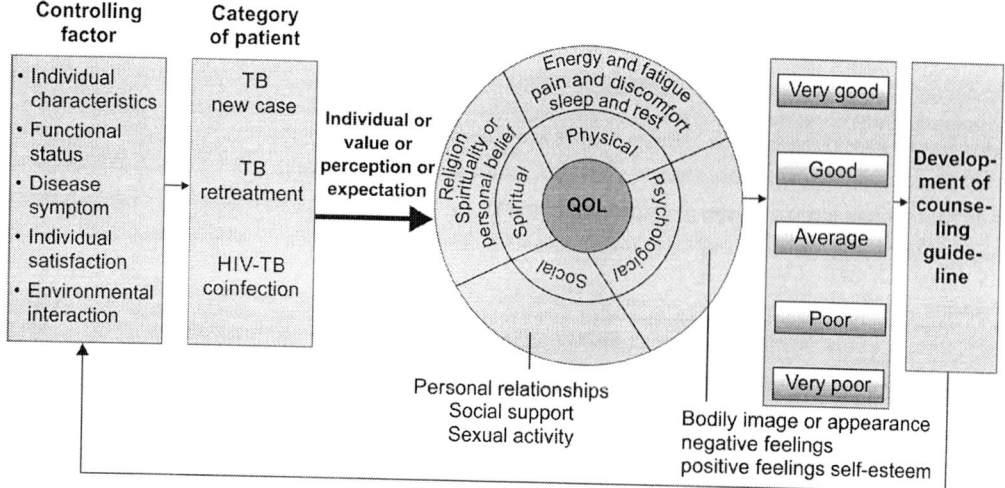

Fig. 5.8: Conceptual framework of quality of life-based on Wilson and Clary HRQOL, Felce and Perry's theory of QOL.

- **Individual value/perception/expectation:** This is otherwise expressed as individual's frame of reference. It implies that what is important is the 'life status' of the individual as compared to some normative standard and his satisfaction with his or her 'life status'. It can vary according to his age, cultural background, etc.
- **Quality of life:** It is a product of livability of environment and individual's ability to make use of opportunities afforded by environment. It shows how much the individual is satisfied or dissatisfied life experiences and personal frame of references. It has six domain, i.e., physical health, psychological, level of independence, social relationships, environment and spirituality. For convenience it has grouped into four broad domain.
    - **Physical:** Energy and fatigue, pain and discomfort, sleep and rest, mobility, activities of daily living, work capacity.
    - **Social**: Personal relationships, social support and sexual activity.
    - **Psychological:** Bodily image and appearance, negative feelings, positive feelings, self-esteem, thinking, learning, memory and concentration.
    - **Spiritual:** Religion/spirituality/personal beliefs.
    - **Outcome:** The QOL is measured by using a 5-point rating scale and the result will be grouped as very good, good, average, poor and very poor.
- **Development of counseling guideline:** After statistical analysis of result the investigator will develop a counseling guideline for development of QOL among these three categories of TB patients.

SUMMARY

- Theory models and primary mechanism based on which a researcher can conduct a study. Theories are constructed in order to explain, predict and master phenomena (e.g., relationships, events, or the behavior). A theory makes generalizations about observations and consists of an interrelated, coherent set of ideas and models.
- A theory is a set of interrelated concepts, which structure a systematic view of phenomena for the purpose of explaining or predicting. A theory is like a blueprint, a guide for modeling a structure. A blueprint depicts the elements of a structure and the relation of each element to the other, just as a theory depicts the concepts, which compose it and the relation of concepts with each other.
- Theories are located on the ladder of abstraction relative to their scope. Based on the level of abstraction the theories can be classified as grand theory, middle-range theories and situation specific theories. Based on the goal orientation, theories can be classified as descriptive theories and prescriptive theories.
- The nursing theories provide direction and guidance for structuring professional nursing practice, education, and research. It also differentiates the focus of nursing from other professions. They serve to guide assessment, intervention, and evaluation of nursing care.
- A theoretical framework consists of concepts and, together with their definitions and reference to relevant scholarly literature, existing theory that is used for your particular study. It refers to the theory that a researcher chooses to guide him or her in his or her research.
- Generally, researcher may opine that his or her research problem cannot meaningfully be researched in reference to only one theory, or concepts resident within one theory. In such cases, the researcher may have to 'synthesize' the existing views in the literature concerning a given situation—both theoretical and from empirical findings. The synthesis may be called

a *model* or *conceptual framework*, which essentially represents an 'integrated' way of looking at the problem.
* Conceptual framework logically constructed concepts to provide general relationship between the concepts of research study without using a single theory.

QUESTIONS TO TEST YOUR KNOWLEDGE

Q1. Explain the concept, characteristics and classification of theories. (2 + 3 + 10)

Q2. Write down the use of nursing theories in nursing research. (10)

Q3. What do you mean by theoretical framework? How it will be developed and applied in research? Enumerate with example. (3 + 12)

Q4. Explain the concept of conceptual framework. What are the purposes of conceptual framework? How it will be developed and applied? Explain with examples. (3 + 3 + 9)

Q5. Multiple choice questions:

I. Logically constructed concepts to provide general relationship between the concepts of research study without using a single theory:
   a. Theoretical framework
   b. Conceptual framework
   c. Theoretical model
   d. Both a and b

II. A highly abstract phenomenon that cannot be directly observed but must be inferred by certain concrete or less abstract indicators of the phenomenon:
   a. Framework
   b. Proposition
   c. Construct
   d. Theory

III. Concerned with the values and beliefs of a discipline and with the values and beliefs held by members of the discipline is called:
   a. Ethics
   b. Philosophy
   c. Self-discipline
   d. Phenomenon

IV. A word picture or mental idea of a phenomenon is:
   a. Theory
   b. Concept
   c. Construct
   d. Conceptual framework

V. When a researcher developing a framework by using single theory it is called:
   a. Theoretical framework
   b. Conceptual framework
   c. Theoretical construct
   d. Conceptual model

VI. King's theory of goal attainment is an example of which of the following theories:
   a. Grand theories
   b. Middle-range theories
   c. Situation specific theories
   d. Prescriptive theories

VII. _____ is a set of related statements that describes or explains phenomena in a systematic way.
   a. Framework
   b. Proposition
   c. Construct
   d. Theory

VIII. Which of the following theories are the most concrete and narrow in scope?
   a. Grand theories
   b. Middle-range theories
   c. Situation specific theories
   d. Descriptive theories

IX. When very little is known about a phenomena to explore these which of the following theories can applied?
   a. Prescriptive theories
   b. Middle-range theories
   c. Situation specific theories
   d. Descriptive theories

X. When the researcher follows two or more theories and develops a framework it is called:
   a. Theoretical framework
   b. Conceptual framework
   c. Theoretical model
   d. All of the above

ANSWERS				
I. b	II. c	III. b	IV. b	V. a
VI. a	VII. a	VIII. c	IX. d	X. b

Chapter 6

Ethics in Research

Learning Objectives

After completion of this chapter, the students will be able to:
- Explain the concept and importance of ethics in nursing research.
- Explore the historical background of ethics in nursing research.
- Enumerate the codes of ethics and ethical principles in nursing research.
- Describe ethical responsibilities of a nurse researcher.
- Identify the dilemma in nursing research.

INTRODUCTION

Ethics are the rules for correct behavior. Professional ethics for nurses will state the ideal ways in which a nurse should behave in all relationships including those with the patient, patient's relatives, coworkers, members of other professions and the public. The discussion of the professional adjustment is complete only when ethics are included. So ethics is a branch of philosophy dealing with values related to human conduct with respect to the rightness and wrongness of certain actions and to the goodness and badness of the motives and ends of such actions. Ethical considerations cover all aspects of research, but they are foregrounded when the subject of the research are humans or animals. Research involving human subjects in the medical, social and behavioral sciences poses complex ethical issues which requires careful thought and consideration on the part of both researchers and research participants. Ethics in research are very important when we are going to conduct an experiment.

DEFINITION

- Ethics is defined as, 'laws of human conduct and duties.' —Haven, 1870
- Ethics is an account of human actions and the goal of ethical deliberations is to judge human actions. —John, 1969
- Ethics is concerned with doing well and avoiding harm. —Bandman L Elsie, 1995

Ethics in nursing research can be defined as the act of moral principles that the researchers have to follow while conducting nursing research to ensure the right and welfare of individuals, groups or communities under study.

Basic assumptions about how research should be conducted?
- Subjects should be protected from harm.
- Subjects should have their identity protected.
- Subjects should be fully informed about the research study.
- Participation is voluntary.
- Study procedures should show respect for cultural values and beliefs.

IMPORTANCE OF ETHICS IN NURSING RESEARCH

Nursing research usually deals with the human being where implication of the ethics becomes very essential. Some of the important reasons to support importance of ethics in nursing research are:
- Protect the vulnerable group and other study participants from harmful effects of the experimental interventions.
- Safeguard the participants from exploitation of researchers.
- Establish the risk-benefit ratio for the study subject.
- Ensure the fullest respect, dignity, privacy, disclose of information and fair treatment for the study subject.
- Build the capability of subject to accept or reject participation in study and have to access to informed or written consent for participation in research study.

HISTORICAL BACKGROUND

Human experimentation has been conducted even before 18th century. However, the ethical attitudes of researchers drawn the interest of society only after 1940's because of human exploitation in several cases. The Nazi program of research involved the use of prisoners of war and racial 'enemies' in numerous experiments designed to test the limits of human endurance and human reaction to diseases and untested drugs. The studies were unethical not only because they exposed the participants to permanent physical harm and even death but also because the subjects were not given an opportunity to refuse participation. Some recent examples of ethical transgression have also occurred in the United States. For instance, between 1932 and 1972, a study known as the Tuskegee Syphilis Study, sponsored by the US Public Health Service, investigated the effects of syphilis among 400 men from a poor Black community. Medical treatment was deliberately withheld to study the course of untreated disease. Another well known case of unethical research involved the injection of live cancer cells into elderly patients at the Jewish Chronic Disease Hospital in Brooklyn, without the consent of those patients. In 1993, the US federal agencies, such as the Atomic Energy Commission, have sponsored radiation experiments since the 1940s on hundreds of people, many of them were prisoners or elderly hospital patients. In Los Angel, California, between, 1989 and 1991 approximately 900 children who were mostly Black of Hispanic, were given an experimental measles vaccine called EZ (Edmonston Zagreb). The researchers never told the parents about the experiment because the vaccine was unlicensed. In 2005, it was revealed that government funded researchers tested experimental AIDS drug on hundreds of foster children without providing these children with an independent advocate (Solomon, 2005). These children who were mostly poor or from minority group, received cutting age treatment at the government expenses. In some cases their lives were extended. However, many children experienced side effects, such as rashes, vomiting and sharp drops in infection fighting blood cells. They had no advocate, the weigh, the advantages and disadvantages of their participation in research.

CODES OF ETHICS IN NURSING RESEARCH

Professional codes and laws were introduced since then in order to prevent scientific abuses of human lives. The Nazi experiments led to the Nuremberg Code (1947) which was the leading code for all subsequent codes made to protect human rights in research. This code focuses on voluntary informed consent, liberty of withdrawal from research, protection from physical and mental harm, or suffering and death. It also emphasizes the risk-benefit balance. The only weak point of this code was the self-regulation of researchers which can be abused in some research studies. All declarations followed, forbade nontherapeutic research. It was only in 1964 with the declaration of Helsinki that the need for nontherapeutic research was initiated. The declaration emphasized the protection of subjects in this kind of research and strongly proclaimed that the well-being of individuals is more important than scientific and social interests. In terms of Nursing the first inquiry was the 'Nightingale Pledge' (1983). Since then there has been a significant development of professional codes in conduct and research. The American Nurses' Association (ANA) Guidelines for Research, the Human Rights Guidelines for nurses in clinical and other research (1985) and the Royal College of Nursing Code for nurses in research (1977) provide a strong assistance to professional nurses as well as reassurance to patients, the public and society, of professionals' intentions. The 'ANA' published other set up guidelines in 1995, ethical guidelines in the conduct, dissemination and implementation of nursing research.

An especially important code of ethics was adopted by the National Commission for the Protection of Human Subjects of Biomedical and Behavioral Research (1978). The commission established by the National Research Act (Public Law 93–348), issued a report in 1978 that served as the basis for regulations affecting research sponsored by the federal government. The report sometime called as the Belmont Report. This report articulated three primary ethical principles on which standards of ethical conduct in research are based.

Nuremberg code is concerned with several criteria for research including the following:
* Research must inform subjects
* Research must be for the good of society
* Research must be based on animal experiments, if possible
* Research must try to avoid injury to research subjects
* Research must be qualified to conduct research
* Subject or the researchers can stop the study if problems occur.

ETHICAL PRINCIPLES IN NURSING RESEARCH

The major ethical principles that should be considered in designing or reviewing the research studies are (Fig. 6.1):
* Beneficence
* Respect of human dignity
* Justice

Principles of Beneficence

The ethical principle of beneficence refers to the Hippocratic 'be of benefit, do not harm'. Beauchamp and Childress, suggest that *'the principle of beneficence includes the professional mandate to do effective and significant research so as to better serve and promote the welfare of our constituents.'* This is the most important ethical principles in nursing research, where every researcher must ensure the following:
* Freedom from harm
* Freedom from exploitation
* Benefits from research
* The risk-benefit ratio

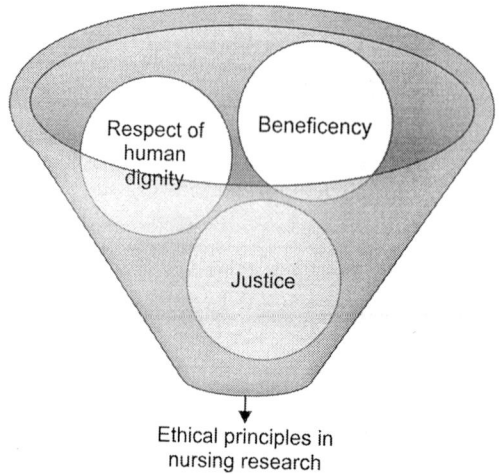

Fig. 6.1: Ethical principles in nursing research.

Freedom from Harm

Exposing research participants to experiences that result in serious or permanent harm is unacceptable. Discomfort and harm can be physiological, emotional, social and economic in nature. To minimize harm research should only be conducted by scientifically qualified people, especially if potentially dangerous technical equipment or specialized procedure. The research should be conducted with minimal risk which is defined as risks anticipated to be no greater than those ordinarily encountered in daily life or during routine physical or psychological tests or procedures. Varda and Behnke (2000) studied the effect of the timing of an initial bath (1 hour versus 2 hours after birth) on newborn temperature. To minimize risks, the researchers excluded all infants with conditions (infection, fetal distress, etc.) that could predispose them to temperature instability. The researchers must be prepared at any time during the study to terminate the research if there is reason to suspect that continuation would result in injury, disability, undue distress, or death to participant. If the study is likely to cause emotional arousal, we must make provisions to refer participants to a mental health professional for counseling.

Freedom from Exploitation

Involvement in research study should not place subjects at a disadvantage or expose them to situation for which they have not been explicitly prepared. Here the researcher has to maintain the confidentiality of the subject. The issue of confidentiality and anonymity is closely connected with the rights of beneficence, respect for the dignity and fidelity. ANA suggests anonymity is protected when the subject's identity cannot be linked with personal responses. If the researcher is not able to promise anonymity he has to address confidentiality, which is the management of private information by the researcher in order to protect the subject's identity. The researcher is responsible to 'maintain confidentiality that goes beyond ordinary loyalty'. By maintaining confidentiality a researcher can protect a subject from exploitation. Subject need to be assured that their participations or the information that might provide to the researchers will not be used against them. A participant reporting drug abuse should not fear exposure to criminal authorities. A prostitute study participant telling where she works and gets his/her customers should not fear exposure to criminal authorities.

Benefits from Research

Subjects agree to participate in scientific investigations for a number of reasons. They may perceive that there are some direct personal benefits. More often, however, any benefits from the research accrue to society in general or to other individuals. Thus, many subjects may participate in a study out of a desire to be helpful. Prospective participants must be given adequate information on potential benefits of their involvement to allow them to make informed decisions.

The Risk-Benefit Ratio

The risk-benefit ratio should also be considered in terms of whether the risk to research subject are commensurate with the benefits to society and the nursing profession in terms of the knowledge produced. The general guideline is that the degree of risk to be taken by those participating in the research should never exceed the potential humanitarian benefits of the knowledge to be gained. Thus the first step in ensuring that research is ethical. All research involves some risk, but in many cases, the risk is minimal. Minimal risk according to federal guidelines, is defined as an anticipated risk that are no greater than those ordinarily encountered in daily life or during the performance of routine physical or psychological tests or procedures. When the risks are not minimal, the researchers must proceed with great caution, taking every step possible to reduce risk and maximize benefits. If the perceived risks and costs to subject outweigh the anticipated benefits of the research, the research should be either abandoned or redesigned. Some of the major potential benefits and costs of research to participants are:

Major Potential Benefits

- Access to an intervention to which they otherwise may not have access.
- Comfort in being able to discuss their situation or problem with an objective and nonjudgmental researcher.
- Increased knowledge about themselves or their conditions, either through opportunity for introspection or through direct interaction with the researcher.
- Enhanced self-esteem resulting from special attention or treatment.
- Escape from normal routine, excitement of being part of a scientific study and satisfaction of curiosity about what it is like to participate in a study.
- Knowledge that the information subjects provide may help others with similar problems or conditions.
- Direct monetary or material gain.

Major Potential Cost

- Physical harm, including unanticipated side effects.
- Physical discomforts, fatigue or boredom.
- Psychological or emotional distress resulting from self-disclosure, introspection, fear of the unknown or interacting with strangers, fear of eventual repercussions, anger all the types of questions being asked and so on.
- Loss of privacy.
- Loss of time.
- Monetary costs (e.g., for transportation, baby sitting, time lost from work, or charges for additional procedures and tests associated with the research).

Principles of Respect for Human Dignity

Respect for the human dignity of subjects is the second ethical principles. This principles includes the right to self-determination and the right to full disclosure.

The Right to Self-determination

The ethical principle right to self-determination is otherwise known as autonomy which means that each person should be given the respect, time and opportunity necessary to make his or her own decisions. Human should be treated as autonomous agents, capable of controlling their own activities and destinies. The principles of self-determination mean that prospective subjects have the right to voluntarily decide whether or not to participate in a study, without the risk of incurring any penalties or prejudicial treatment. Participants have full right to question the researcher for any additional information or clarification of doubts and they have right to quit from the study at any stage of the research study.

The Right to Full Disclosure

The principle of respect for human dignity encompasses people right to make informed voluntary decision about their participation in a study. Such decision cannot be made without full disclosure. Full disclosure means that the researcher has fully described the nature of the study, the subject right to refuse participation, the researcher's responsibilities, and the likely risk and benefits that would be incurred. Full disclosure is normally provided to subject before their participation in a study either in a debriefing session or in written communication. A fully informed consent must be taken from the participant. In case of the fetus, infant, toddlers, younger child or psychological, neurological or physical inability to give informed consent this can be obtained from parents or legal guardians. In case of a child aged between 7 and 18 years an assent must be obtained.

The Principles of Justice

The principles of justice are the third ethical principles. The principles include the subject' *right to fair treatment and the right to privacy.*

The Right to Fair Treatment

To fair and nondiscriminatory selection of the participants, such as any risk and benefits will be equally shared by study participants. Participant selection should be based on research requirement and not on convenience, gullibility, or compromised position of certain types of people. The nonprejudicial treatment of individuals who decline to participate or who withdraw from the study after agreeing to participate. The honoring of all agreements made between the researcher and the subject, including adherence to the procedure outline in advance and the payment of any promised stipend. Subject' assess to research personnel at any point in the study to clarify information. Subject' assess to appropriate professional assistance if there is any physical or psychological damage. Debriefing, if necessary, to divulge information that was withheld before the study. Respectful and courteous treatment at all times.

The Right to Privacy

This principle of the entitled 'A Patient's Bill of rights' document published in 1975 by the American Hospital Association (AHA), affirm the patient's right of privacy. According to Levine: 'privacy is the freedom an individual has to determine the time, extent, and general circumstances under which private information will be shared with or withheld from others, assign an identification (ID) number to each subject and attach the ID number rather than other identifiers to the actual research information, maintain any identification information and lists of ID numbers with corresponding identifying information in a locked file. Some researcher believes that an invasion of privacy happens when private information, such as beliefs, attitudes, opinions and records, is shared with others, without the patients knowledge or consent. Whenever subjects refuse to report personal information as they regard it an invasion of privacy, the researcher ought to respect their views. This may even apply to report of age, income, marital status, and other details that the subject may regard intimate. They also imply that privacy can be invaded when researchers study certain groups without their knowledge and without identifying themselves.

INFORM CONSENT

When people are invited to take part, they should be given a verbal explanation of the study, including details, such as its purpose and duration, the required procedures and an explanation of the risks, burdens and potential benefits. They should then be given a written information sheet and have a set period in which to consider whether they want to participate before written consent can be given. Informed consent is the major ethical issue in conducting research. According to Armiger 'it means that a person knowingly, voluntarily and intelligently, and in a clear and manifest way, gives his consent research should, as far as possible, be based on participants' freely volunteered informed consent. This implies a responsibility to explain fully and meaningfully what the research is about and how it will be disseminated. It is one of the means by which a patient's right to autonomy is protected. Participants should be aware of their right to refuse to participate; understand the extent to which confidentiality will be maintained; be aware of the potential uses to which the data might be put; and in some cases be reminded of their right to renegotiate consent. Informed consent seeks to incorporate the rights of autonomous individuals through self-determination. It also seeks to prevent assaults on the integrity of the patient and protect personal liberty and veracity.

Major Elements of Informed Consent (Fig. 6.2)

Vulnerable Participants

Vulnerability increases the need for justification for the use of such subjects. An intense analysis of potential risks and benefits should be the first step of starting such a research and careful approach should exist both in acquiring consent and during the research procedure itself. Persons with diminished autonomy are also more vulnerable to invasion of privacy, since their right to privacy is limited in contrast to other's right to know. In the case of mentally ill, family as well as employers and colleagues have the right to know while patients may not be able to see the testimony of others in their own record. Children, the elderly, the mentally ill may be incapable of understanding information that would enable them

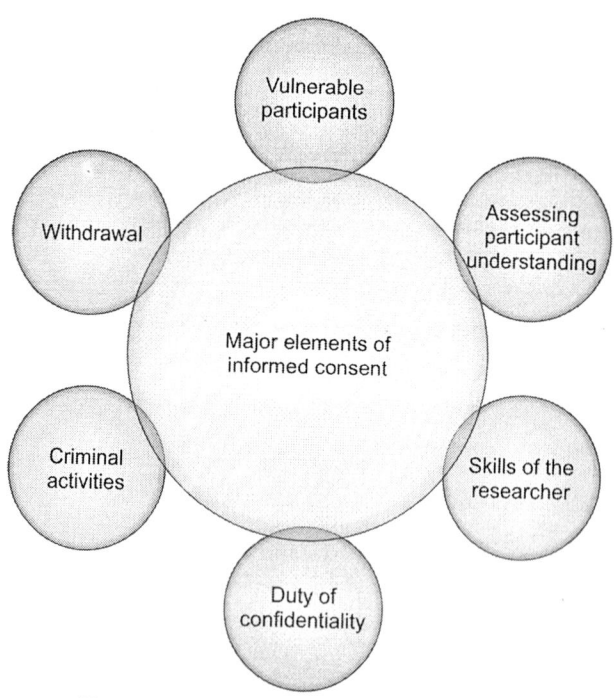

Fig. 6.2: Major elements of informed consent.

to make an informed decision about study participation are potentially vulnerable participants. Consequently, careful consideration of their situation and needs is required, and extra care must be taken to protect them. For example, how will you assess the diminished capacity of an elderly individual, who will be the guardian, and how and when will you involve another individual as guardian in the process.

Assessing Participant Understanding

The participants may not have the experience or educational background in order to fully understand the implications of the research. So for participating in research an important part of the process is for the researcher to ensure that the participants understands the research, their role in it, and any risks they may be taking. During discussion the use of open-ended and nondirective questions (i.e., those that begin with words such as 'what,' 'where,' 'how often,' 'when,' and 'please describe') is most effective at doing this.

Skills of the Researcher

The nurse researchers should have the necessary skills and knowledge for the specific investigation to be carried out and be aware of the limits of personal competence in research. Any lack of knowledge in the area under research must be clearly stated. Inexperienced researchers should work under qualified supervision which has to be reviewed by an ethics committee.

Duty of Confidentiality

The duty of confidentiality may be negotiable in that it requires the confidant not to disclose information unless authorized to do so and only in ways agreed. Authorization is based upon an undertaking or understanding about the ways in which the information will be used (e.g., if I tell you a secret, I expect you not to pass it on), for what purposes, and to whom it will be disclosed. A breach of confidentiality may occur, if the information is used in any other way. Although undertakings can be verbal, there are advantages in a written record.

Methods for Protecting Confidentiality

Responses must be anonymous (as feasible). ANA suggests anonymity is protected when the subject's identity cannot be linked with personal responses. If the researcher is not able to promise anonymity he has to address confidentiality, which is the management of private information by the researcher in order to protect the subject's identity.

All information that can be attributed to individuals is kept confidential. Fictional names are often used in qualitative analysis or code numbers are assigned to individuals for conducting the analysis. Respondents may be referred to using terms that do not indicate name/characteristics of individuals such as 'respondent' or 'participant'. In small samples, care should be taken not to reveal much about personal characteristics of respondents such as ethnicity or job title, if it would help readers identify individual respondents.

- A coding system can be used to track returned surveys or case records. However, the coding system should be kept in a secured location separate from the responses.
- The responses are also kept in a secure location; only the researcher will have access.
- Any instruments that could identify a respondent should be destroyed after data analysis if it cannot be kept in a secure location. This includes tape recordings.
- Information about individual respondents should not be shared with agencies or supervisors.

Criminal Activities

There is no legal obligation to disclose information received relating to criminal activities unless legal proceedings or an investigation are underway. Even then, the confidant will only be guilty of perverting the course of justice if a researcher deliberately evades questioning. Researchers are therefore unlikely to be under a legal duty to disclose unless actually approached by the police with regards to the specific information or case in question. Participants should be aware of this before they reveal possibly incriminating information.

Withdrawal

Always stress the fact that participation is voluntary and that the participant can withdraw at any time state that refusing to participate will involve no penalty or decrease in benefits to which the participant is otherwise entitled. Emphasize that the individual may discontinue participation at any time without penalty or loss of benefits. If there are limitations or risks involved in withdrawal, such as a danger to the participant's well-being, these must also be clearly explained.

The process of obtaining inform consent is as follows:
- Researcher is identified and credentials presented
- Subject selection process is described
- Purpose is described
- Study procedures are discussed
- Compensation, if any is discussed
- Potential risks are described
- Potential benefits are described
- Alternative procedures if any are disclosed
- Anonymity or confidentiality is assured
- Right to refuse to participate or to withdraw from study without penalty is assured
- Offer to answer all question is made
- Means of obtaining study result is presented

Reasons for Limiting Information

The most common reason for limiting information is that valid data could not be obtained if the participants were fully informed about the purposes and procedures of the research. Methodological requirements of the research may demand that the participants remain unaware of the specific hypotheses under investigation. In other situations, incomplete information or misinformation may have to be provided to elicit the behavior of a naive individual or to create psychological reality under conditions that permit valid inference. Fully informed consent cannot be obtained in some kinds of research without the possibility that the results may be biased. In those circumstances where a methodological requirement may necessitates the use of concealment or deception, the researcher has a special responsibility:
- To determine whether the use of such techniques is justified by the study's prospective scientific, educational, or applied value.
- Whether alternative procedures are available that do not use concealment or deception.
- That the participants are provided with sufficient explanation as soon as possible.

These issues should be explored before undertaking the research with colleagues, supervisor(s) and the school/departmental ethics committee.

ETHICAL RESPONSIBILITIES OF A NURSE RESEARCHER

Some of the essential ethical responsibilities of nurse researchers are:
- Ensure the respect of individual's autonomy in consenting to participate in research and also take care for adequate protections are in place to protect study subjects from any potential harm.

- An adequate protection of the vulnerable groups in study, such as children, elderly, pregnant women, mentally ill patients, physically disabled, terminally ill and institutionalized people, etc.
- The nurse researchers must ensure the optimum balance between risk-benefit ratio through ensuring minimizing potential harms and to maximizing the possible benefits for all subjects enrolled in study.
- The benefits and risk associated with the study must be equally distributed among identifying prospective study subjects.
- The privacy, confidentiality and anonymity must be promised and protected during entire study period.
- Maintaining competence in identified research area to maintain proficiency in research methods.

DILEMMA IN NURSING RESEARCH (FIG. 6.3)

Ethical dilemma is defined as a situation requiring a choice between two equally desirable or undesirable alternatives.

- **Fallibility of disciplined research:** Each research question can be solved by different approaches, depending on several factors. Therefore it is always confusing to decide a best approach for solving a research question.
- **Handling multiple variables:** Most of the research studies in the field of nursing usually focus on the measurement of the multiple variables in single attempt. This attempt of handling multiple data in single instance not only causes the data collection, analysis, and interpretation problems, but also needs lots of time, energy, any money to handle these multiple numerical data.

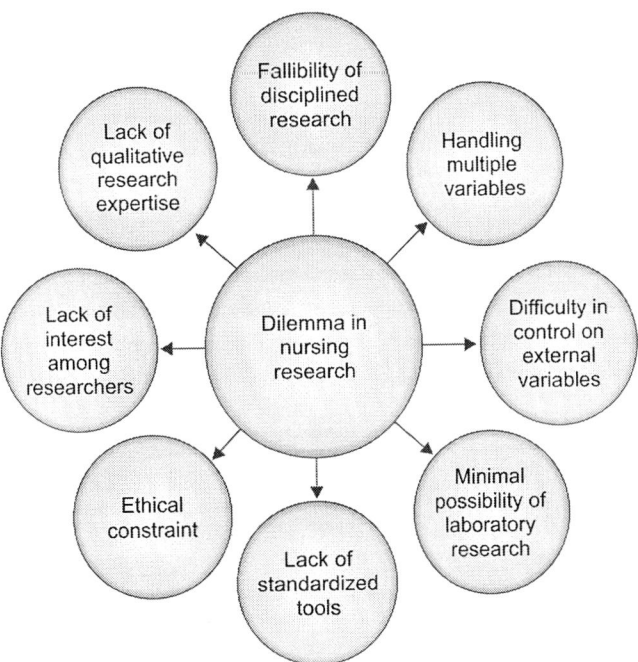

Fig. 6.3: Ethical dilemma in nursing research

- **Difficulty in control on external variables:** Research in nursing usually conducted in natural setting. Therefore, it becomes very difficult to exert control over external variables while measuring the effect of independent variable on dependent variable. For instance, a researcher wants to assess the efficacy of an antibiotic in treatment of an infection where patient's biochemical parameters, diet, lifestyle, consumption of other drugs, etc., are the external variables, which are ethically difficult to control.
- **Minimal possibility of laboratory research:** Research in nursing usually deals with phenomena related to humans, where ethically as well as practically it becomes very difficult to conduct research studies in laboratory. Most of the researches in these disciplines are conducted outside laboratory, in natural setting.
- **Lack of standardized tools:** Research in nursing deals with natural phenomena where valid and reliable standardized tools needed to generate empirical evidences. However, it is evident that there is significant lack of valid and reliable tools to measure variables in nursing.
- **Lack of interest among researchers:** It is generally observed that people in the field of nursing experiences lack of interest because of several reasons like lack of government funding, research training and motivation.
- **Ethical constraint:** Research studies in nursing deals with human beings where safeguarding their rights become an important issue. Moreover, several problems cannot be studied only because of the ethical constraint.
- **Lack of qualitative research expertise:** Qualitative research methods are considered to be best to study phenomena in the field of nursing but there is a significant dearth of experts equipped with the knowledge of qualitative research. But now the researchers take ethical concern.

ETHICAL COMMITTEE IN RESEARCH

A research ethics committee (REC) is a group of people appointed to review research proposals to assess formally if the research is ethical. This means the research must conform to recognized ethical standards, which includes respecting the dignity, rights, safety and well-being of the people who take part. An ethics committee in hospital is an advisory group appointed by the hospital medical executive board. The multidisciplinary ethics committee represents the hospital and the community it serves. Most hospitals have an ethics committee, made up of doctors, nurses, social workers, patient relation liaison, lawyers, a chaplain, medical ethical professional and lay person from the community.

In order to make sure that participants are protected, all studies must be reviewed by human subjects/ethics review committee. Any research projects must be reviewed by ethical committee and the committees have an important role to play in ensuring the ethical standards and scientific merit of research involving human subjects.

There are three important obligations placed on the ethics committee. Firstly, and most importantly, the ethics committee must ensure that the rights of research participants are protected. This is achieved by ensuring that individuals receive sufficient information, which can be easily understood, and ensuring that appropriate strategies are in place to protect participants from potential adverse consequences of the research. Secondly, the REC has an obligation to society which provides the resources for research and will ultimately be affected by the results. Thirdly, the REC has an obligation to the researcher. The research proposal should be treated with respect and consideration. The REC should strive to meet each of these obligations. All researchers should welcome the contribution made by REC to the research process because they help to ensure that research meets the high ethical and scientific standards expected by society.

Why are Research Ethics Committee Needed?

Research is essential for protecting and improving health and well-being, as well as for achieving modern, effective care services. At the same time, research can sometimes involve an element of risk, because research can involve trying something new. It is important that any risks are minimized and do not compromise the dignity, rights, safety and well-being of the people who take part. Ethical committees can helps to ensure that service users and the public can have confidence in, and benefit from, high-quality, ethical research.

Researchers must satisfy a REC that the research they propose will be ethical and worthwhile. The committee has to be assured that any anticipated risks, burdens or intrusions will be minimized for the people taking part in the research and are justified by the expected benefits for the participants or for science and society REC aim to protect people who take part in research. This helps promote public confidence about the conduct of researches and the dignity, rights, safety and well-being of research participants. As a result, more people will be encouraged to take part in research. This in turn leads to more, better and quicker improvements in health and social care.

Research ethics committee review complements researchers' own consideration of the ethical issues raised by their research and their involvement of service users, care professionals, methodologists and statisticians, academic supervisors, data protection officers, etc., at the design stage.

Role of Research Ethics Committees

There are three important obligations placed on the ethics committee.

Protection of Research Participants

Whatever the research context, the interests of participants come first. Most importantly, the ethics committee must ensure that the rights of research participants are protected. This is achieved by ensuring that individuals receive sufficient information, which can be easily understood, and ensuring that appropriate strategies are in place to protect participants from potential adverse consequences of the research. Their dignity, rights, safety and well-being must be the primary consideration in any research proposal, as well as in REC review. RECs must be assured that there are proportionate safeguards to protect people taking part in research.

Society

The research ethics committee has an obligation to society which provides the resources for research and will ultimately be affected by the results. Why the research has been undertaken? The result of the research must be provide benefit to the society.

Researchers

The research ethics committee has an obligation to the researcher. The research proposal should be treated with respect and consideration. All researchers should welcome the contribution made by research ethics committees to the research process because they help to ensure that research meets the high ethical and scientific standards expected by society.

Over all the REC take into account of the interests and safety of the researchers, as well as the public interest in reliable evidence affecting health and social care, and enables ethical and worthwhile research of benefit to participants or to science and society. The benefits and risks of taking part in research, and the benefits of research evidence for improved health and social care, should be distributed fairly among all social groups and classes. Selection criteria in research protocols should not unjustifiably exclude potential participants, for instance on the basis of economic status, culture, age, disability, gender reassignment, marriage and civil partnership, pregnancy and maternity, race, religion or belief, sex or sexual orientation. RECs should take these considerations into account in reviewing the ethics of research proposals, particularly those involving under-researched groups.

Composition of Research Ethics Committees

Nature of Membership

The membership of a REC should allow for a sufficiently broad range of experience and expertise so that the rationale, aims, objectives and design of the research proposals that it reviews can be effectively reconciled with the dignity, rights, safety and well-being of the people who are likely to take part.

RECs are expected to reflect current ethical norms in society as well as their own ethical judgment. REC members may come from groups associated with particular interests but they are not representatives of those groups. REC members are appointed in their own right to participate in the work of a REC as equal individuals of sound judgment, relevant experience and adequate training in research ethics and REC review.

A REC should contain a mixture of people who reflect the currency of public opinion ('lay' members), as well as people who have relevant formal qualifications or professional experience that can help the REC understand particular aspects of research proposals ('expert' members).

The research ethics service as a whole should reflect the diversity of the adult population of society, taking account of age, disability, gender reassignment, marriage and civil partnership, pregnancy and maternity, race, religion or belief, sex and sexual orientation. This applies to both the lay and expert membership.

Expert and Lay Members

Each REC should have expert members to ensure methodological and ethical expertise about research in care settings and in relevant fields of care, as well as professional expertise as care practitioners. This expertise should be appropriate to the types of research proposal the REC reviews.

Lay members are people who are independent of care services, either as employees or in a nonexecutive role. Their primary professional interest is not care-related research. At least a third of each REC's membership should be lay. At least half the lay membership should comprise people who have never been care professionals, researchers in a care field, or chairs, members or directors of care service bodies or organizations providing care.

The research ethics service should adopt and publish operational definitions of expert and lay members, taking into account other applicable requirements and support RECs and their appointing authorities to ensure an appropriate balance of members.

Chapter 6: Ethics in Research

SUMMARY

* Ethics are the rules for correct behavior. Professional ethics for nurses will state the ideal ways in which a nurse should behave in all relationships including those with the patient, patient's relatives, co-workers, members of other professions and the public. Ethics is defined as, 'laws of human conduct and duties. Ethics is an account of human actions and the goal of ethical deliberations is to judge human actions.
* Nursing research usually deals with the human being where implication of the ethics becomes very essential.
* Human experimentation has been conducted even before 18th century. However, the ethical attitudes of researchers drawn the interest of society only after 1940's because of human exploitation in several cases.
* Professional codes and laws were introduced since then in order to prevent scientific abuses of human lives. The Nazi experiments led to the Nuremberg Code (1947) which was the leading code for all subsequent codes made to protect human rights in research.
* The major ethical principles that should be considered in designing or reviewing the research studies are beneficence, respect of human dignity and justice. There is essential ethical responsibilities of nurse researchers which they have to follow during conducting research.
* There is some ethical dilemma which confuses nurse researchers. Ethical dilemma is defined as a situation requiring a choice between two equally desirable or undesirable alternatives.

QUESTIONS TO TEST YOUR KNOWLEDGE

Q1. What do you mean by ethics? Enumerate the importance of ethics in nursing research. Describe the codes of ethics in nursing research. (3 + 5 + 7)

Q2. Explain the ethical principles applied in nursing research. (15)

Q3. Write short notes on following: (5 × 3)
   a. Ethical dilemma
   b. Ethical responsibilities of a nurse researcher
   c. Elements of informed consent

Q4. Multiple choice questions:
   I. The Right to Self-determination is an example of which of the following ethical principle:
      a. Principle of beneficence
      b. Principle of respect of human dignity
      c. Principle of justice
      d. None of the above
   II. The set of principles and guidelines that help us to uphold the things we value is known as:
      a. Concepts
      b. Rules
      c. Ethics
      d. Assumptions
   III. One of the important reasons to take inform consent is:
      a. Build the capability of subject to accept or reject participation in study
      b. Protect study participants from the harmful effects of the experimental interventions
      c. Protect the vulnerable from the harmful effects of experimental interventions
      d. All of the above
   IV. Research participants must give what before they can participate in a study?
      a. Guidelines
      b. A commitment
      c. Informed consent
      d. Private information

V. Ethic means:
  a. The rules for correct behavior
  b. Act of moral principles
  c. Concerned with doing well and avoiding harm
  d. All of the above

VI. Freedom from exploitation is an example of which of the following ethical principle:
  a. Principle of beneficence
  b. Principle of respect of human dignity
  c. Principle of justice
  d. None of the above

VII. Which of the following organization served as the basis for regulations affecting research sponsored by the federal government?
  a. National commission for the protection of human subjects of biomedical and behavioral research
  b. Commission of biomedical and behavioral research
  c. International commission to protect human subjects of biomedical and behavioral research
  d. None of the above

VIII. When there is confusion to select the best possible tool to conduct a research this situation is called:
  a. Ethical principle
  b. Ethical dilemma
  c. Ethical standard
  d. Ethical belief

IX. Protection of research participants is the role of:
  a. Ethical committee members
  b. Researcher
  c. Participants
  d. Both a and b

ANSWERS				
I. b	II. c	III. d	IV. c	V. d
VI. a	VII. a	VIII. b	IX. d	

Chapter 7

Concept of Research Design

Learning Objectives

After completion of this chapter, the students will be able to:
- Describe the concept of research design and factors affecting selection of research design.
- Explain major classification of research design.
- Explain different types of experimental and nonexperimental research design in detail.
- Explain the characteristics and types of qualitative research studies.

INTRODUCTION

A research design can be described as a conceptual structure within which research is going to be carried out. It comprises the blueprint for the collection, measurement and analysis of data. Decisions with regards to what, where, when, how much, by what means concerning an enquiry or a research design are taken. A research design is the arrangement of conditions for collection and evaluation of data in a fashion which is designed to combine relevance to the research purpose with economy in process. A research design is the detailed outline of how an investigation will take place, how data is to be collected, what instruments will be employed, how the instruments will be used and the intended means for analyzing data collected. The design of a study defines the type of research undertaken. It is the framework that has been created to seek answers to research questions. It is the arrangement of conditions carry out research in a manner that aims to combine relevance to the research purpose with economy in procedure. Research design stands for advance planning of the methods to be adopted for collecting the relevant data and the techniques to be used in their analysis, keeping in view the objective of the research and the availability of staff, time and money. Preparation of the research design should be done with great care as any error in it may upset the entire project. Proper selection of research design can minimizes bias and maximizes the reliability of the data. It also yields maximum information, gives minimum experimental error, and provides different aspects of a single problem. A research design depends on the purpose and nature of the research problem. Thus, one single design cannot be used to solve all types of research problem and a particular design is suitable for a particular problem.

DEFINITIONS

The design of a study is the end result of a series of decisions made by the researcher concerning how the study will be conducted. The design is closely associated with the framework of the study and guides planning for the implementation (**Burn and Grove, 1997**). Research design refers to the plan, structure, and strategy of research—the blueprint that will guide the research process. Decisions regarding what, where, when, how much, by what means concerning an inquiry or a research study constitute a research design.

MEANING OF RESEARCH DESIGN

A research design is the arrangement of conditions for collection and analysis of data in a manner that aims to combine relevance to the research purpose with economy in procedure.
It is the logical and systematic plan, structure and strategy of investigation used:
- To answer the research question
- To control the variance
- The function of a research design is to ensure that the evidence obtained enables us to answer the initial question as unambiguously as possible.

ELEMENTS

The key elements of good research design includes the following:
- It is a plan which identifies the sources and kinds of information strongly related to the research problem.
- It is a strategy indicating which method is going to be employed for collecting and analyzing the data.
- Additionally, it consists of the time and cost budgets because most research is done under these two constraints. In a nutshell a research design must contain:
  - A clear statement of the research problem.
  - Methods and techniques to be utilized for gathering information from the population to be researched.
  - Approach to be utilized in processing and analyzing data.

FACTORS AFFECTING SELECTION OF RESEARCH DESIGN

A good design is often characterized by adjectives like flexible, appropriate, efficient, economical and so on. Generally, the design which minimize bias and maximize the reliability of the data collected and analyzed is considered a good research design. There are different factors affecting in selecting research design which are described below (Fig. 7.1):

Level of Knowledge about the Phenomena

Research is always searching for new which is still in curious. Before selecting any research design it is very important to verify the level of knowledge explored regarding that phenomenon.

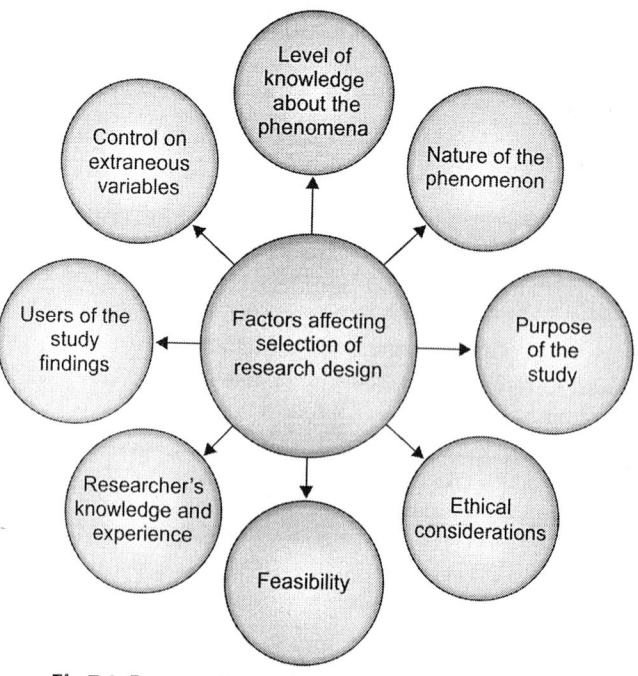

Fig 7.1: Factors affecting selection of research design.

How much people understood that and what needs to be identified. Whether the other researcher had conducted the same study or not how many researcher had conducted and what's their views, etc. Everything should be explored.

Nature of the Phenomenon

Nature of the phenomenon means nature of the research process. This is the most important factor, which helps the researcher to decide about the selection of a research design. Based on the nature of research process or phenomenon, researchers decide whether it should be investigated through an experimental, quasi-experimental, or nonexperimental approach.

Purpose of the Study

The selection of research design is mainly depends upon the purpose of the study. Study may be conducted for the purpose of prediction, description exploration, or correlation of the research variables. Exploratory study carried out when not much is known about the problem at hand, or no details are available on how similar problems or research issues have been solved in the past.

Descriptive study carried out as a way to determine and be able to describe the characteristics of the variables of interest in a situation characteristics of the variables of interest in a situation.

Studies which engage in hypotheses testing generally explain the nature of certain relationships, or establish the differences among groups or the independence of two or more factors in a situation.

Ethical Considerations

The incorporation and application of ethical and legal principles in the research design are essential. It is a major factor in selection of research design. This includes moral obligations, such as respect for participants and their rights, informed consent, and protection from harm, including any adverse effects to educational progress, health and well-being. Selection of a research design is significantly influenced by the ethics of the research study. For example, a researcher may be willing to conduct a research study through a certain experimental approach, but problems of ethical approval may stop the researcher to do so and he or she may have to settle for another available possible research design.

Feasibility

In selection of research design feasibility is a major factor in which affecting selection. Feasibility means practically possibility. All the researches are not feasible in every situation. Feasibility also depends upon availability of the study subjects, availability of facility and equipment time, money, availability of scientific information and sufficient data, top management's support, manpower availability and ability, knowledge, skill, technical understanding and technical background of the researcher, etc. Based on the feasibility of research the researcher can select research design.

The Number and Availability of Study Subjects

The number and availability of study subjects may influence the selection of research design. If only few subjects are involved, an in-depth qualitative researcher may be carried out. For descriptive research design a large sample size is required. Without appropriate study subjects the conduction of studies is not possible. For example, for a comparative study like 'comparison of quality life of adolescent girls between urban slum and rural area' or for descriptive study like 'a study to assess the quality life of adolescent girls in urban slum' for these type of studies large sample size is required. According to the study type the sample size may varies.

Resources

None of the researcher can conduct any without resources, such as money, equipment, facilities, and support from colleagues. However, some of the studies require more amounts of resources as compared to others. Therefore, the selection of a research design may be affected by the availability of resources for the research study.

Researcher's Knowledge and Experience

Selection of research design is largely influenced by the researcher's knowledge and experience, because researcher use to avoid using those designs wherein they lack confidence, relevant knowledge, or experience. Researcher's interest and motivation are also important in selecting research design. Interest and motivation levels help researchers decide about the particular research design(s). Motivated researchers always analyze most aspects of research design before selecting one or a combination, while casual and callous researchers may choose research design.

Time

Time is also a major deciding factor for the selection of research design. For example, a researcher needs more time to conduct longitudinal studies, while cross-sectional studies may be conducted in shorter time. Therefore, time is also a significant contributing factor in selection of a research design.

Users of the Study Findings

A research design decides to use the various methods of data collection and data analysis. Therefore, while choosing a research design, researcher must ensure that research design is as appropriate for the users of the study findings as possible, so that maximum advantage of the results can be obtained.

Possible Control on Extraneous Variables

An efficient design can maximize result, decrease errors, and control pre-existing or impaired conditions that may affect the outcome of the study. The maximized efforts of the researcher should maximize control. Therefore, possible control over the extraneous variables may affect the selection of a research design. For example, a researcher wants to conduct a study through true-experimental design but because of inability to control of extraneous variables, other similar design has to be opted for, such as quasi-experimental or pre-experimental research.

CLASSIFICATION OF RESEARCH DESIGN

Quantitative

Quantitative research is generally associated with the positivist or postpositivist paradigm. It usually involves collecting and converting data into numerical form so that statistical calculations can be made and conclusions drawn. Formal, objective, systematic process to describe, test the relationships and examine the cause-effect interaction among variables. Researchers will have one or more hypotheses. These are the questions that they want to address which include predictions about possible relationships between the things they want to investigate (variables). In order to find answers to these questions, the researchers will also have various instruments and materials (e.g., paper or computer tests, observation checklists, etc.) and a clearly defined plan of action.

Data is collected by various means following a strict procedure and prepared for statistical analysis. Nowadays, this is carried out with the aid of sophisticated statistical computer packages. The analysis enables the researchers to determine to what extent there is a relationship between two or more variables. This could be a simple association (e.g., people who exercise on a daily basis have lower blood pressure) or a causal relationship (e.g., daily exercise actually leads to lower blood pressure). Statistical analysis permits researchers to discover complex causal relationships and to determine to what extent one variable influences another.

The results of statistical analyzes are presented in journals in a standard way, the end result being a P value. For people who are not familiar with scientific research jargon, the discussion sections at the end of articles in peer reviewed journals usually describe the results of the study and explain the implications of the findings in straightforward terms.

Principles

- ❖ Objectivity is very important in quantitative research. Consequently, researchers take great care to avoid their own presence, behavior or attitude affecting the results (e.g., by changing the situation being studied or causing participants to behave differently). They also critically examine their methods and conclusions for any possible bias.
- ❖ Researchers go to great lengths to ensure that they are really measuring what they claim to be measuring. For example, if the study is about whether background music has a positive impact on restlessness in residents in a nursing home, the researchers must be clear about what kind of music to include, the volume of the music, what they mean by restlessness, how to measure restlessness and what is considered a positive impact. This must all be considered, prepared and controlled in advance.
- ❖ External factors, which might affect the results, must also be controlled for. In the above example, it would be important to make sure that the introduction of the music was not accompanied by other changes (e.g., the person who brings the CD player chatting with the residents after the music session) as it might be the other factor which produces the results (i.e., the social contact and not the music). Some possible contributing factors cannot always be ruled out but should be acknowledged by the researchers.
- ❖ The main emphasis of quantitative research is on deductive reasoning which tends to move from the general to the specific. This is sometimes referred to as a top down approach. The validity of conclusions is shown to be dependent on one or more premises (prior statements, findings or conditions) being valid. Aristotle's famous example of deductive reasoning was: All men are mortal 'Socrates is a man, Socrates is mortal'. If the premises of an argument are inaccurate, then the argument is inaccurate. This type of reasoning is often also associated with the fictitious character Sherlock Holmes. However, most studies also include an element of inductive reasoning at some stage of the research (*see* Section on Qualitative research for more details).
- ❖ Researchers rarely have access to all the members of a particular group (e.g., all people with dementia, carers or healthcare professionals). However, they are usually interested in being able to make inferences from their study about these larger groups. For this reason, it is important that the people involved in the study are a representative sample of the wider population or group. However, the extent to which generalizations are possible depends to a certain extent on the number of people involved in the study, how they were selected and whether they are representative of the wider group. For example, generalizations about

psychiatrists should be based on a study involving psychiatrists and not one based on psychology students. In most cases, random samples are preferred (so that each potential participant has an equal chance of participating) but sometimes researchers might want to ensure that they include a certain number of people with specific characteristics and this would not be possible using random sampling methods. Generalizability of the results is not limited to groups of people but also to situations. It is presumed that the results of a laboratory experiment reflect the real life situation which the study seeks to clarify.

When looking at results, the P value is important. P stands for probability. It measures the likelihood that a particular finding or observed difference is due to chance. The P value is between 0 and 1. The closer the result is to 0, the less likely it is that the observed difference is due to chance. The closer the result is to 1, the greater the likelihood that the finding is due to chance (random variation) and that there is no difference between the groups or variables.

Qualitative

Qualitative research is the approach usually associated with the social constructivist paradigm which emphasizes the socially constructed nature of reality. It is about recording, analyzing and attempting to uncover the deeper meaning and significance of human behavior and experience, including contradictory beliefs, behaviors and emotions. Researchers are interested in gaining a rich and complex understanding of people's experience and not in obtaining information which can be generalized to other larger groups, focus on the whole of the human experience and the meaning given by the individuals experiencing it. Gives a broader understanding and deeper insight into the complex human behavior.

The approach adopted by qualitative researchers tends to be inductive which means that they develop a theory or look for a pattern of meaning on the basis of the data that they have collected. This involves a move from the specific to the general and is sometimes called a bottom-up approach. However, most research projects also involve a certain degree of deductive reasoning (*see* Section on Quantitative research for more details).

Qualitative researchers do not base their research on predetermined hypotheses. Nevertheless, they clearly identify a problem or topic that they want to explore and may be guided by a theoretical lens—a kind of overarching theory which provides a framework for their investigation.

The approach to data collection and analysis is methodical but allows for greater flexibility than in quantitative research. Data is collected in textual form on the basis of observation and interaction with the participants, e.g., through participant observation, in-depth interviews and focus groups. It is not converted into numerical form and is not statistically analyzed.

Data collection may be carried out in several stages rather than once and for all. The researchers may even adapt the process midway, deciding to address additional issues or dropping questions which are not appropriate on the basis of what they learn during the process. In some cases, the researchers will interview or observe a set number of people. In other cases, the process of data collection and analysis may continue until the researchers find that no new issues are emerging.

Principles

- ❖ Researchers will tend to use methods which give participants a certain degree of freedom and permit spontaneity rather than forcing them to select from a set of predetermined responses (of which none might be appropriate or accurately describe the participant's thoughts, feelings, attitudes or behavior) and to try to create the right atmosphere to enable people to express themselves. This may mean adopting a less formal and less rigid approach than that used in quantitative research.
- ❖ It is believed that people are constantly trying to attribute meaning to their experience. Therefore, it would make no sense to limit the study to the researcher's view or understanding

of the situation and expect to learn something new about the experience of the participants. Consequently, the methods used may be more open-ended, less narrow and more exploratory (particularly when very little is known about a particular subject). The researchers are free to go beyond the initial response that the participant gives and to ask why, how, in what way, etc. In this way, subsequent questions can be tailored to the responses just given.

❖ Qualitative research often involves a smaller number of participants. This may be because the methods used such as in-depth interviews are time and labor intensive but also because a large number of people are not needed for the purposes of statistical analysis or to make generalizations from the results.

❖ The smaller number of people typically involved in qualitative research studies and the greater degree of flexibility does not make the study in any way 'less scientific' than a typical quantitative study involving more subjects and carried out in a much more rigid manner. The objectives of the two types of research and their underlying philosophical assumptions are simply different. However, as discussed in the section on 'philosophies guiding research', this does not mean that the two approaches cannot be used in the same study.

Table 7.1 shows differences between quantitative and qualitative research design.

Table 7.1: Differences between quantitative and qualitative research design.

Quantitative	Qualitative
• Subject/study participant/respondent • Researcher/investigator/ scientist • Naturalistic setting— controlled laboratory setting • What is investigated?—concept/construct/variable • System of organizing concepts—theory, theoretical framework, conceptual framework, conceptual model • Numerical data • Functional or cause-effect relationship is studied • Deductive reasoning (general to particular)	• Study participant/key informant • Researcher/investigator • Naturalistic setting—field work • What is investigated?—concept or phenomena • System of organizing concepts—theory, conceptual framework, sensitizing framework • Narrative description of facts or experiences • Pattern of association is studied • Inductive reasoning (particular to generalization) • Assumptions • Objectivity of reality • Variables can be identified • Relationships measured • Etic (outside's point of view)
Assumptions • Objectivity of reality • Variables can be identified • Relationships measured • Etic (outside's point of view)	**Assumptions** • Reality is subjective • Variables are complex, interwoven • Difficult to measure • Emic (insider's point of view)
Purpose • Generalizability • Prediction • Causal explanations	**Purpose** • Contextualization • Interpretation • Understanding actors' perspectives
Approach • Begins with hypotheses and theories • Manipulation and control • Uses formal instruments • Experimentation • Deductive • Component analysis • Reduces data to numerical	**Approach** • Ends with hypotheses and grounded theory • Emergence and portrayal • Researcher as instrument • Naturalistic • Inductive • Searches for patterns • Makes minor use of numerical
Researcher role • Detachment • Objective	**Researcher role** • Personal involvement • Empathic understanding

The quantitative research design is formal, objective, systematic process for obtaining quantifiable information about the world, presented in numerical form, and analyzed through the use of statistics, used to describe and to test relationships and especially used to examine the cause-and-effect of relationships. Quantitative researchers attempt to remain detached from the study, and from the sample (in studies where the sample is made up of human beings). They strive to maintain objectivity—in other words they try not to influence it with their own personal values, feelings, and experiences. This is because quantitative researchers believe that researchers' involvement in the study could bias it. By 'bias it', they mean that they do not want to sway the study towards the perceptions and values of the researchers' rather than allowing the hard scientific facts to hold sway. Biasing a research study is considered by scientists as being poor scientific technique—and is definitely a no-no in quantitative research. This of course is totally different to the attitude of many qualitative researchers, who whilst not wanting to bias their research still maintain that they cannot approach a study without considering their own perceptions and values, feelings and experiences, etc.

In quantitative research your aim is to determine the relationship between one thing (an independent variable) and another (a dependent or outcome variable) in a population. Quantitative research designs are either descriptive (subjects usually measured once) or experimental (subjects measured before and after a treatment). A descriptive study establishes only associations between variables. An experiment establishes causality.

For an accurate estimate of the relationship between variables, a descriptive study usually needs a sample of hundreds or even thousands of subjects; an experiment, especially a crossover, may need only tens of subjects. The estimate of the relationship is less likely to be biased if you have a high participation rate in a sample selected randomly from a population. In experiments, bias is also less likely if subjects are randomly assigned to treatments, and if subjects and researchers are blind to the identity of the treatments. In all studies, subject characteristics can affect the relationship you are investigating. Limit their effect either by using a less heterogeneous sample of subjects or preferably by measuring the characteristics and including them in the analysis. In an experiment, try to measure variables that might explain the mechanism of the treatment. In an unblinded experiment, such variables can help define the magnitude of any placebo effect. Studies aimed at quantifying relationships are of two types—descriptive and experimental.

EXPERIMENTAL RESEARCH DESIGN

In a descriptive study, no attempt is made to change behavior or conditions. A researcher measure things as they are. In an experimental study a researcher take measurements, try some sort of intervention, then take measurements again to see what happened. Experimental research seeks to determine if a specific treatment influences an outcome. This impact is assessed providing a specific treatment to one group and withholding it from another and then determining how both groups scored on an outcome.

Characteristics of Experimental Research Design

There are three essential characteristics of experimental research design.
1. **Control:** Researcher introduces one or more control over the experimental situation including the use of control group. Extraneous variables must be controlled for in experimental studies. Extraneous variables are participant or environmental variables that 'confuse relationships among the variables being studied'. Participant variables that act as extraneous variables include both intervening variables and organismic variables. Intervening variables include

variables that are not directly observable (e.g., anxiety, boredom) and must be controlled by researchers. While organism variables cannot be altered by researchers, as they include variables, such as participants gender, they too can be controlled. Experimenters can best control for extraneous variables by using randomization. Randomization requires that researchers randomly select study participants as well as randomly assign participants to treatment groups. Researchers can employ a variety of practices to ensure that extraneous variables are controlled for through random selection and random assignment such as by using a table of random numbers. By using either a table of random numbers or simply flipping a coin, researchers can be certain that participants were selected and assigned to groups by pure chance and, thus differences amongst participants should be equally distributed between treatment groups. Randomization is an integral element of experimental research as it allows researchers to create treatment groups that are relatively equal, thus, any differences noted after the researcher has implemented the experimental treatment can be attributed to the treatment.

In situations where researchers are prevented from randomly selecting participants, researchers should at least randomly assign participants to groups. When researchers are not able to use either random selection or random assignment, researchers should at least randomly select which group will receive the treatment and which group will act as the control group.

Additional methods exist that researchers can utilize to control for extraneous variables. One such method is to hold certain variables constant throughout an experiment for both the control and treatment group. This practice is often utilized with certain environmental variables such as the learning materials used, participants 'prior exposure to certain variables, and the place and time the experiment occurs.

For instance, if a principal tutor of school of nursing is interested in studying the effectiveness of two different types structure teaching program, the principal might control for extraneous variables by holding certain variables constant for both. The control and treatment group by selecting two groups to act as a control and treatment group should be away from each other. The selection process is random selection from all the class. They will teach at same time in morning by using two different well-structured plan. This will allow the principal to reduce the influence of extraneous variables by assigning same time. The principal will be certain that any differences noted in learning between the treatment group and control group are not due to the time of the morning and evening during which the instruction was taught and cannot be due to one class of students being less alert than the other class. The principal might also decide to control for extraneous variables by holding another variable constant the learning topic content used by the teachers will be same but two different module will be prepared by the researcher.

2. **Randomization:** Randomization is 'the process of assigning individuals at random to groups or to different groups in an experiment'. The purpose of random assignment is to insure that groups receiving different treatments are as reasonably equal or similar in any way that could possibly impact the outcome (or dependent variable). Thus, random assignment helps increase the likelihood that any personal characteristic that could bias. A study's outcomes are evenly distributed among groups of participants. The process of evenly distributing potential bias is referred to as equating the groups. Such characteristics that could bias the outcome measured by a study are referred to as extraneous variables. Since personal characteristics that could bias a study's outcome can never be completely eliminated, the process of randomly assigning participants to groups also serves to randomly distribute any potential bias. It is important to note that random assignment and random selection

do not refer to the same process. Rather, random selection refers to the process of selecting individuals so each individual has an equal chance of being selected. Random selection, which serves a different purpose in research, often is not utilized during experimental research as it is not always a logical possibility.

3. **Manipulation:** Experimental research requires the manipulation of at least one independent variable. Manipulation means intervention. The researcher will provide a new intervention to the experimental group. This basically means that researchers decide which variable will serve as the independent variable to be manipulated and which group of participants will receive this treatment. Some of the standard notation and its meaning are used in research they are:

- O   Observation
- O_1 1st observation
- O_2 2nd observation
- R   Randomization
- X   Experimental manipulation or intervention
- E   Experimental group
- C   Control group

True Experimental Design

In true experimental design, the study should be fully under the control of the researcher. Here all the characteristics of the experimental research design will strictly follow like manipulation, control-randomization.

Advantages

- Powerful to establish cause-effect relationship.
- Greater degree of purity of observation due to control.
- Time factor can be reduced using laboratory settings.
- Free from real world constraints.
- Enables the investigator to control for changes in the instrumentation.
- Randomization decreases selection bias and maturation.

Disadvantages

- Laboratory experiment cannot be replicated in real life of human due to ethical issues or control may not be absolute.
- Control of extraneous variables is difficult.
- Confounding factors may affect the study results.
- Getting cooperation from subjects is difficult.

There are different varieties of research design (**Fig. 7.2**).

Pretest-Post-test Control Group Design

Pretest-post-test control group design is considered a strong experimental design for several reasons. First, the design includes the usage of both a control and treatment group. Second, the design also requires that a pretest and post-test be administered to both the control and treatment group. This obviously serves to ensure that participants in both groups are as equivalent as possible on certain variables prior to the implementation of the treatment for the treatment group. Participants are randomly assigned to either the control or experimental group while the treatment is only given to the experimental group. Both the control and experimental

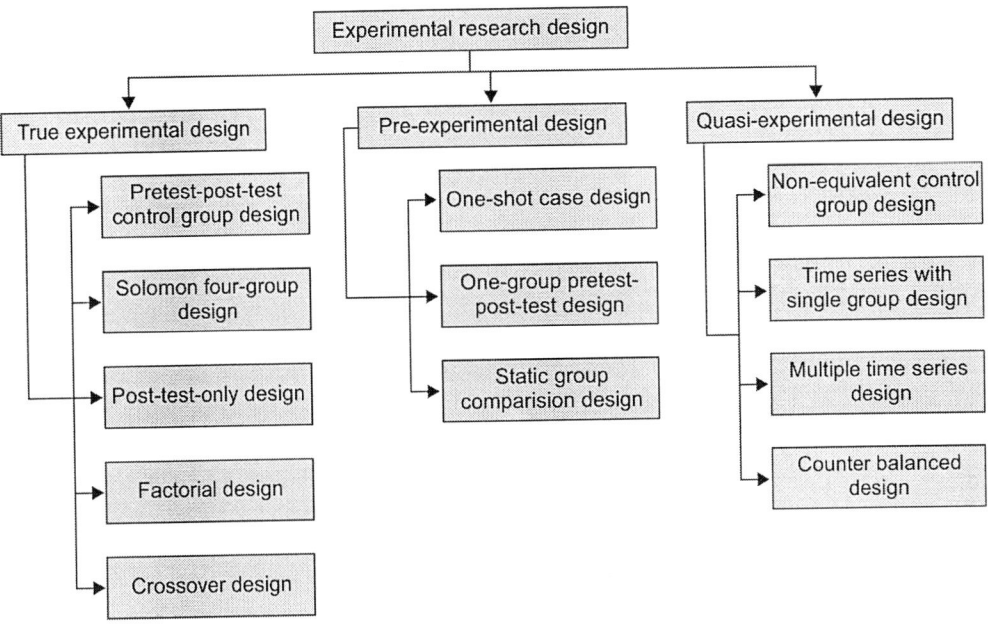

Fig. 7.2: Classification of experimental research design.

groups are then again tested. This is an excellent research design because it includes a control or comparison group and has random assignment. This design controls for all of the standard threats to internal validity. Differential attrition may or may not be a problem depending on what happens during the conduct of the experiment.

Note that while this design is often presented as a two group design, it can be expanded to include a control group and as many experimental groups as are needed to test your research question.

$$RO_1 \quad X \quad O_2 \text{ experimental group}$$
$$RO_1 \quad \quad \quad O_2 \text{ control group}$$

Post-test Only Control Group Design

The post-test only control group design is a research design in which the research participants are randomly assigned to an experimental and control group and then post tested on the dependent variable after the experimental group has received the experimental treatment condition. This is an excellent research design because it includes a control or comparison group and has random assignment. Just like the previous pretest-post-test control group design, it controls for all of the standard threats to internal validity. Differential attrition may or may not be a problem depending on what happens during the conduct of the experiment. This design does not include a pretest of the dependent variable, but this does not detract from its internal validity because it includes the control group and random assignment which means that the experimental and control groups are equated at the outset of the experiment. Helpful in situations where pretesting the subjects is not possible.

$$R \text{ expt}_1 \quad X \quad O_2$$
$$R \text{ contr}_1 \quad \quad O_2$$

For example, effect of handout regarding stress incontinence on subsequent help seeking behavior of mothers after normal vaginal delivery.

Solomon Four-group Design

It is also one type of true experimental design. Here four groups (two experimental and two control groups) are selected. The main criteria for this design is all subjects for four groups are randomly assigned. The first two groups of the Solomon four group design are designed and interpreted in exactly the same way as in the pretest-post-test design, and provide the same checks upon randomization. Next two groups are interpreted as post-test only control group design. Use this design when it is suspected that, in taking a test more than once, earlier tests have an effect on later tests, e.g., by learning or priming effects. In addition to the basic pretest/treatment/post-test design, do three additional tests, one without the treatment, one without the pretest and one without both pretest and treatment **(Table 7.2)**.

Table 7.2: Numerical presentation of Solomon four-group design.

Group		Pretest	Treatment	Post-test
A	R	O_1	X	O_2
B	R	O_1		O_2
C	R		X	O_2
D	R			O_2

In a test where there is no priming or learning effect, the pretest and scores without treatment will all be similar. Where there is a priming or learning effect, then repeated tests without the treatment will show a significant change, whilst posts-tests without a pretest will give results dissimilar to the basic pretest and posttest design. Pretest and posttest are common ways of determining change caused by a treatment, but they are subject to improvement effects. Priming occurs when the pretest helps the subject predict what to expect in the posttest. Learning occurs when the pretest acts as a practice, such that the subject increases skill at doing this type of test. The Solomon design applies different variations of the test, omitting various elements and thus allowing the effects of these omissions to be assessed.

Advantages

- The Solomon four-group design is one of the three primary designs recommended for use with true experimental research, but can also be used in quasi-experimental studies.
- This design is a combination of the pretest–post-test control group design and the post-test only design. It has the advantages of these other two designs with the additional advantage of being able to test and control for instrument reactivity.
- Researchers using this design are in a position to examine both the main effects of testing and the interaction of testing and treatment. The researcher is also in a position to examine the combined effect of maturation and history by comparing the post-test only control group and the pretest control group.
- Using the Solomon four-group design, subjects are randomly assigned to one of four different groups. Two of the groups receive the treatment (i.e., intervention) and two do not (i.e., control). Only one of the treatment groups is administered the pretest; however, all four groups are post-tested. Some researchers also use a modified version of this design in which there is only one control group instead of two, and that group is given a pretest and a post-test.

- This design is the only type of experimental design that is able to assess the presence of pretest sensitization. In other words, the post-test measure may be affected not only by the treatment or intervention, but could also be distorted by exposure to the pretest.
- Braver and Braver discuss the general lack of concern investigators have for pretest sensitization, but this interaction may significantly limit the generalizability of the research. The Solomon four-group design allows the researcher to test for this and separate out the effects of the pretesting and the treatment.
- Use of this design enables the researcher to have more confidence in inferring causal relationships because experimental designs have a higher degree of internal validity than other methods. There is also a reduction in between subject variation, which increases the power of the study to determine true treatment effects.

Limitations

Despite the advantages in strengthening both internal and external validity of research, the Solomon-four group design is seldom used. While its rigor is an advantage, it may deter researchers who are not aware of how it can be utilized in various and creative ways.
- Large number of subjects needed.
- Difficulty in introducing the treatment simultaneously for all groups.
- Difficulty of randomizing subjects to one of the four groups.
- Complex statistical analysis.

Factorial Design

A factorial design is a design in which two or more independent variables are simultaneously investigated to determine the independent and interactive influence which they have on the dependent variable. It also has random assignment to the groups. Each combination of independent variables is called a 'cell.' Research participants are randomly assigned to as many groups are there are cells of the factorial design if both of the independent variables can be manipulated. The research participants are administered the combination of independent variables that corresponds to the cell to which they have been assigned and then they respond to the dependent variable. The data collected from this research give information on the effect of each independent variable separately and the interaction between the independent variables.

The effect of each independent variable on the dependent variable is called a main effect. There are as many main effects in a factorial design as there are independent variables. If a research design included the independent variables of gender and type of instruction, then there would potentially be two main effects, one for gender and one for type of instruction.

An interaction effect between two or more independent variables occurs when the effect which one independent variable has on the dependent variable depends on the level of the other independent variable. In factorial design, two or more treatments are implemented simultaneously to find the main effect as well as the interaction effect due to the treatment. In this design testing of multiple hypotheses is done in a single experiment. Here subjects are assigned at random a specific combination of. For example, a nurse researcher conducted a study. The effect of diet and exercises on reducing the weight of obese person, here diet therapy and exercises are administered separately and combine to observe the individual effects and combine effects, consider the relationship of diet and exercise. While dieting might allow an individual to lose four pounds or exercise without dieting might decrease a person's body weight by three pounds, the combination (or interaction effect) of diet and exercise will result in the greatest weight loss, seven pounds or more. In this case, the sum is greater than the parts; however, an interaction effect can also occur when the sum is less than its parts.

Crossover Design

In this type of design the subjects are serving as their own control group. In this study among two groups with randomly selected subjects two or more treatments are done but in different order for different groups. Here both the groups are considered as experimental groups and two experiments are performed for both the groups but in reverse order. In this design two treatments given to participants are, one being the experimental treatment (XE), the other a control or reference treatment (XC). The subjects are randomly assigned to one of two groups. One group receives the experimental treatment first and the other group receives the experimental group second. After a period of time, sufficient to allow for any treatment effect to wash out (W), the treatments are crossed over. Multiple crossover designs involve several treatments. For example, a nurse researcher is conducting a study on the effectiveness of self-instructional module and structure teaching module on knowledge of nursing students on prevention of infection in labor room. Here both the module administered separately both the group and vice versa.

$$R \; expt_1 \quad X1 \quad X2 \quad O_2$$
$$R \; expt_2 \quad X2 \quad X1 \quad O_2$$

Useful when >1 IV is there, i.e., for complex hypothesis studies.

Pre-experimental Design

Pre-experimental designs are so named because they follow basic experimental steps but fail to include a control group. In other words, a single group is often studied but no comparison between an equivalent nontreatment group is made. It is the simplest form of research design. In a pre-experiment either a single group or multiple groups are observed subsequent to some agent or treatment presumed to cause change. In this design there is only experimental group, no control group and no randomization.

One-shot Case Study or Single Case Study

The one-shot case study, as with other pre-experiments is considered a pre-experiment (or a weak experiment) because the design lacks essential components of a true experiment: random assignment of participants and control group. One-shot case studies occur when a researcher selects a single group of participants to act as the treatment group, implements a treatment, and then administers a post-test. This research design is problematic as no threats to validity, such as maturation, history, and mortality, are controlled for. As a pretest measure is absent in this type of research design, it is impossible to tell where participants were performing prior to the implementation of the treatment. Recommends that, 'if you have a choice between using this design and not doing a study—select another study'. This design is diagrammed as shown:

Group 1 → treatment implemented → post-test administered.

$$X \, O_1$$

Disadvantages

- A total lack of control. Also, the scientific evidence is very weak in terms of making a comparison and recording contrasts.
- There is also a tendency to have the fallacy of misplaced precision, where the researcher engages in tedious collection of specific detail, careful observation, testing etc., and misinterprets this as obtaining solid research. However, a detailed data collection procedure should not be equated with a good design. In the chapter on design, measurement, and analysis, these three components are clearly distinguished from each other.

❖ History, maturation, selection, mortality, and interaction of selection and the experimental variable are potential threats against the internal validity of this design.

One-group Pretest-Post-test Design

It is the simplest type of pre-experimental design, where only the experimental group is selected and a pretest observation of the dependent variables is made before study subjects. Implementation of the treatment to the selected group is administered and finally a post-test observation of dependent variables is carried out. This is a wide accepted research design used to assess the effect of treatment on the group. There is an argue for this design as subtype of quasi-experimental research design. However, in absence of both randomization and control group. This design ethically cannot be placed under the classification of quasi-experimental research design.

There are several disadvantages to this type of experimental design. First, the absence of a control group does not allow researchers to make comparisons between groups. Another problematic component of the one-group pretest-post-test design is the possible impact of the pretest on students 'post-test scores'. Finally, researchers cannot be certain that observed changes in post-test scores cannot be contributed to extraneous variables.

$$O_1 \quad X \quad O_2$$

Static-group Comparison Design

Another weak pre-experiment design is the static-group comparison design. While you may not be familiar with its name, you likely are familiar with research that has employed the static-group comparison design. There are two elements of true experimental designs that are absent in studies that utilize the static-group comparison design. First, this design does not include the administration of pretest to ensure that participants in the control and treatment groups are similar on specific variables. Secondly, and perhaps most problematic, this design does not require that participants are randomly assigned to either the control or treatment group. Rather, intact groups of participants are selected to act as the control and treatment group without any certainties that the groups are similar prior to the implementation of treatment on the outcome variable. This is what the name of the design refers to with 'static'; specifically, that groups are already intact or inactive prior to the experiment.

$$X \quad O_1 \quad \text{Group 1}$$
$$X \quad O_2 \quad \text{Group 2}$$

i.e., intervention, post-test of Group 1
versus
intervention, post-test of Group 2

The static group that has experienced the independent variable is compared with one that has not.

Advantages

❖ Very simple and convenient to conduct these studies in natural settings especially in nursing.
❖ Most suitable design for the beginners in the field of experimental research.

Quasi-experimental Design

Quasi-experimental, like true-experimental designs, examine cause and effect relationships between or among independent and dependent variables, but they specifically lack the element of random assignment to treatment or control. Instead, quasi-experimental designs typically allow the researcher to control the assignment to the treatment condition, but using some criterion other than random assignment. In some cases, the researcher may have control over assignment to treatment. Quasi-experiments are subject to concerns regarding internal validity, because the treatment and control groups may not be comparable at baseline. With random assignment, study participants have the same chance of being assigned to the intervention group or the comparison group. As a result, differences between groups on both observed and unobserved characteristics would be due to chance, rather than to a systematic factor related to treatment (e.g., illness severity). Randomization itself does not guarantee that groups will be equivalent at baseline. Any change in characteristics postintervention is likely attributable to the intervention. With quasi-experimental studies, it may not be possible to convincingly demonstrate a causal link between the treatment condition and observed outcomes. This is particularly true if there are confounding variables that cannot be controlled or accounted for. Although quasi-experimental designs are useful in testing the effectiveness of an intervention and are considered closer to natural settings, these research designs are exposed to a greater number of threats of internal and external validity, which may decrease confidence and generalization of study's findings.

Advantages

- Since quasi-experimental designs are used when randomization is impractical and/or unethical, they are typically easier to set up than true experimental designs, they can be very useful in generating results for general trends.
- Utilizing quasi-experimental designs minimizes threats to external validity as natural environments do not suffer the same problems of artificiality as compared to a well-controlled laboratory setting.
- Since quasi-experiments are natural experiments, findings in one may be applied to other subjects and settings, allowing for some generalizations to be made about population. Also, this experimentation method is efficient in longitudinal research that involves longer time periods which can be followed up in different environments.
- Quasi-experimental design is often integrated with individual case studies; the figures and results generated often reinforce the findings in a case study, and allow some sort of statistical analysis to take place.
- In addition, without extensive prescreening and randomization needing to be undertaken, they do reduce the time and resources needed for experimentation.

Disadvantages

- Quasi-experimental estimates of impact are subject to contamination by confounding variables.
- The lack of random assignment in the quasi-experimental design method also poses many challenges for the investigator in terms of internal validity. This deficiency in randomization makes it harder to rule out confounding variables and introduces new threats to internal validity.
- Disadvantages also include the study groups may provide weaker evidence because of the lack of randomness.
- Using unequal groups can also be a threat to internal validity. If groups are not equal, which is not always the case in quasi-experiments, then the experimenter might not be positive what the causes are for the results.
- Lack of control over extraneous variables.

- Threat to internal validity and selection bias.
- Less reliable.

Nonequivalent Pretest-Post-test Control Group Design

Sometimes a researcher needs a particular type of participant or they only have access to a certain group of participants. This means that the researcher collects participants in a group that cannot or should not be divided up, or more simply, the researcher cannot randomly assign the participants and the researcher can apply nonequivalent pretest-post-test control group design. The nonequivalent pretest-post-test control group design is identical in many ways to the pretest-post-test control group design except that subjects are not randomly (NR) assigned to groups. Both groups are pretested (O) and post-tested (O). However, only the experimental group is exposed to a treatment (X).

O_1 X O_2 experimental group
O_1 O_2 control group

Time Series Design with the Single-Group

A quasi-experimental research design in which periodic measurements are made on a defined group of individuals both before and after implementation of an intervention. This design is useful when the experimenter wants to measure the effects of a treatment over a long period. The experimenter would continue to administer the treatment and measure generally its effects repeatedly at a particular period interval for a number of times during the course of the experiment. It is a single-subject research, in which the researcher carries out an experiment on an individual or on a small number of individuals, by alternating between administering and then withdrawing the treatment to determine the effectiveness of the intervention.

The researcher measures only one group repeatedly both before and after exposure to a treatment. To examine the effect of a new, government-funded meal program on school children, a nutritional scale is administered to a sample of school children receiving this program. The nutritional scale is measured once before the program, and then three months after the program, and at the end of one year following program implementation. The outcomes at different time points are compared to assess the program effect. Another example can be consider as the effectiveness of yoga on reducing dysmenorrhea.

Expt $O_1 O_2 O_3 O_4 O_5$ X $O_6 O_7 O_8 O_9 O_{10}...$

Multiple Time Series Design

Multiple time series design groups are measured or tested repeatedly on the same variable over time. Again, there is no random assignment (NR) to groups. The experimental group is exposed to a treatment (X) at some point in the series and there is a control group which is not exposed to treatment.

Experimental $O_1 O_2 O_3 O_4 O_5$ X $O_6 O_7 O_8 O_9 O_{10}$
Control $O_1 O_2 O_3 O_4 O_5$ $O_6 O_7 O_8 O_9 O_{10}$

Counterbalanced Design

The counterbalanced design is similar to the crossover experimental design except that subjects are not randomly assigned (NR) to the different groups. All groups are exposed to all treatments. The most common counterbalanced design is the *Latin square*, where four different treatments are applied to four naturally assembled groups or individuals. Each of the groups or individuals is post-tested after each treatment. The number of treatment and groups must be equal. The

Latin square is shown here.

Gr. A X_1 O X_2 O X_3 O X_4 O
Gr. B X_2 O X_4 O X_1 O X_3 O
Gr. C X_3 O X_1 O X_4 O X_2 O
Gr. D X_4 O X_3 O X_2 O X_1 O

(Where X is the treatment and O is the observation)

NONEXPERIMENTAL RESEARCH DESIGN

Nonexperimental research design is the label given to a study when a researcher cannot control, manipulate or alter the predictor variable or subjects, but instead, relies on interpretation, observation or interactions to come to a conclusion. Typically, this means the nonexperimental researcher must rely on correlations, surveys or case studies, and cannot demonstrate a true cause-and-effect relationship. Nonexperimental research tends to have a high level of external validity, meaning it can be generalized to a larger population. As nonexperimental designs do not have random assignment, manipulation of variables, or comparison groups. The researcher only to observes what occurs naturally without intervening in any way.

Cause of Using Nonexperimental Research Design

- Number of human characteristics or independent variables are not subject to experimental manipulation or randomization.
- Some variables cannot ethically be manipulated.
- In some instances, independent variables have already occurred, so no control over them is possible. Researcher collects data and describes a phenomena as they exist without any intervention.
- For some research, it is not practical to conduct a true experiment or manipulate variables.
- For some situations, it is more realistic to explore phenomena in more natural manner.
- No scope for experimental research.

Classification

Figure 7.3 shows the classification of nonexperimental research.

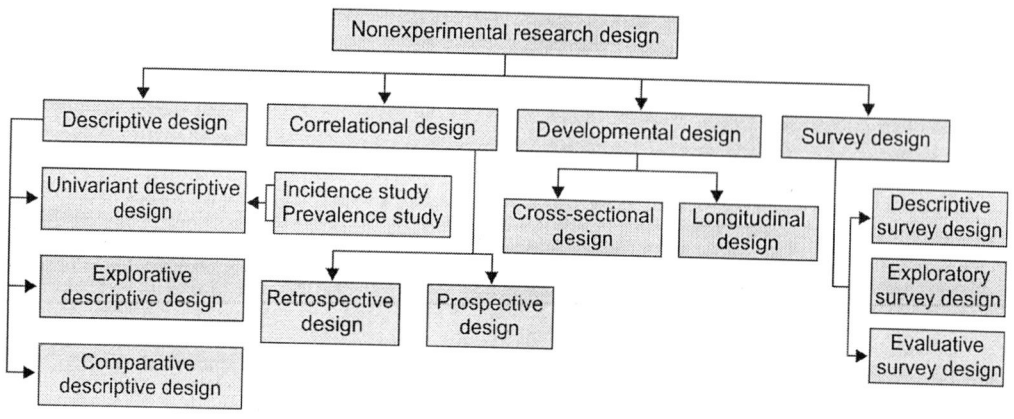

Fig. 7.3: Classification of nonexperimental research design.

Descriptive Design

Descriptive studies are used when little is known about a particular phenomenon. The researcher observes, describes, and documents various aspects of a phenomenon. There is no manipulation of variables or search for cause and effect related to the phenomenon. Descriptive designs describe what actually exists, determine the frequency with which it occurs, and categorizes the information. This design is used to gain more information about characteristics within a particular field of study and it may also used to develop theories. These are mainly of three types, they are univariate study, exploratory descriptive design and comparative descriptive design. Univariate study again classified as prevalence studies and incidence studies.

Univariate Studies

As the meaning of the term says univariate studies not necessarily focused on only one variable. There may be multiple variables but the primary purpose is to describe the status of all and not to relate them to one another.

Prevalence studies: These studies determine the prevalence rate of some conditions at a particular point in time. These are cross-sectional studies showing total current existing cases.

Incidence studies: These are used to measure the frequency of developing new cases. Mainly longitudinal designs are needed to determine incidence rates. The incidence rate is generally calculated for one year.

Exploratory Descriptive Design

Exploratory descriptive design is used to identify, explore, and describe the existing phenomenon and in other words, it is not only a simple description or the frequency of occurrence of a phenomenon, but its in-depth exploration its related factors. For example, an exploratory study to assess the multifactorial dimensions of falls a study of its related factors to improve further understanding about a less-understood phenomenon and home safety measures for elderly people living in selected communities in the city.

Comparative Descriptive Design

Comparative descriptive design involves comparing and this design is used to compare two distinct groups on the basis of selected attributed such as knowledge level, perceptions or any other attributes. In comparative design, researcher can contrast two or more samples of study subjects on one or more variables, often at a single point of time and attitudes; physical or psychological symptoms. For example, a comparative study on health problems among rural and urban older people in district Ganjam, Odisha. Comparative studies are used to describe the variables and to examine the differences between two or more groups that occur naturally in a setting. The results obtained from these analyzes are frequently not generalized to a population.

Correlational Design

Correlational design is a procedure in which subjects' scores on two variables are simply measured, without manipulation of any variables, to determine whether there is a relationship exist between them. So, correlational research examines the relationship between two or more nonmanipulated variables. In correlational studies, the researchers examine the strength of

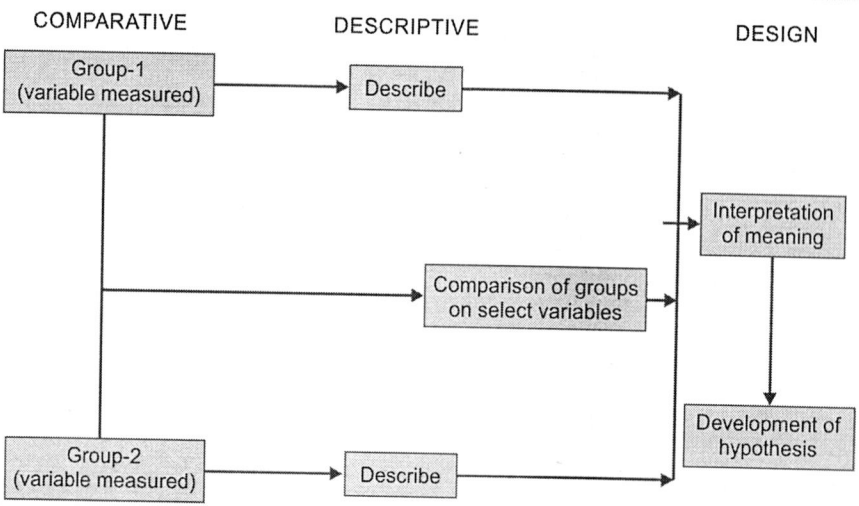

Fig. 7.4: Diagrammatic representation of correlational design.

relationships between variables by determining how change in one variable is correlated with change in the other variable. *Correlational design* describes only the existing relationship without fully understanding or explaining the complex causal pathway that exists. It is a relationship that is not causal in nature. It is an associative relationship **(Fig. 7.4)**.

What is the relationship between: (1) Height and weight? (2) Birth order and years of education? (3) Cigarettes smoked per day and health care costs? This design was used for a correlational study on the effect of smoking on lung cancer among people. In other words, it is a research design where researchers study the relationship of two or more variables without any intervention. This is a nonexperimental design, where researcher examines the relationship between two or more variables in a natural setting without manipulation or control.

In correlational studies, the researchers examine the strength of relationships between variables by determining how change in one variable is correlated with change in the other variable. Generally, correlational studies have independent and dependent variables, but the effect of independent variable is observed on dependent variable without manipulating the independent variable. In some correlational studies, identification of the independent and dependent variables is difficult; however, in most correlational studies, the independent variable is identified, which, without any intervention, influences the dependent variable. For example, this design was used in a correlational investigation of the study habits and visual acuity among school children studying in selected schools of city Berhampur, Ganjam, Odisha. In this study, study habits are the independent variable, while visual acuity is the dependent variable. In epidemiological language these studies are known as cause and effect study, where cause and effect relationship is investigate in natural settings without imposing experimental interventions. This cause and effect relationship can be investigated either in forward manner, i.e., from cause to effect (prospective) or backward manner, i.e., effect to cause (retrospective).

Types of Correlational Research Design

- ❖ Based on the type of relationship it is classified as:
  - **Prospective research design:** Prospective studies start with a presumed cause. A design in which the researcher relates the present to the future is a prospective research

design. Starts from the present, when a researcher observes that a group of population is exposing to a particular condition, which may have a long-term effect then he/she will observe that group to assess that long-term effect. For example, a researcher wants to assess the effects of occupational hazards on the health of the occupational workers, here she has to work prospectively. Prospective designs are often longitudinal, but may also be cross-sectional. In this research design, researcher observes phenomenon from cause to effect.

For example, a researcher conducting a prospective correlational study on effect of maternal infection during pregnancy on fetal development and in this study, the researcher starts by collecting data from pregnant women regarding any history of infection among women during their current pregnancies, next observes fetal development and pregnancy outcome, and finally analyzes the relationship of maternal infection during pregnancy and fetal development and pregnancy outcome. In this the researcher links the present phenomenon with the past events.

- **Retrospective research design:** A design in which the researcher studies the current phenomenon by seeking information from past is a retrospective research design. In other words, the researcher has a backward approach to study a phenomenon, where he or she moves from effect to identify the cause. For example, this design was used in a retrospective correlational study on substance-abuse-related high-risk factors among traumatic head injury patients admitted in Neurosurgery ICU of MKCG Medical College, Berhampur and in this study, the researcher first approached head injury patients and then tried to identify the number of head injuries that occurred under the influence of substances.

Based on the depth of relationship it is classified as:

- **Explanatory design:** Research looks for simple associations between variables and investigates the extent to which the variables are related. It is conducted when researchers want to explore the extents to which two or more variables covary, i.e., where changes in one variable are reflected in changes in the other. When conducting an explanatory correlational study, researchers typically collect data at one time as their focus is not based on future or past performance of participants. Thus, when analyzing the findings of explanatory correlation research, researchers analyze participants as a single group rather than creating subcategories of participants. Finally, in this type of study researchers collect two scores from each participant as each score represents each variable being studied.
- **Prediction design:** Research designed to identify variables that will positively predict outcomes. Prediction design is used by researchers when the purpose of the study is to predict certain outcomes in one variable from another variable that serves as the predictor. Prediction designs involve two types of variables: a predictor variable and a criterion variable. While the predictor variable is utilized to make a forecast or prediction, the criterion variable is the anticipated outcome that is being predicted. The time at which variables are measured also differs in prediction studies as the predictor variable is typically measured at one time while the criterion variable is usually measured at a later date. Prediction studies also include a forecast of anticipated future performance, as well as advanced statistical procedures including multiple regression. For further information about multiple regressions see (link to statistics portion of site).

Characteristics of Correlational Research

Any time a researcher has at least two scores, a graph called a scatter plot can be used to provide a visual representation of the data that has been collected. Each point on a scatter plot represents two scores provided by one person. Researchers must select the scores for one variable to be plotted on the x-axis (the horizontal axis of the graph) while scores for the second variable are plotted on the y-axis (the vertical axis of the graph). Scatter plots are vitally important to correlational research as they allow researchers, as well as research consumers to determine the following by looking at patterns within the entire group of data points (Creswell, 2008; Lodico, et al. 2006):

- ❖ The form of the relationship
- ❖ The type of association
- ❖ The existence of extreme scores
- ❖ The direction of the relationship
- ❖ The degree of the relationship

Developmental Research Design

Developmental research designs are generally used as adjunct research designs with other research designs, such as cross-sectionaldescriptive, longitudinal-correlational research designs. Developmental research design examines the phenomenon with reference to time.

Cross-sectional Research Design

Cross-sectional research design is one in which researcher collects data at particular point of time (one period of data collection) and more convenient to carry out. Here the researcher interacts only once to collect data from the study subject. These studies based on a single examination of a cross section of population at one point in time. The results of the study are applied on the whole population. The cross section of the population is sampled carefully so that it is representative of the whole population. Prevalence studies are the examples of this design. Cross-sectional studies are useful for detailed community assessment, study of morbidity and underlying factors especially chronic diseases, e.g., study of diabetes or hypertension by personal characteristics and lifestyle. These studies are economical and comparatively quick to perform.

Longitudinal Research Design

In longitudinal research design the researcher conduct the study for a period of time. The study may extends towards the past or future or past. For example, a researcher is interested in the perception of nursing students towards nursing profession from the beginning of nursing program to its end. Its value is in its ability to demonstrate change over a period of time. Longitudinal research design is used to collect data over an extended time period (long-time study). In this example, it is appropriate to use the longitudinal research design to study this phenomenon. Retrospective and prospective studies are the examples. Longitudinal studies are generally classified into three types: (i) Trend studies, (ii) Panel studies, and (iii) Follow-up studies.

1. **Trend studies:** These help to investigate a sample from a general population over a time with respect to some phenomenon.

    Trend studies permit researchers to examine pattern and rate of changes and to make prediction about future direction based on previously identified patterns and rates of changes.

2. **Panel studies:** In panel studies, same people are involved. A panel in research is referred to the sample of people involved in a study, and over a period of time they become more informative on the phenomenon than the subjects in trends studies because the researcher cannot only examine the patterns of change, and but also the reasons for change. The same selected people are contacted for two or more times to collect further data.
3. **Follow-up studies:** These are undertaken to determine the subsequent states of subject(s) with a specific condition or those who have received a specific intervention.

Survey Design

Definition

Technique of descriptive research that seeks to determine present practices or opinions of a specified population. A *survey* is defined as a brief interview or discussion with individuals about a specific topic.

The term survey is often used to mean 'collect information.' Survey research is often used to assess thoughts, opinions, and feelings. Survey research can be specific and limited, or it can have more global, widespread goals. Today, survey research is used by a variety of different groups. *Survey research* involves the collection of information from a sample of individuals through their responses to questions. Survey research can be classified as field studies with a quantitative orientation. Only rarely, however, do survey researchers study whole populations; they study samples drawn from populations. From these samples they infer the characteristics of the defined population or the universe. Sample surveys attempt to determine the incidence, distribution, and interrelations among sociological and psychological variables, and in so doing, usually focus on people, the vital facts of people, and their beliefs, opinions, and attitudes. Survey research may be classified according to the purposes descriptive, explanatory, and exploratory and comparative.

Descriptive surveys are used to gather information largely on what people do and think. Thus a researcher might use this type of survey to find out what young people think about drugs, what drugs they might use, and with what frequency.

Analytic surveys are used to answer research questions or to test hypotheses. A researcher might collect data from the general population which detailed information on health habits, e.g., diet, exercise, smoking and so on. This information might then be used to make predictions concerning the state of health of the population at some future date. For example, it might be possible to predict the amount of heart disease in a population ten years hence, based on this sort of data.

According to the Span of Time Involved

The span of time needed to complete the survey brings us to the two different types of surveys:
1. **Cross-sectional surveys:** Collecting information from the respondents at a single period in time uses the cross-sectional type of survey. Cross-sectional surveys usually utilize questionnaires to ask about a particular topic at one point in time. For instance, a researcher conducted a cross-sectional survey asking teenagers' views on cigarette smoking as of May 2010. Sometimes, cross-sectional surveys are used to identify the relationship between two variables, as in a comparative study. An example of this is administering a cross-sectional survey about the relationship of peer pressure and cigarette smoking among teenagers as of May 2010.

2. **Longitudinal surveys:** When the researcher attempts to gather information over a period of time or from one point in time up to another, he is doing a longitudinal survey. The aim of longitudinal surveys is to collect data and examine the changes in the data gathered. Longitudinal surveys are used in cohort studies, panel studies and trend studies.

QUALITATIVE RESEARCH DESIGN

Qualitative research is designed to reveal a target audience's range of behavior and the perceptions that drive it with reference to specific topics or issues. It uses in-depth studies of small groups of people to guide and support the construction of hypotheses. The results of qualitative research are descriptive rather than predictive. The qualitative approach to research is a unique grounding—the position from which to conduct research—that fosters particular ways of asking questions and particular ways of thinking through problems. The questions asked in this type of research usually begin with words like *how, why,* or *what*. Qualitative research is aimed at gaining a deep understanding of a specific organization or event, rather than a surface description of a large sample of a population. It is also called ethnomethodology or field research. Qualitative data collection methods vary using unstructured or semistructured techniques. Some common methods include focus groups (group discussions), individual interviews, and participation or observations. The sample size is typically small, and respondents are selected to fulfill a given quota.

Qualitative research does not introduce treatments or manipulate variables, or impose the researcher's operational definitions of variables on the participants. Rather, it lets the meaning emerge from the participants. It is more flexible in that it can adjust to the setting. Concepts, data collection tools, and data collection methods can be decided as the research progresses.

Aims

- To get a better understanding through first-hand experience, truthful reporting, and quotations of actual conversations.
- To understand how the participants derive meaning from their surroundings, and how their meaning influences their behavior.
- To provide an explicit rendering of the structure, order, and broad patterns found among a group of participants.
- To generates data about human groups in social settings.
- To gain an understanding of underlying reasons, opinions, and motivations and provides insights into the problem or helps to develop ideas or hypotheses for potential quantitative research.
- To uncover trends in thought and opinions, and dive deeper into the problem.

Characteristics (Fig. 7.5)

Focus on Natural Settings

Qualitative researchers often collect data in the field at the site where participants experience the issue or problem under study. They do not bring individuals into a laboratory (a contrived situation), nor do they typically send out instruments for individuals to complete, such as in

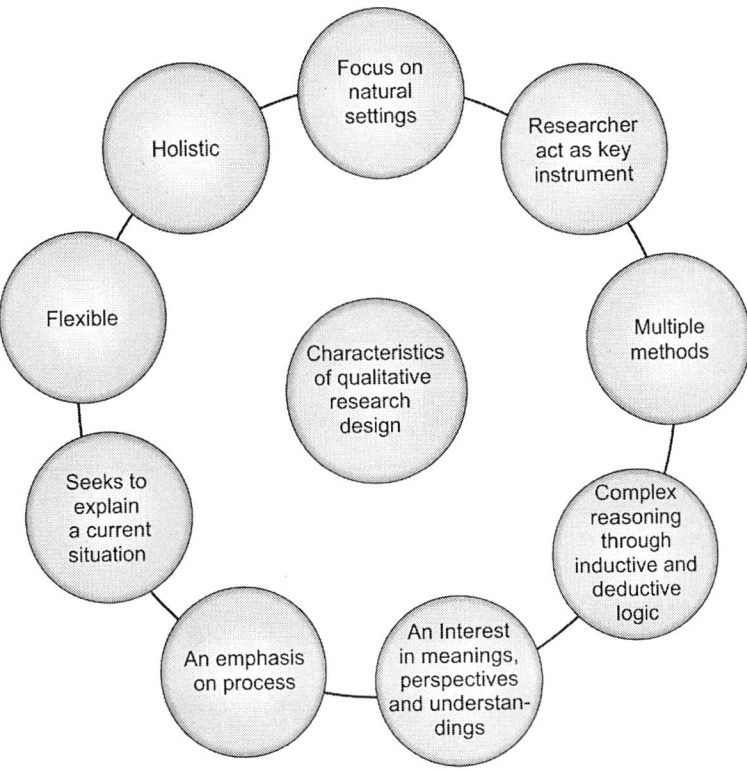

Fig. 7.5: Characteristics of qualitative research design.

survey research. Instead, qualitative researchers gather up-close information by actually talking directly to people and seeing them behave and act within their context. In the natural setting, the researchers have face-to-face interaction over time. In order to gain access to deeper levels, the researcher needs to develop a certain rapport with the subjects of the study, and to win their trust. Needless to say, this must not be abused later when the researcher leaves the field.

Researcher Act as Key Instrument

The qualitative researchers collect data themselves through examining documents, observing behavior, and interviewing participants. They may use an instrument, but it is one designed by the researcher using open-ended questions. They do not tend to use or rely on questionnaires or instruments developed by other researchers.

Multiple Methods

Qualitative researchers typically gather multiple forms of data, such as interviews, observations, and documents, rather than rely on a single data source. Then they review all of the data and make sense of it, organizing it into categories or themes that cut across all of the data sources.

Complex Reasoning through Inductive and Deductive Logic

Qualitative researchers build their patterns, categories, and themes from the 'bottom up,' by organizing the data inductively into increasingly more abstract units of information. This inductive process involves researchers working back and forth between the themes and the database until they establish a comprehensive set of themes.

An Interest in Meanings, Perspectives and Understandings

The qualitative researcher seeks to discover the meanings that participants attach to their behavior, how they interpret situations, and what their perspectives are on particular issues. The participant may be behave differently at different situation. The researcher should understood why this is happening. Research methods employed have to be sensitive to the perspectives of all participants. In addition, the methods must pick up the interaction between perspectives and situation to see how they bear on each other.

Researchers therefore work to obtain 'inside' knowledge of the social life. If they have to understand people's outlooks and experiences, they must be close to individuals and to groups, live with them from day-to-day, look out at the world through their viewpoints, see them in various situations and in various moods, appreciate the inconsistencies, ambiguities and contradictions in their behavior, explore their interests, understand their relationships among themselves and with other groups. The researcher has to understand the culture of groups, learn their own language and use it, and also engage in highly symbolic nonverbal activity.

An Emphasis on Process

There is a focus on how things happen, how they develop, on becoming. Everyday life is an everchanging picture, there is no settled state. Action is a continuous process of meaning attribution, which is always emerging, in a state of flux, and subject to change. Typical subjects for enquiry might be how a group culture forms and develops, how particular roles are perceived and performed and how transitions are managed, etc.

When an researcher observing the tribal people, their culture, custom and tradition he or she has to observe whether there is any change in their lifestyle and what factors are influencing on these.

Flexible

Qualitative research is flexible and elastic in nature. It is not rigid and does not follow any strict protocol. It depends upon the situation and researchers interest. It is a subjective way to look at life as it is lived and an attempt to explain the studied behavior. Rather than design an experiment and artificially control the variables, qualitative researchers use anthropological and ethnographic methods to study the participants. It is capable in adjusting to what is being learned during the period of data collection.

Seeks to Explain a Current Situation

Instead of providing a broad view of a phenomenon that can be generalized to the population, qualitative research seeks to explain a current situation and only describes that situation for that group. Since only a current situation is observed, all qualitative research is done in the field. A possible exception is the focus group, which is conducted with 3–10 persons and uses a script of questions. The moderator asks the questions and the recorder records the responses. Although a focus group is conducted in a controlled environment, the open-ended questions and lack of rigid sample selection make it seem more like a field exercise.

Holistic

Qualitative research design striving for an understanding of the whole. It generally use open-ended questions which can be answered a number of way as the participants want by addressing their whole situation.

Classifications

The qualitative research design is classified in **Figure 7.6**.

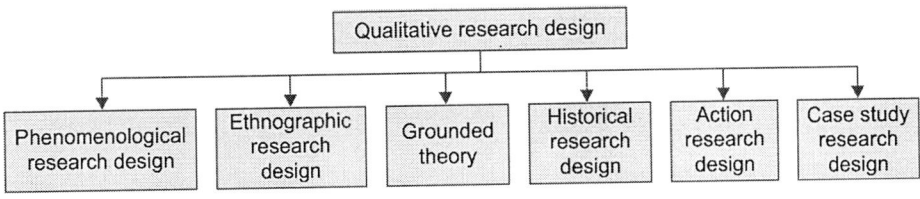

Fig. 7.6: Classification of qualitative research design

Ethnography

Ethnography is the systematic study of people and cultures. It is designed to explore cultural phenomena where the researcher observes society from the point of view of the subject of the study. An ethnography is a means to represent graphically and in writing the culture of a group. It is usually based on participant-observation and resulting in a written account of a people, place or institution. The term ethnography has come to be equated with virtually any qualitative research project where the intent is to provide a detailed, in-depth description of everyday life and practice.

An ethnographic understanding is developed through close exploration of several sources of data. Using these data sources as a foundation, the ethnographer relies on a cultural frame of analysis. The value of ethnographic research conducted in a variety of social, cultural, and physical contexts is that it can encourage us as social scientists to be open to possibilities and to imagine new ways of thinking about what might appear too familiar to be worthy of in-depth consideration. This is another reason why I value the ethnography of everyday life. It is in neglected details of day-to-day life that real insight into the meaning of social and cultural change is most powerfully and relevantly expressed.

Ethnographers generate understandings of culture through representation of what we call an *emic* perspective, or what might be described as the 'insider's point of view.' The emphasis in this representation is thus on allowing critical categories and meanings to *emerge* from the ethnographic encounter rather than imposing these from existing models. An *etic* perspective, by contrast, refers to a more distant, analytical orientation to experience.

Focused Ethnography and its Relevance for Nursing

Focused ethnography is an applied research methodology that 'has been widely used in the investigation of fields specific to contemporary society which is socially and culturally highly differentiated and fragmented' (Knoblauch, 2005). It is particularly useful in evaluating or eliciting information on a special topic or shared experience (Richards and Morse, 2007). Knoblauch (2005) noted an increasing interest in the use of focused ethnographies among those whose focus of study is limited to small elements of society. It is of particular value to nurse researchers who emphasize a distinct issue, situation or 'problem within a specific context among a small group of people' living in a bigger society (Roper and Shapira, 2000). They may target shared features of individuals in groups, so that they can focus on common behaviors and experiences (Richards and Morse, 2007). Because of its nature, focused ethnography allows the researcher to better understand the complexities surrounding issues from the participants' perspectives (emic view) while bringing the outsider's framework to the study (etic view) (Roper and Shapira, 2000). This has contributed to the development of knowledge relevant to nursing.

The ethnographic approach to qualitative research comes largely from the field of anthropology. The emphasis in ethnography is on studying an entire culture. Originally, the idea of a culture was tied to the notion of ethnicity and geographic location (e.g., the culture of the Trobriand Islands), but it has been broadened to include virtually any group or organization. That is, we can study the 'culture' of a business or defined group (e.g., a Rotary club).

Focused Ethnography in Nursing Research

The three main purposes of focused ethnographies for nursing research outlined by Roper and Shapira (2000) are to: (i) Discover how people from various cultures integrate health beliefs and practices into their lives. (ii) Understand the meaning that members of a subculture or group assign to their experiences. (iii) Study the practice of nursing as a cultural phenomenon. The following exemplars will demonstrate how nurses have applied these uses of focused ethnography in various research contexts. Discovering how people from various cultures integrate health beliefs and practices into their lives Kilian, et al. (2008) used a focused ethnography to examine the perceptions of older adults and their adult children regarding risk and falls. Use of focused ethnography allowed them to meaningfully contextualize the issue of falling and the risks involved from multiple perspectives, and to consider personal, interpersonal and societal influences. The authors conducted semistructured interviews, each lasting 35–90 minutes, over a period of four and a half months. The theoretical perspectives of Denzin and Lincoln (2005), Fetterman (1998), and Guba and Lincoln (1989) guided analysis.

Schwandt (2007) defined ethnography as 'the process and product of describing cultural behavior'. According to Roper and Shapira (2000), 'Ethnography is a research process of learning about people by learning from them.' Ethnography provides a truthful account of people's stories in their own words and local context as researchers immerse themselves in the social world of the participants to better grasp the meanings behind participants' social behavior in their culture (Roper and Shapira, 2000, Fetterman, 2010). Through written descriptions, researchers generate accounts of people's experiences and culture (Wolf, 2007). Ethnography generally employs three data collection strategies: (i) Participant observation, (ii) Formal and informal interviews, and (iii) Examination of relevant documents. These strategies are essential in helping the researcher to gain a better understanding of the culture being studied. Participant observation is a strategy in which the researcher actively becomes involved in participants' life events in their natural settings (Roper and Shapira, 2000). It is an opportunity for the researcher to become immersed in the culture being studied (Fetterman, 2010). Interviews, whether formal or informal, were regarded by Fetterman (2010) as the 'ethnographer's most important data-gathering technique'. By conducting semistructured individual or focus-group interviews, the researcher is able to map participants' responses, which are essential to subsequent coding and analysis. Collection and analysis of documents such as 'maps, policies, procedures, patient records, results of tests, biographical material, and census figures [can help to] understand the community and to validate participant observations and interview findings' (Roper and Shapira, 2000). The amount, variety and depth of relevant information obtained from these sources provide valuable data that can be used by the researcher to make sense of the culture being investigated.

Ethnography is an extremely broad area with a great variety of practitioners and methods. However, the most common ethnographic approach is participant observation as a part of field research. The ethnographer becomes immersed in the culture as an active participant and records extensive field notes. As in grounded theory, there is no preset limiting of what will be observed and no real ending point in an ethnographic study.

Phenomenology

Phenomenology is sometimes considered a philosophical perspective as well as an approach to qualitative methodology. It has a long history in several social research disciplines including psychology, sociology and social work. Phenomenology is a school of thought that emphasizes a focus on people's subjective experiences and interpretations of the world. That is, the phenomenologist wants to understand how the world appears to others.

Meaning of Phenomenology

Phenomenology coined from Greek word *phainómenon* means 'that which appears' and *lógos* means 'study'. So it is the philosophical study of the structures of experience and consciousness. It is a 'science whose purpose is to describe particular phenomena or the appearance of things as lived experience.

Phenomenology offered by different scholars focus that it is phenomenology that has the potential to penetrate deep to the human experience and trace the essence of a phenomenon and explicate it in its original form as experienced by the individuals. In simple words, it is the study of the lived experiences of persons.

Importance of Phenomenology

Phenomenology focus on a concept or phenomenon which is really a part of human experience that is love, anger, betrayal, happiness, caring, undergoing coronary bypass surgery, what it means to be/experience being underweight, and so on. It focuses on universal essence rather than individual experience by using bracketing. Bracketing means keeping aside of personal experience. The focus of phenomenological inquiry is what people experience in regard to some phenomenon or other and how they interpret those experiences.

Fields often using phenomenology are social sciences, health sciences, psychology, and nursing education. Phenomenology is well-suited to studying research questions involving affective, emotional and often intense human experiences.

Phenomenological Research

A phenomenological research study is a study that attempts to understand people's perceptions, perspectives and understandings of a particular situation (or phenomenon). In other words, a phenomenological research study tries to answer the question '*What is it like to experience such and such?*' By looking at multiple perspectives of the same situation, a researcher can start to make some generalizations of what something is like as an experience from the 'insider's' perspective. The research is carried out through following steps:
- ❖ Identification of a shared experience
- ❖ Attempt to locate universal nature of an experience

- Attempt to identify shared experience among various individuals experiencing shared phenomena
- Attempt to locate essence of an experience
- What was experienced and how he/she experienced.

Phenomenology Types

Phenomenological tradition under three major headings. They are:
1. **Hermeneutic phenomenology:** it is a qualitative research methodology that arose out of and remains closely tied to phenomenological philosophy, a strand of continental philosophy and reflecting on lived experiences with interpretation by the researcher. Basic themes of hermeneutic phenomenology are 'interpretation,' 'textual meaning,' 'dialogue,' 'preunderstanding,' and 'tradition.'
2. **Transcendental phenomenology:** in philosophy, the adjective transcendental and the noun transcendence convey the basic ground concept from the word's literal meaning (from Latin), of climbing or going beyond, albeit with varying connotations in its different historical and cultural stages. It especially focus less on the researcher's interpretation and more on the describing experiences of participants.
3. **Existential phenomenology:** Existential phenomenology, oriented to lived experience, the embodied human being in the concrete world. Basic themes of existential phenomenology are 'lived experience,' 'modes of being,' 'ontology,' and 'lifeworld.'

Assumptions of Phenomenology

- First, it rejects the concept of objective research. Phenomenologist prefer grouping assumptions through a process called phenomenological epoche.
- Second, phenomenology believes that analyzing daily human behavior can provide one with a greater understanding of nature.
- Third assumption is that persons, not individuals, should be explored. This is because persons can be understood through the unique ways they reflect the society they live in.
- Fourth, phenomenologists prefer to gather 'capta,' or conscious experience, rather than traditional data. Finally, phenomenology is considered to be oriented on discovery, and therefore phenomenologists gather research using methods that are far less restricting than in other sciences.

Methodology

A phenomenological study often involves the four steps that's are bracketing, intuiting, analyzing and describing.
1. **Bracketing:** The process of setting aside the researcher's experiences with the phenomenon to better examine the consciousness itself. Setting aside one's own understanding of the phenomenon to look at how other people experience the phenomenon.
2. **Intuiting:** It requires the researcher to become totally immersed in the phenomena under the investigation and the process whereby the researcher to know about the phenomenon as described by the participants. Intuiting involves the 'researcher as instrument' in the interview process the researcher becomes the tool for data collection and listen to the indescription of quality of life through the interview process. The investigator's intuition is 'fed' by more and more data through attentive listening, deep critical reflection about commonalities across participants, and a concerted effort to understand.

3. **Analyzing:** Analyzing involves the identifying the essence of the phenomenon under the investigation based on data obtained and how the data are presented.
4. **Describing:** The aim of describing operation is to communicate and bring to retain and verbal description distinct critical elements of the phenomenon. The description is based on classification of grouping.

Historical Studies

Historical research involves a systematic collection and a critical evaluation of data relating to past occurrences of a particular phenomenon. Nurses are increasingly interested in establishing a body of nursing knowledge and defining the role of professional nurses. One means of achieving these aims is to examine the roots of nursing through historical research. Historical studies concern the identification, location, evaluation and synthesis of data from the past. Historical research seeks not only to discover the events of the past but to relate these past happenings to the present and to the future. Leininger (1985) wrote, 'Without a past, there is no meaning to the present, nor can we develop a sense of ourselves as individuals and as members of groups'. Although there is a need for historical research in nursing, a limited number of nurse researchers have chosen it. The purpose of historical research is to gain a clear understanding of the impact of the past on the present and future events related to the life process. It involves detailed analysis of what has been written or done and is used to describe, explain or interpret these events.

Meaning

The process of learning and understanding the background and growth of a chosen field of study or profession can offer insight into organizational culture, current trends and future possibilities. The historical method of research applies to all fields of study because it encompasses there: Origins, growth, theories, personalities, crisis, etc.

Source of Data

The sources of historical data are frequently referred to as primary and secondary sources.
- *Primary sources* are those that provide firsthand information or direct evidence. Oral histories, original documents, such as written records or diaries, eyewitnesses, pictorial sources, and physical evidence, relics, remains artifacts, etc. Suppose a nurse researcher wished to examine the practices of nurse midwives during the 1940s. An oral history might be obtained from an older member of the nursing profession who had practiced as a nurse midwife during that time.
- *Secondary sources* are secondhand information or sometimes third or fourth hand like information provided by a person who did not directly observe the event, object, or condition. For example, a letter written by Florence Nightingale about nursing care during the Crimean War would be considered a primary source of data. If a friend summarized the information about nursing care during the Crimean War based on a letter she received from Florence Nightingale, this source of information would be considered a secondary source. Other secondary sources are textbooks, encyclopedias, newspapers, periodicals review of research and other references.

Criticism

The data for historical research should be subjected to two types of evaluation. These evaluations are called external criticism and internal criticism. *External criticism* is concerned with the authenticity or genuineness of the data and should be considered first. *Internal criticism* examines the accuracy of the data and is considered after the data are considered to be genuine. Whereas external criticism establishes the validity of the data, internal criticism establishes the reliability of the data.

Steps of Conducting of Historical Research

- **Choose a subject:** Choose a subject usually it will be relevant by the class, or limited by the instructor. Probably, you will then need to narrow your topic down and often define your research paper by gaining a working hypothesis and a thesis.
- **Find sources:** Source may be primary or secondary. One can use both internet and libraries to find your sources. The best sources are still those that are found in libraries or archives, so do NOT limit your searches to the web, even if it is easier.
- **Learn from your sources:** Historians usually distinguish between three kinds of sources, tertiary, primary, secondary. You can use sources to find more sources. Reading tertiary sources like encyclopedias, dictionaries, and handbooks can give you the general outline of subjects and their problems. They often have useful bibliographies (lists of books used), that are sources you can use. Secondary sources (professional historical books, scholarly articles) also have bibliographies that should lead you to more information. Primary sources, the immediate records of the past, should be used whenever possible.
- **Evaluate your sources:** While you are researching, you should be carefully judging each source. Take careful notes from your sources, always recording carefully from where you got what information.
- **Start writing, while you research:** You can, and should, begin writing as soon as possible. Do not wait until you have collected all your information. Prewriting can be based on good notes. You should be shaping your thesis in writing. To get there, if you started with a broad subject, along the way you should have been refining your subject into an arrow topic or a hypothesis. Writing as you go helps you to clarify your ideas, measure the length of parts of your argument and finish the paper sooner.
- **Write a rough draft:** Write your rough draft as if it were your finished paper. Put it aside, and go over it again carefully. You might use the checklist provided by the instructor.
- **Have other people critique your draft:** It is best to talk to the person, but written comments, perhaps according to a checklist, are also good. Rewrite until you have a polished draft. The more you rewrite, the better it will be.
- **Submit your final draft:** Notice that the end product is called a draft. Do the best you can.

Case Studies

Case studies are in-depth examinations of people or groups of people. A case study could also examine an institution, such as hospice care for the dying. The case method has its roots in sociology and has also been used a great deal in anthropology law and medicine. In medicine, case studies have frequently been concerned with a particular disease. In nursing, the case study approach might be used to answer a question such as 'How do the nurse and patient manage nausea associated with chemotherapy?'

A case study may be considered as quantitative or qualitative research depending on the purpose of the study and the design chosen by the researcher. As is true of other types of qualitative studies, for a case study to be considered as a qualitative study, the researcher must be interested in the meaning of experiences to the subjects themselves, rather than in generalizing results to other groups of people. Case studies are not used to test hypotheses, but hypotheses may be generated from case studies.

Patricia Benner is a qualitative researcher who has been interested in how a nurse moves from being a novice to an expert nurse. She has used the case study approach extensively. She contended that case studies help us formalize experiential knowledge and thus promote quality nursing care.

Data may be collected in case studies through various means, such as questionnaires, interviews, observations, or written accounts by the subjects. A nurse researcher might be interested in how people with diabetes respond to an insulin pump. One person or a group of people with diabetes could be studied for a time to determine their responses to the use of an insulin pump. Diaries might be used for the day-to-day recording of information. The nurse researcher would then analyze these diaries and try to interpret the written comments. Content analysis is used in evaluating the data from case studies.

Content Analysis

It involves the examination of communication messages. The researcher searches for patterns and themes. After reading the diaries of the individuals who are using insulin pumps, the nurse researcher might come up with themes such as: 'freedom from rigid schedule,' 'more normal life,' and 'release from self-inflicted pain.' When subjects are chosen for case studies, care must be taken in the selection process. In the previously discussed example, the researcher should avoid choosing only those clients who are expected to respond favorably or unfavorably to the insulin pump.

Case studies are time consuming and may be quite costly. Additionally, subject dropout may occur during this type of study. Whenever a study is carried out over an extended period, loss of subjects must be considered. A person may move from the locality or simply decide to discontinue participation in the study.

Action Research Studies

Action research is a type of qualitative research that seeks action to improve practice and study the effects of the action that was taken solutions are sought to practice problems in one particular hospital or health care setting. There is no goal of trying to generalize the findings of the study, as is the case in quantitative research studies. In action research, the implementation of solutions occurs as an actual part of the research process. There is no delay in implementation of the solutions.

Action research became popular in the 1940s. Kurt Lewin (1946) was influential in spreading action research. He came interested in helping social workers improve their practice. Although many of you may have heard of Lewin and his contribution to change theory, his involvement in action research is not as well-known.

Participatory Action Research

Participatory action research (PAR) is a special kind of community-based action research in which there is collaboration between the study participants and the researcher in all steps of the study: determining the problem, the research methods to use, the analysis of data, and how the study results will be used. The participants and the researcher are co-researchers throughout the entire research study. According to Kelly (2005), PAR provides an opportunity for involving a community in the development and assessment of a health program.

Grounded Theory

Grounded theory is a qualitative research approach that was originally developed by Glaser and Strauss in the 1960s. The self-defined purpose of grounded theory is to develop theory about phenomena of interest. But this is not just abstract theorizing they are talking about. Instead the *theory* needs to be *grounded* or rooted in observation—hence the term.

Grounded theory is a complex *iterative* process. The research begins with the raising of *generative questions* which help to guide the research but are not intended to be either static or confining. As the researcher begins to gather data, *core theoretical concept(s)* are identified. Tentative *linkages* are developed between the theoretical core concepts and the data. This early phase of the research tends to be very open and can take months. Later on the researcher is more engaged in verification and summary. The effort tends to evolve toward one *core category* that is central.

There are several key analytic strategies:

- *Coding* is a process for both categorizing qualitative data and for describing the implications and details of these categories. Initially one does *open coding*, considering the data in minute detail while developing some initial categories. Later, one moves to more *selective coding* where one systematically codes with respect to a core concept.
- *Memoing* is a process for recording the thoughts and ideas of the researcher as they evolve throughout the study. You might think of memoing as extensive marginal notes and comments. Again, early in the process these memos tend to be very open while later on they tend to increasingly focus in on the core concept.
- *Integrative diagrams and sessions* are used to pull all of the detail together, to help make sense of the data with respect to the emerging theory. The diagrams can be any form of graphic that is useful at that point in theory development. They might be concept maps or directed graphs or even simple cartoons that can act as summarizing devices. This integrative work is best done in group sessions where different members of the research team are able to interact and share ideas to increase insight.

SUMMARY

- The design of a study is the end result of a series of decisions made by the researcher concerning how the study will be conducted. The design is closely associated with the framework of the study and guides planning for the implementation.
- There are varieties of factors affecting in selecting research design. The factors are knowledge about the phenomena, nature of the phenomenon, purpose of the study, ethical considerations, feasibility of the study and researcher's knowledge and experience, etc.
- Research design is classified as qualitative and quantitative research design then each design is classified in various ways. Quantitative research design is classified as experimental and nonexperimental research design.
- The quantitative research design is formal, objective, systematic process for obtaining quantifiable information about the world, presented in numerical form, and analyzed

through the use of statistics, used to describe and to test relationships and especially used to examine the cause-and-effect of relationships.
* There are three essential characteristics of experimental research design. That's are control, randomization and manipulation. The experimental design is classified as true experimental, quasi experimental and pre-experimental.
* Solomon four-group design is also one type of true experimental design. Here four groups (two experimental and two control groups) are selected randomly.
* Time series design is a type of quasi-experimental design where the researcher measures repeatedly both before and after exposure to a treatment. It may be a single group or within multiple groups.
* Qualitative research is designed to reveal a target audience's range of behavior and the perceptions that drive it with reference to specific topics or issues. It uses in-depth studies of small groups of people to guide and support the construction of hypotheses.

QUESTIONS TO TEST YOUR KNOWLEDGE

Q1. What do you mean by research design? Write the elements and enumerate the factors affecting selection of research design. Draw a diagram of classification of research design.   (3 + 3 + 5 + 4)

Q2. Enumerate briefly the classification of true experimental research design.   (14)

Q3. Explain the classifications of qualitative research design.

Q4. Write short notes on followings: (5 × 5)
  a. Correlational design
  b. Time series design
  c. Solomon four-group design
  d. Developmental research designs
  e. Survey design

Q5. Multiple choice questions: (1 × 11)
  I. In which type of research design researcher will follow randomization, use control group and do manipulation:
    a. Quasi experimental design
    b. True experimental design
    c. Descriptive design
    d. Correlational design
  II. When there is manipulation but lack of at least one of the two other properties like randomization or control group is called:
    a. Experimental research design
    b. Quasi experimental research design
    c. Descriptive research design
    d. Time series design
  III. A community health nurse conducts a study on the perception of people regarding utilization of ASHA service. What research design is appropriate to use in this study?
    a. Quasi-experiment
    b. Exploratory
    c. Descriptive
    d. Experimental
  IV. Which is not a direct threat to the internal validity of a research design?
    a. History
    b. Testing
    c. Sampling error
    d. Differential selection
  V. Studies in which the independent variable or presumed is identified at the present time and then subjects are followed for sometime in the future to observe the dependent variable or effect is known as:
    a. Prospective studies
    b. Retrospective studies
    c. Concurrent studies
    d. Prevalence studies

VI. True experimental design that minimizes threats to internal and external validity is:
   a. Pretest-Post-test control group design
   b. Post-test only control group design
   c. Solomon four group design
   d. Factorial design

VII. A research design where two or more independent variables are simultaneously investigated to determine the independent and interactive influence which they have on the dependent variable is:
   a. Pretest-post-test control group design
   b. Post-test only control group design
   c. Solomon four group design
   d. Factorial design

VIII. A type of research design the subjects are serving as their own control group.
   a. Post-test only control group design
   b. Solomon four group design
   c. Crossover design:
   d. Factorial design

IX. Research studies that involve the collection and analysis of data about cultural groups is:
   a. Phenomenology
   b. Grounded theories
   c. Ethnographic studies
   d. Case studies

X. The researcher is hearing a repetition of themes or ideas as additional participants are interviewed in a qualitative study:
   a. Maturation
   b. Saturation
   c. Triangulation
   d. Manipulation

XI. Combining both qualitative and quantitative methods in one study is called:
   a. Maturation
   b. Saturation
   c. Triangulation
   d. Manipulation

ANSWERS

I. b	II. b	III. b	IV. c	V. a
VI. c	VII. d	VIII. c	IX. c	X. b
XI. c				

Chapter 8

Sampling and its Design

> **Learning Objectives**
>
> After completion of this chapter, the students will be able to:
> - Explain the concept of population sample and sampling.
> - Enumerate principles of sampling and sampling process.
> - Discuss the importance and limitations of sampling technique.
> - Identify sampling and nonsampling errors and characteristics of good sample.
> - Describe different types of probability sampling and non-probability technique.
> - Distinguish between probability sampling and non-probability technique with their advantage and disadvantages.

INTRODUCTION

When a researcher gathers data from the entire population (even in relatively small populations) it is difficult to include everyone in the population. The data collection may take too long. In statistics for quality assurance, and survey methodology, sampling is concerned with the selection of a subset of individuals from a statistical population to estimate characteristics of the whole population. It is important to keep in mind that the primary point of sampling is to create a small group from a population that is as similar to the larger population as possible. Because it can be generally presumed that in a survey or any other form of research when all items are covered, no element of chance is left and highest accuracy is obtained. But in practice this may not be true. Even the slightest element of bias can get larger and larger as the number of observation increases. So the researcher has to be very careful during collection of data. For collection of data from the whole population is time consuming and sometimes impossible because it should be within the resource available and feasible. So in general for conducting any study we have to select a small group of the population which will be the representative of the entire population. Thus it is clear that one of the features we look for in a sample is the degree of representativeness means how well does the sample represent the larger population from which it was drawn and how closely do the features of the sample resemble those of the larger population.

CONCEPT OF POPULATION

A population is the entire aggregation of cases in which researcher is interested. For example, a nurse researcher interested to conduct a study on the 'attitude of GNM students towards patient care in emergency situation in Odisha'. There the population meant all the nursing students undergoing GNM course in India. Population is not restricted to human subjects, it may be all hospital records, blood samples, institutions or other different units. But when the researcher is selecting any population group he/she has to establish some criteria to determine whether a person qualifies as a member of the population or not. That criteria are called as eligibility criteria or inclusion criteria of population. For making selection easy the researcher can also develop some exclusion criteria when he/she defines the populations sometimes in terms of characteristics that people must *not* possess. For the above study the inclusion criteria are:

❖ The nursing students undergoing GNM course.
❖ They are the citizen of Odisha.
❖ Here the researcher can develop the exclusion criteria as only the nursing students residing in hostel because it is difficult for her to follow-up day scalars.
❖ Similarly, if a researcher wants to conduct a study on the antenatal mothers attending antenatal clinic and develop a tool on local language Odia then her exclusion criteria is the mothers who are unable to speak Odia.

DEFINITION OF POPULATION

Population is a complete set of elements (persons or objects) that possess some common characteristics defined by the eligibility criteria established by the researcher.

ELIGIBILITY CRITERIA OF POPULATION DURING SELECTION

Before selection of population the researcher selects some predetermine criteria based on which the population will be selected. The exact criteria by which it could be decided whether an individual would or would not be classified as a member of the population is known as inclusion criteria. Inclusion criteria that specify the population characteristics or sometimes which criteria is not included or excluded during selection is termed as exclusive criteria. Some factors which affects eligibility criteria are as follows **(Fig. 8.1)**:

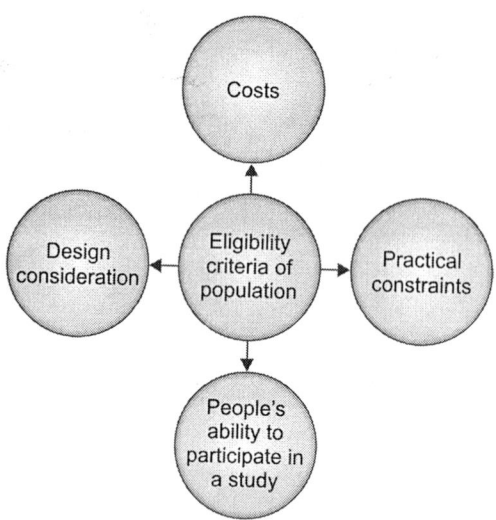

Fig. 8.1: Eligibility criteria of population during selection.

Costs

Some criteria reflect cost constraints. The research should be based on the budgetary panning prepared by the researcher. Researcher sometimes unable to take large sample due to cost constraints or sometime the researcher select specific people also for this reason. For example, when we exclude people from our population who cannot speak specific language, it does not mean that the researcher is not interested in them rather than he cannot afford to hire translators or multilingual data collectors.

Practical Constraints

Sometimes practical constraint also affecting the selection of sample process. Practical constraint include not accessibility and availability of sample or lack of time or unwillingness of participants, etc. For example, difficulty in including the people who are laborer because they are not available during visiting of the researcher or a researcher is conducting a study on the effects of consanguineous marriage of the couples on their off-springs here he/she has to search the couples having consanguineous marriage which may difficult to get.

People's Ability to Participate in a Study

The health conditions of some people may be an obstacle for their participation in the study. For example, people with mental retardation, who is medically unstable, cannot be included in the study.

Design Considerations

When we are selecting a sample from a group of population we have to check the homogeneity of the population from which we will draw the sample and it is very difficult to do that because there is a huge individual difference between them, but it is sometimes advantageous to studies the internal validity or to define a homogeneous population as a mean of controlling confounding variables. Some time some population can be excluded from study who are not having the characteristics of homologous group or threatening of internal validity and not making control over extraneous variables.

PROCESS OF SELECTION OF SAMPLE (FIG. 8.2)

The population generally composed of two groups—target population and accessible population.

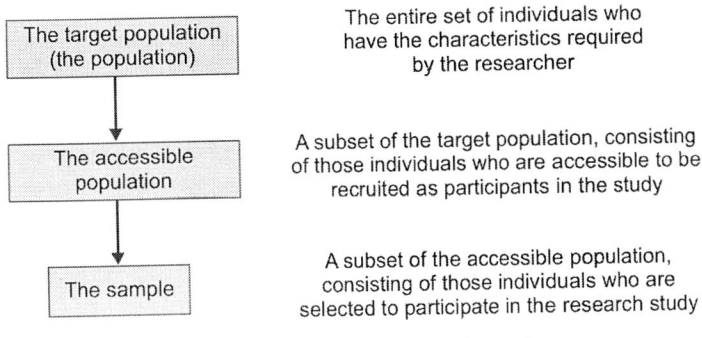

Fig. 8.2: Process of selection of sample.

Target Population

Target population is the entire group of people or objects to which the researcher wishes to generalize the study findings which meet set of criteria of interest to researcher. The target population is the collection of elements or objects that possess the information sought by the researcher and about which inferences are to be made. The target population should be defined in terms of elements (respondents), sampling units, extent, and time.

Accessible Population

The portion of the population to which the researcher has reasonable access; may be a subset of the target population may be limited to region, state, city, county, or institution. This population is a subset of the target population and is also known as the study population. It is from the accessible population that researchers draw their samples. Let us consider a problem statement 'A study to assess the effectiveness of video-assisted teaching module (VATM) regarding prevention of malnutrition among under-fives on knowledge of the mothers in selected rural communities, Odisha'.

For this problem statement the target population is mothers of under-five children in rural communities and accessible population mothers of under-children in rural communities, Odisha from which the sample can be drawn. Process of selection of sample is shown in **Figure 8.2**.

CONCEPT OF SAMPLE

A sample is 'a smaller (but hopefully representative) collection of units from a population used to determine truths about that population'.

A sample is simply a subset of the population. The concept of sample arises from the inability of the researchers to test all the individuals in a given population. The sample must be representative of the population from which it was drawn and it must have good size to warrant statistical analysis.

The main function of the sample is to allow the researchers to conduct the study to individuals from the population so that the results of their study can be used to derive conclusions that will apply to the entire population. It is much like a give-and-take process. The population 'gives' the sample, and then it takes conclusions, from the results obtained from the sample.

SAMPLING

Sampling is the process of selecting units (e.g., people, organizations) from a population of interest so that by studying the sample we may fairly generalize our results back to the population from which they were chosen. It is a process of selecting subjects who are representative of population events, behaviors or other elements with which to conduct study. In research studies it is always not possible to study an entire population; therefore the researcher draws a representative part of a population through sampling process.

Definitions

Sampling is a process of selecting a part of the assigned population to represent the entire population. Sampling process entails the formulation of specific criteria for selection, which ensures that the characteristics of phenomenon of interest will be present in all the units being studied.

It is the act, process, or technique of selecting a representative part of a population for the purpose of determining parameters or characteristics of the whole population.

Sampling is the selection of some part of an aggregate or a whole on the basis of which judgments or inferences about the aggregate or mass is made.

Three factors that influence sample representativeness are sampling procedure, sample size and anticipation (response). For selecting sample properly the sample should be properly-selected.

Principles of Sampling (Fig. 8.3)

Based on the Objectives

The sample selection process is depends upon the objectives of the study, for example, in case of a descriptive study the objective of the research is to describe the phenomenon for which a large sample is needed. Similarly when the objective of a study is to assess the effectiveness of any nursing intervention, our sample size is less because we have to control over the extraneous variable and it is difficult if sample size is large. Generally, probability sampling technique is the standardized sampling technique, but in some cases a researcher deciding to select nonprobability sampling technique like any accidental cases or purposefully a researcher went to do some study like move to the rehabilitation center where malnourished children are available to conduct his study on evaluating the effectiveness of diet therapy on treating malnutrition among under-five children. Similarly, he/she can select any type of probability sampling technique based on the study objectives.

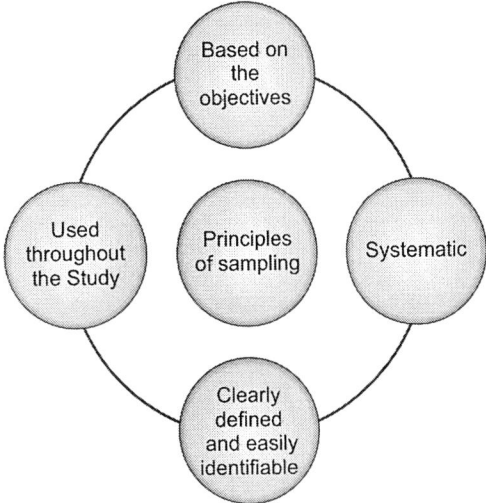

Fig. 8.3: Principles of sampling.

Systematic

Sampling is the selected elements (people or objects) chosen for participation in a study and the sampling process is a systematic process consists of a series of steps through which the researcher has to move. The proper selection of sample gives more accurate result.

Clearly Defined and Easily Identifiable

The characteristics of the sample, sampling techniques, and sampling size should be predetermined and should be clearly defined by which the selection of sample will become easy. Sample reflects the characteristics of the population, so those sample findings can be generalized to the population. Before entering to the study the characteristics of population should be determined and the sampling technique should be clear which helps in identifying the sample easily.

Used Throughout the Study

The main principle of sampling is, the sampling technique should be same throughout in study. Sometimes the study will continue for a long time and it is difficult to get the subject by using same sampling technique but in any longitudinal studies the sampling technique should not be changed.

The sample selection process should based on two basic principles.

Law of Statistical Regularity

This law comes from the mathematical theory of probability. According to King, 'law of statistical regularity says that a moderately large number of the items chosen at random from the large group are almost sure on the average to possess the features of the large group.' According to this law the units of the sample must be selected by random sampling technique.

Law of Inertia of Large Numbers

According to this law, when the larger the size of the sample; the more accurate the results are likely to be. There is a relationship between the size of a sample and its accuracy. Within the human being there is individual difference even though in same homogeneous group. The larger the sample the greater would be the accuracy reason for this is the sample will be more representative of the population.

Sampling is very complex and technical task in research. The opportunity to study the entire population of these people, places and things is an endeavor that most researchers do not have the time and money to undertake. It is almost impossible to collect data from the entire population because of amount of people, places, or things within population.

Characteristics of Good Sample

There are various qualities and characteristics features that make a sample good. The characteristics are as follows:

- **Representative:** Representative is one of the key characteristics of selecting sample. The sample should be the representative of whole population. By following appropriate sampling technique a researcher can able to fulfill this characteristics. This helps in generalizing the research findings for the population.
- **Free from bias and errors:** A good sample should have minimum sampling error and bias. Generally, random sampling technique from the homogeneous group with appropriate sample size make the sample having less sampling errors or sampling bias.
- **No substitution and incompleteness:** A sample is said to be good if once a subject is selected for the study, is neither be replaced nor incomplete in any aspect of researcher's interest. The sample should fulfill all the inclusive criteria for selection of sample.
- **Appropriate sample size:** It is believed that in quantitative studies the larger the sample size provide better probability of the result. The sample size should be analyzed before proceeding to the study. Appropriate sample size estimation will save lot of time, money and other research-related expense and give unbiased result.

Importance of Sampling (Fig. 8.4)

The sampling serves many purposes in research, which includes:

Economical

In most cases, it is not possible and economical for researchers to study an entire population. With the help of sampling, the researcher can save lot of time, money, and resources to study a phenomenon. Furthermore, data collected through a carefully selected sample are highly accurate measures of the larger population. So sampling provides an economical option for the researcher to generate empirical evidences. Well-designed sampling techniques will help to save lot of time, money, and other expenditure related to selection of sample.

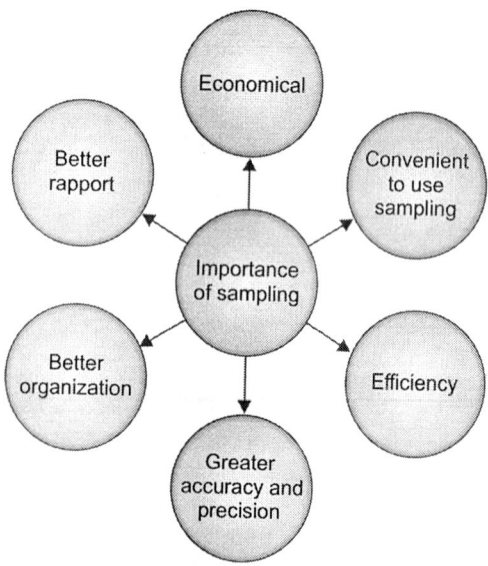

Fig. 8.4: Importance of sampling.

Convenient to Use Sampling

It is convenient to use sampling to collect data from small proportion of population than studying whole population. Selecting whole population is troublesome and not feasible in terms of time, money, machine and man. Observations are easier to collect and summarize with a sample than with a complete count.

Efficiency

The suitable sampling techniques will improve the speed of data collection which is another important step of research. Sometimes highly trained personnel or specialized equipment limited in availability which may be used to obtain the data. By sampling using of scarce resources is possible.

Greater Accuracy and Precision of Data

Selecting whole population will be difficult to handle than handling the information of a small portion of the population. It is easier to maintain quality of data with small samples investigation rather than selecting the whole population.

Better Organization

Dealing with the whole population will be difficult to organize resources, such as time, money, printing facilities, vehicles, etc., so sampling helps to overcome the problem of disorganization of resources and help organization of project.

Better Rapport

It is challenging task for a researcher to maintain rapport with whole population. Selecting representative sample will help the researcher to maintain one-to-one rapport and seek objective information, which is one of the important objectives of research.

Limitations of Sampling

- **Chances for errors and bias:** Sampling bias is consistent error that arises due to faulty sampling technique. Generally in probability sampling the chance of error and bias are less. But if the group is not a homogeneous one then also there is chance of sampling error. Generally, there is a difference between population mean and sample mean which may be minimized by proper sampling technique.
- **Difficulty of getting the representative sample**: Sample size and representativeness are two related, but different issues. Large unrepresentative samples can perform as badly as small unrepresentative samples. So representative of sample is very important, and for getting representative of sample the researcher should not left any part of population and he/she has to check the homogeneity of the population, but there are so many constraints which act as barriers to do this. Hence it is a big limitation for sampling.
- **Untrained manpower:** Proper training is very essential to the personnel recruited for collecting data before going for data collection. Otherwise the researcher will not get a proper representative of sample.
- **Absence of the informants:** Absences of the subject or informant is a big limitation of sampling because in absence of any part of population can cause sampling error.

SAMPLING PROCESS (FIG. 8.5)

Identify the Population of Interest

A population is the group of people that the researcher want to make assumptions about. Once the decision to sample has been made, the first question related to sample, concerns identifying the target population, that is the complete group of specific population elements related to research project. It is important to carefully define the target population. So the first step of sampling process is identification of the population who are fulfilling the predetermining criteria set by the researcher must be carried out. Knowledge about target and accessible population is important to access a representative sample in a study. First the researcher has to select the target population from which accessible population will be selected based on the researcher's convenience. For example, a study on effectiveness of Mid-day Meal Programme in India, the target population is all government schools in India whereas the accessible population is the selected schools where the researcher able to reach based on his convenience where he can draw the sample.

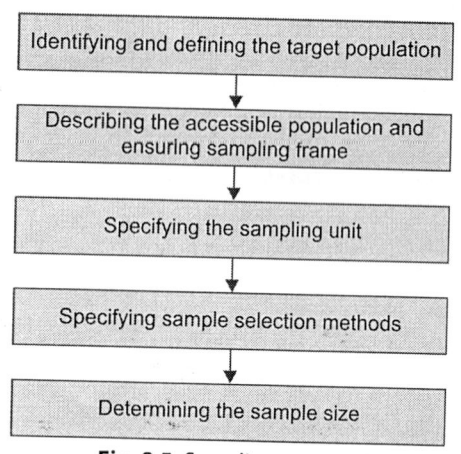

Fig. 8.5: Sampling process.

Describing the Accessible Population and Specifying a Sampling Frame

It is always not possible to have access to each subject included in the target population. So, researcher must establish a description about the accessible population, from which sampling frame developed. Accessible population is determined from the target population based on their availability and accessibility. Sampling frame is the list of elements from which a sample may be drawn. It has the property that we can identify every single element in population and include in our sampling unit. A decision has to be taken concerning a sampling unit before selecting sample. Sampling unit may be based on a geographical area one such as state, district, village, or a hamlet, etc., or a construction unit such as house, flat, etc., or if it is in the school the sampling may be each class. Basically, a sampling frame is a complete list of all the members of the population that we wish to study. To give an example, if we wish to study the underlying factors that cause patients to be admitted into hospital following an acute asthmatic attack in a given area, then we would need to know the names of all the people in that area who have been admitted into hospital for this reason.

From a list of these names, randomly we can then select an appropriate number as representatives of the population whom we can invite to take part in the research as sample. If we do not have such a sampling frame, then we are restricted to less satisfactory forms of samples which cannot be randomly selected, because not all individuals within that population will have the same probability of being selected for the sample.

Specify a Sampling Method

There are basically two ways to choose a sample from a sampling frame: (i) Randomly or (ii) nonrandomly. There are benefits to both. Basically, if sampling frame is approximately the same demographic makeup as the population, then the sampling technique is random sampling technique, perhaps by flipping a coin or drawing names out of a hat. But what if your sampling frame does not really represent your population? For example, if the area where researcher conducting her study has a lot more men than women and a lot more Whites than minority races? In the population of every college student in the world, there might be more of a balance. In that case, she might want to nonrandomly select her sample in order to get a demographic makeup that is closer to that of her population or otherwise first she will make her population homogeneous groups and then collect the data randomly from each homogeneous groups. Some time the researcher has to conduct a study by purposefully going to a place or accidentally she has to conduct a study, there she has to select nonprobability sampling technique. In this step sampling method has specified.

Determine the Sample Size

In general, larger samples are better, but they also require more time and effort to manage. No sample will be perfect for a study, so it is need to decide how much error to allow. The confidence interval determines how much higher or lower than the population mean, you are willing to let your sample mean fall has to make choices and find a balance between what will give her good data and what is practical. The sample size is an important feature of any empirical study in which the goal is to make inferences about a population from a sample. In practice, the sample size used in a study is usually determined based on the cost, time, or convenience of collecting the data, and the need for it to offer sufficient statistical power. In different studies there may be different sample sizes. For example, in a stratified survey there would be different sizes for each stratum based on the number of individuals. In purposive sampling technique we are taking the whole accessible population as our sample hence the intended sample size is equal to the population. In experimental design, where a study may be divided into different treatment groups, there may be different sample sizes for each group. Sample sizes may be chosen in several ways:

- Using experience—small samples, though sometimes unavoidable, can result in wide confidence intervals and risk of errors in statistical hypothesis testing.
- Using a target variance for an estimate to be derived from the sample eventually obtained, i.e., if a high precision is required (narrow confidence interval) this translates to a low target variance of the estimator.
- Using a target for the power of a statistical test to be applied once the sample is collected.
- Using a confidence level, i.e., the larger the required confidence level, the larger the sample size (given a constant precision requirement).

Implement the Plan

Once researcher know the population, sampling frame, sampling method, and sample size, she/he can use all that information to choose the sample. Two general approaches to sampling are used in research *probability* and *nonprobability*. In probability samples, each member of the population has a known nonzero probability of being selected which means all elements in the population have some opportunity of being included in the sample, and the mathematical probability that any one of them will be selected can be calculated.

Nonprobability sampling or *judgment* sampling depends on subjective judgment. The nonprobability method of sampling is a process where probabilities cannot be assigned to the units objectively, and hence it becomes difficult to determine the reliability of the sample results in terms of probability. In nonprobability sampling, members are selected from the population in some nonrandom manner. They selected on the basis of their availability (e.g., because they volunteered) or because of the researcher's personal judgment that they are representative. The consequence is that an unknown portion of the population is excluded. These sampling types include convenience sampling, judgment sampling, quota sampling, and snowball sampling. The advantage of probability sampling is that sampling error can be calculated. Sampling error is the degree to which a sample might differ from the population. When inferring to the population, results are reported plus or minus the sampling error. In nonprobability sampling, the degree to which the sample differs from the population remains unknown.

SAMPLING ERRORS

There may be fluctuations in the values of the statistics of characteristics from one sample to another, or even those drawn from the same population. The selected sample may vary in some characteristics to other samples and the population as well. For example, imagine that you want to measure the average height of men in earth. This average height exists but obviously it is very difficult to measure such a large population so what you can do is measure hundreds or thousands of people and calculate the average height of these people. But the average height of these people is probably not exactly equal to the average height of men on earth. So the difference between the quantity you want to know and the quantity you found is sampling error.

Sampling errors occur as a result of calculating the estimate (estimated mean, total, proportion, etc.) based on a sample rather than the entire population. This is due to the fact that the estimated figure obtained from the sample may not be exactly equal to the true value of the population. Since the sample does not include all members of the population, statistics on the sample, such as means and quintiles, generally differ from parameters on the entire population. Even the statistics based on samples drawn from the same population always vary from each other (and from the true population value) simply because of chance. These variations in the possible sample values of a statistic can theoretically be expressed as sampling errors although in practice the exact sampling error is typically unknown. The measure used to estimate the sampling error is the standard error. Since sampling is typically done to determine the characteristics of a whole population, the difference between the sample and population values is considered a sampling error exact measurement of sampling error is generally not feasible since the true population values are unknown; however, sampling error can often be estimated by probabilistic modeling of the sample. The likely size of the sampling error can generally be controlled by taking a large enough random sample from the population.

Reasons of the Sampling Errors

- ❖ Sampling process error occurs because researchers draw different subjects from the same populations, but the subjects have individual differences.
- ❖ The most frequent cause of the said error is a biased sampling procedure. Every researcher must seek to establish a sample that is free from bias and is representative of the entire population. In this case the researcher is able to minimize or eliminate sampling error.
- ❖ Another possible cause of error is chance. The process of randomization and probability sampling is done to minimize, sampling process error but it is still possible that all the randomized subjects are not representative of the population.
- ❖ The most common results of sampling error is systematic error where in the results from the sample differ significantly from the result from the entire population. It follows logic that if

the sample is not representative of the entire population the results from it will most likely differ from the results taken from the entire population.

NONSAMPLING ERRORS

The accuracy of an estimate is also affected by errors arising from causes, such as incomplete coverage and faulty procedures of estimation, and together with observational errors, these makeup what are termed nonsampling errors. The aim of a survey is always to obtain information on the true population value. The idea is to get as close as possible to the latter within the resources available for survey. The discrepancy between the survey value and the corresponding true value is called the observational error or response error. Response non-sampling errors occur as a result of improper records on the variety of interests, careless reporting of the data, or deliberate modification of the data by the data collectors and recorders to suit their interests. Nonresponse error occurs when a significant number of people in a survey sample are either absent; do not respond to the questionnaire; or, are different from those who do in a way that is important to the study.

SAMPLING BIAS

Sampling bias also called systematic bias or systematic variance. Although judgment sampling is quicker than probability sampling, it is prone to systematic errors. Sampling bias usually occurs when randomization is not used. The difference between sample data and population data that can be attributed to faulty sampling of the population. Sampling bias is a possible source of sampling errors. It leads to sampling errors which either have a prevalence to be positive or negative.

SAMPLING TECHNIQUE (FIG. 8.6)

Sampling is concerned with choosing a subset of individuals from a statistical population to estimate characteristics of a whole population. Sampling technique is the process of selection of sample for conducting a study. There are mainly two types of sampling technique:
1. Probability sampling technique
2. Nonprobability sampling technique

Probability Sampling Technique

Probability sampling is based on the theory of probability. It is also known

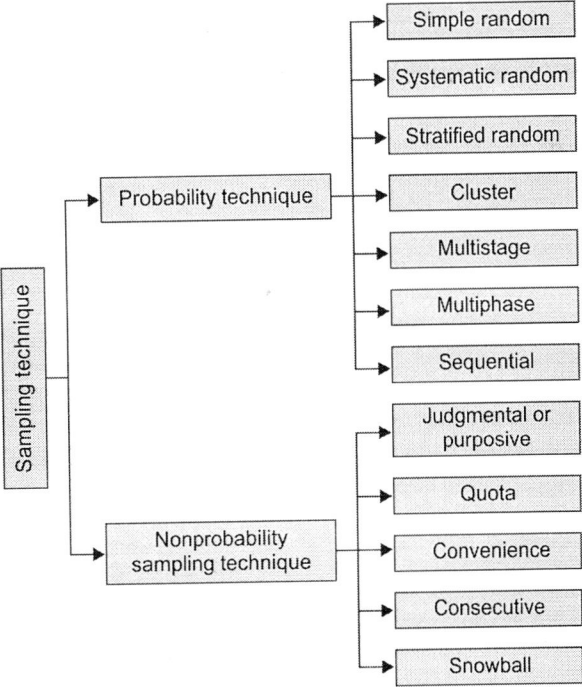

Fig. 8.6: Classification of sampling technique.

as random probability. The primary characteristics of probability sampling is the random selection of elements from the population. It provides a known nonzero chance of selection for each equal and independent chance of being included in the sample.

The sampling units are selected as random (by chance) and neither investigator nor the population element have any conscious influence on what is included in the sample. In probability sampling every population has a chance is known as probability. The closeness of a sample to the population can be determined by estimating sampling bias or error. Though randomization, the danger of unknown sampling bias can be minimized. Hence probability sampling is preferable. Cost and time required for probability sampling may be large.

Definition of Probability Sampling Method

Probability sampling one those in which the sample elements are automatically selected by some scheme under which a particular sample of given size from a specified population has some known probability being selected.

Features of Probability Sampling

- Probability sampling is a technique wherein the samples are gathered in a process that gives all the individuals in the population equal chances of being selected.
- In this sampling techniques the researcher must guarantee that every individual has an equal opportunity for selection and this can be achieved only if the researcher utilizes randomization.
- The advantage of using a random sample is the absence of both systematic and sampling bias. If random selection is done properly, the sample is representative of the entire.
- The effect of this is a minimal or absent systematic bias, which is a difference between the results from the sample and those from the population. Sampling bias is also eliminated since the subjects are randomly chosen.

Types of the Probability Sampling

Probability sampling techniques are further classified in following subtypes:
- Simple random sampling
- Systematic random sampling
- Stratified random sampling
- Cluster sampling
- Multistage sampling
- Multiphase sampling
- Sequential sampling

Simple Random Sampling Technique

Simple random sampling is a basic type of sampling, since it can be a component of other more complex sampling methods. The principle of simple random sampling is that every object has the same probability of being chosen. Each individual is chosen randomly and entirely by chance, such that each individual has the same probability of being chosen at any stage during the sampling process. Conceptually, simple random sampling is the simplest of the probability sampling techniques. It requires a complete sampling frame, which may not be available or feasible to construct for large populations. Even if a complete frame is available, more efficient approaches may be possible if other useful information is available about the units in the population. Simple random sampling is applicable when population is small, homogeneous and readily available. The list of the subjects in population is called as sampling frame. All subsets of the frame are given an equal probability. Each element of the frame thus has an equal probability of selection. The sample drawn from sampling frame by using following methods.

The Lottery Method

This is most primitive and mechanical method. Each member of the population is assigned a unique number. Each number is placed in a bowl or hat and mixed thoroughly. The blind folded researcher then picks the number tags from the hat. All the individuals bearing the numbers picked by the researcher are the subjects for the study. This may be carried out by using replacement method, where chosen numbers are replaced back in the container or by nonreplacement method, where chosen number are not replaced back in container.

The Use of Table Random Numbers

This most commonly and accurately used method in simple random sampling. Table present several number in rows and columns. Researcher initially prepares a numbered list of the elements, members of the population, and then with a blind fold choose a number are considered until desired numbers of subjects are achieved.

Example (**Table 8.1**)

Table 8.1: Example of a table for table random method.

10	09	73	25	33	76	52	01	
37	54	20	48	05	64	89	47	
08	42	26	89	53	19	64	50	
12	01	90	25	29	09	37	67	
66	80	79	99	70	80	15	73	
31	06	97	08	05	45	57	18	
73	79	64	57	53	03	52	96	

Nowadays random tables may be generated from the computer and subjects may be selected as desired in the use of random table. For population with a small number of members it is advisable to use the first method, but if the population has many numbers a computer- aided random selection is preferred.

Merits

- One of the best things about simple random sampling is the ease of assembling the sample.
- It is also considered a fair way of selecting a sample from a given population since every member is given equal opportunity of being selected.

- ❖ Require minimum knowledge about the population in advance.
- ❖ One of the unbiased probability methods of sampling.
- ❖ Free from sampling errors.

Demerits

- ❖ One of the most obvious limitations of simple random sampling method is the requirement of a complete and up-to-date list.
- ❖ Lots of procedures need to be done before sampling in accomplished.
- ❖ Expensive and time consuming.

Systematic Random Sampling

Systematic random sampling is a little bit different from simple random sampling. It relies on arranging the study population according to some ordering scheme and then selecting elements at regular intervals through that ordered list. Systematic sampling involves a random start and then proceeds with the selection of every kth element from then onwards. In systematic sampling interval size has been selected as $k = N/n$. Let's assume that we have a population that only has $N = 1000$ people in it and that we want to take a sample of $n = 100$. To use systematic sampling, the population must be listed in a random order. The sampling fraction would be $n/N = 100/1000 = 10\%$. In this case, the interval size, k, is equal to $N/n = 1000/100 = 10$. Now, select a random integer from 1–5. In our example, imagine that you chose 4. Now, to select the sample, start with the 4th unit in the list and take every k-th unit (every 10th, because $k = 10$). You would be sampling units 4, 14, 24, 34 and so on to 1000. In order for systematic sampling to work, it is essential that the units in the population be randomly ordered, at least with respect to the characteristics of measuring. Systematic sampling is fairly easy to do and is widely used for its convenience and time efficiency. In many surveys, it is found to provide more precise estimates than simple random sampling. This happens when there is a trend present in the list with respect to the characteristic of interest.

Merits

- ❖ Researcher find this technique convenient and simple to carry out.
- ❖ Distribution of sample is spread evenly over the entire given population.
- ❖ Less cumbersome, time consuming and is cheaper than simple random sampling technique.

Demerits

- ❖ If first subject is not randomly selected then it becomes a nonrandom sampling technique.
- ❖ Sometimes this may result in biased sample.

Stratified Random Sampling

Stratified random sampling is a probability sampling technique wherein the researcher divides the entire population into different subgroups or strata, then randomly selects the final subjects proportionally from the different strata. This method is used for heterogenous population. Here researcher divides the entire population into different homogeneous subgroups or strata. The strata are divided according to selected traits of the population, such as age, gender, religion, socioeconomic status, diagnosis, education, type of care nursing area specialization, site of care, etc., on the basis of information available from a frame.

All units are allocated to strata by placing within the same stratum, those units which are more-or-less similar with respect to the characteristics being measured. If this can be reasonably achieved, the strata will become homogenous, i.e. the unit-to-unit variability within a stratum will be small. It is important to note that the strata must be nonoverlapping. Having overlapping subgroups will grant some individuals higher chances of being selected as subject. Researchers can use various different sample allocation techniques to distribute the samples in the strata. In proportional allocation, the sample size in a stratum is made proportional to the number of units in the stratum. In equal allocation, the same number of units is taken from each stratum irrespective of the size of the stratum. The most common strata used in stratified random sampling are age, gender, socioeconomic status, religion, nationality and educational attainment.

Types of Stratified Random Sampling

Proportionate Stratified Random Sampling

In this proportionate stratified random sampling, the sample size of each stratum in this technique is proportionate to the population size of the stratum when viewed against the entire population. This means that the each stratum has the same sampling fraction.

For example, the researcher has three strata with 100, 200 and 300 population sizes respectively. And the researcher chose a sampling fraction of 1/5. Then, the researcher must randomly sample 20, 40 and 60 subjects from each stratum respectively.

The important thing to remember in this technique is to use the same sampling fraction for each stratum regardless of the differences in population size of the strata. It is much like assembling a smaller population that is specific to the relative proportions of the subgroups within the population.

Disproportionate Stratified Random Sampling

The only difference between proportionate and disproportionate stratified random sampling is their sampling fractions. With disproportionate sampling, the different strata have different sampling fractions.

The precision of this design is highly dependent on the sampling fraction allocation of the researcher. If the researcher commits mistakes in allotting sampling fractions, a stratum may either be overrepresented or underrepresented which will result in skewed results.

Merits

- It ensures representation of all groups in a population.
- Researchers also employ stratified random sampling they want to observe exiting relationships between two or more subgroups.
- This technique has high statistical precision. It also means that it requires a small sample size which can save a lot of time, money and effort of the researchers.

Demerits

- Requires complete information of population.
- Large population is required.
- Chances of faulty classification of strata.

Cluster Sampling

The smallest units into which a population can be divided are called the elements of the population, and groups of elements called as the clusters. Cluster sampling technique is done when simple random sampling is almost impossible because of the size of the population. In random sampling methods when sampling a population that is distributed across a wide geographic region lies in covering a lot of ground geographically in order to get to each of the units sampled is difficult in that cases a researcher can follow cluster sampling technique. The researcher can follow one-stage cluster sampling or two-stage cluster sampling. In one-stage sampling. All of the elements within selected clusters are included in the sample and in two-stage sampling a subset of elements within selected clusters are randomly selected for inclusion in the sample.

The population divided into clusters of homogeneous units, usually based on geographical contiguity. Here the sampling units are groups rather than individuals and among them a sample of a cluster is then selected. All units or selected units from the selected clusters are studied. Cluster sampling is ordinarily conducted in order to reduce costs. The population within a cluster should ideally be as heterogeneous as possible, but there should be homogeneity between cluster means. Each cluster should be a small-scale representation of the total population. The clusters should be mutually exclusive and collectively exhaustive. A random sampling technique is then used on any relevant clusters to choose which clusters to include in the study. In single-stage cluster sampling, all the elements from each of the selected clusters are used. In two-stage cluster sampling, a random sampling technique is applied to the elements from each of the selected clusters.

The main difference between cluster sampling and stratified sampling is that in cluster sampling the cluster is treated as the sampling unit so analysis is done on a population of clusters (at least in the first stage). In stratified sampling, the analysis is done on elements within strata. In stratified sampling, a random sample is drawn from each of the strata, whereas in cluster sampling only the selected clusters are studied.

Advantages

- Cluster sampling technique is a cheaper sampling technique than other due to less travel expenses and administration costs.
- Compiling research information about every household in city would be a very difficult, whereas compiling information about various blocks of the city will be easier.
- Feasibility of sampling from a larger population is easy by this method. This method takes large populations into account. Where deploying other technique would be very difficult task.

Disadvantages

- **Reduced variability:** When estimates are being considered by any other method, reduced variability in results are observed. This may not be an ideal situation every time.
- **Higher sampling error:** Higher sampling error which can be expressed in the so-called 'design effect', the ratio between the number of subjects in the cluster study and the number of subjects in an equally reliable, randomly sampled unclustered study.

❖ **Biased samples:** If the group in population that is chosen as a sample has a biased opinion, then the entire population is inferred to have the same opinion. This may not be the actual case.

Multistage Sampling

Multistage sampling refers to sampling plans where the sampling is carried out in stages using smaller and smaller sampling units at each stage but only the last sample of subject is studied. Multistage sampling involves, combining various probability techniques in the most efficient and effective manner possible. The process of estimation is carried out stage by stage, using the most appropriate methods of estimation at each stage. In cluster sampling technique using all the sample elements in all the selected clusters may be prohibitively expensive or unnecessary. Under these circumstances, multistage cluster sampling becomes useful. Instead of using all the elements contained in the selected clusters, the researcher randomly selects elements from each cluster. Constructing the clusters is the first stage. Deciding what elements within the cluster to use is the second stage. The technique is used frequently when a complete list of all members of the population does not exist and is inappropriate. Multistage sampling represents a more complicated form of cluster sampling in which larger clusters are further subdivided into smaller, more targeted groupings for the purposes of surveying.

Example: For studying the Panchayat raj system in villages (Fig. 8.7)

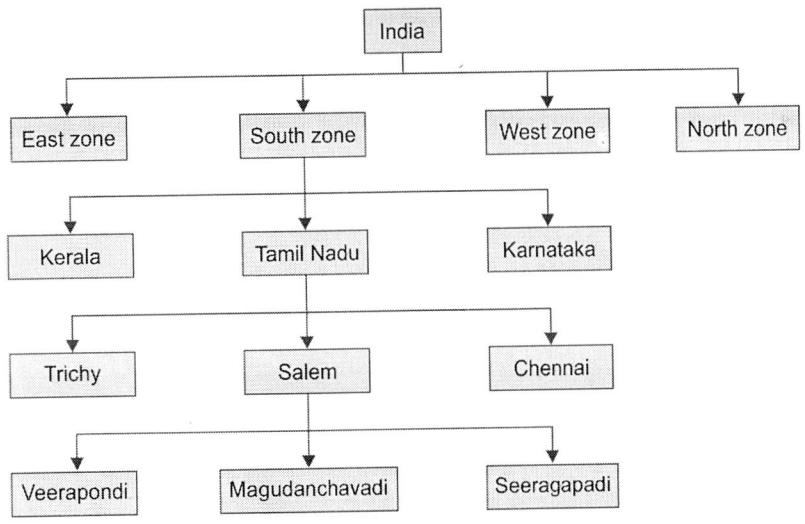

Fig. 8.7: Multistage sampling technique for studying the panchayat raj system.

Multiphase Sampling

This type is same as multistage sampling, however, each sample is adequately studied before another sample is drawn from it. A sampling procedure in which some information is collected from the whole sample and additional information is collected, at the same time or later, from subsamples of the entire. A multiphase sample collects basic information from a large sample of units and then, for a subsample of these units, collects more detailed information sample.

Multiphase sampling is useful when the frame lacks auxiliary information that could be used to stratify the population or to screen out part of the population. Multiphase sampling can be used when there is insufficient budget to collect information from the whole sample, or when doing so would create excessive burden on the respondent, or even when there are very different costs of collection for different questions on a survey. The sampling unit at each phase is the same, but some of them are interviewed in detail or asked more questions than others ask. In other words, all the members of the sample provide basic information and some of them provide more and detailed information, e.g.

- In TB survey MT in all cases: Phase I
- X-ray chest in MT +ve cases: Phase II
- Sputum examination in X-ray +ve cases: Phase III
- Survey by such procedure is less costly, less laborious and more purposeful.

Nonprobabilistic Sampling

Introduction

Nonprobability sampling is a sampling technique where the samples are gathered in a process that does not give all the individuals in the population equal chances of being selected because it does not involve random selection. Nonprobabilistic samples do not depend upon the rationale of probability theory. At least with a probabilistic sample, we know the odds or probability that we have represented the population well. We are able to estimate confidence intervals for the statistic. With nonprobabilistic samples, we may or may not represent the population well, and it will often be hard for us to know how well we have done so. In general, researchers prefer probabilistic or random sampling methods to nonprobabilistic ones, and consider them to be more accurate and rigorous. However, in applied social research there may be circumstances where it is not feasible, practical or theoretically sensible to do random sampling. Here, we consider a wide range of nonprobabilistic alternatives.

Use of Nonprobability Sampling

Nonprobability sampling can be used when:
- Demonstrating that a particular trait exists in the population.
- The researcher aims to do a qualitative, pilot or exploratory study.
- Randomization is impossible like when the population is almost limitless.
- The research does not aim to generate results that will be used to create generalizations pertaining to the entire population.
- The researcher has limited budget, time and workforce.
- An initial study which will be carried out again using a randomized, probability sampling.

Classification of Nonprobability Sampling

Nonprobability sampling technique can be classified in a varieties of sampling methods which are described as follows.

Judgmental Sampling or Purposive Sampling

Judgmental sampling is a nonprobability sampling technique where the researcher selects units to be sampled based on their knowledge and professional judgment. The researcher chooses the sample whom they think would be appropriate for the study. This is used primarily when there is a limited number of people that have expertise in the area being researched. This is used in cases where the speciality of an authority can select a more representative sample that can bring more accurate results than by using other probability sampling techniques. Judgmental sampling design is usually used when a limited number of individuals possess the trait of interest. It is the only viable sampling technique in obtaining information from a very specific group of people. It is also possible to use judgmental sampling if the researcher knows a reliable professional or authority that he thinks is capable of assembling a representative sampling and its design 19 sample. For example, the researcher conducted a study on effectiveness of diet therapy on treatment of severe acute malnutrition among under-five children. For conducting such type of study the researcher has move to an area or institution where he/she will get her sample. Here purposive sampling technique can be applied.

Advantages

- **Economical:** It is less costly and less time consuming.
- **Proper representation:** It ensures proper representation of the universe when the investigation has full knowledge of the composition of the universe and is free from bias.
- **Avoid irrelevant items:** It prevents unnecessary and irrelevant items entering into the sample per chance.
- **Intensive study:** It ensures intensive study of the selected items.
- **Accurate results:** It gives better results if the investigator is unbiased and has the capacity of keen observation and sound judgment.

Disadvantages

- **Personal bias:** There is enough scope for bias or prejudices of the investigator to play and influence the selection.
- **No equal chance:** There is no equal chance for all the items of the universe being included in the sample.
- **No degree of accuracy:** There is no possibility of having any idea about the degree of accuracy achieved in the investigation conducted by this method.
- **No possibility of sample error:** There is no possibility of calculating the sample error the idea of which is based on the mathematical concepts which are no applicable to nonrandom methods of sampling.
- **Unsuitable for large samples:** This method is not suitable for the large samples where the size of both the universe and the sample is considerably large.

Quota Sampling

A quota is established when a researchers are free to choose any respondent they wish as long as the quota is met.

Quota sampling is like stratified sampling in that stratification factors are identified which are thought to be relevant to the survey, but instead of sampling randomly the participants to come from each stratum, the survey samplers themselves choose the people subjectively from each stratum until sufficient people have been chosen and have responded. The main difficulty with this is the subjective choice of participants. Use of quota sampling also disguises nonresponse, as invited participants may decline to take part but the sampling will continue until the quotas are achieved.

For example, an interviewer may be told to sample 200 females and 300 males between the age of 45 and 60 years.

The interviewers might be tempted to interview those who look most helpful. The problem is that these samples may be biased because not everyone gets a chance of selection. This random element is its greatest weakness and quota versus probability has been a matter of controversy for many years.

Quota sampling is useful when time is limited, a sampling frame is not available, the research budget is very tight or when detailed accuracy is not important. Subsets are chosen and then either convenience or judgment sampling is used to choose people from each subset. The researcher decides how many of each category is selected.

Advantages

- Among all nonprobability sampling technique it is more representative of the population being studied. It is considered as nonprobability based equivalent of the stratified random sampling technique.
- Unlike probability sampling techniques, quota sampling is much quicker and easier to carry out because it does not require a sampling frame and the strict use of random sampling techniques.
- The quota sample improves the representation of particular strata (groups) within the population, as well as ensuring that these strata are not over-represented.
- The use of a quota sample, which leads to the stratification of a sample (e.g., male and female students), allows us to more easily compare these groups (strata).

Disadvantages

- In quota sampling, the sample has not been chosen using random selection, which makes it impossible to determine the possible sampling error.
- Indeed, it is possible that the selection of units to be included in the sample will be based on ease of access and cost considerations, resulting in sampling bias.
- It also means that it is not possible to make statistical inferences from the sample to the population. This can lead to problems of generalization.

Convenience Sampling

Convenience sampling is a type of nonprobability sampling which involves the sample being drawn from that part of the population which is close to hand. It is a statistical method of drawing representative data by selecting people because of the ease of their volunteering or selecting units because of their availability or easy access. It is also called accessibility sampling which involves asking a sample of people to respond to a survey. The researcher using such a sample cannot scientifically make generalizations about the total population from this sample because it would not be representative of the total population.

The advantages of this type of sampling are the availability and the quickness with which data can be gathered and which is very economic also. The disadvantages are the risk that the sample might not represent the population as a whole, and it might be biased by volunteers and there is chance of a number of biases.

Consecutive Sampling

Consecutive sampling is very similar to convenience sampling except that it seeks to include all accessible subjects as part of the sample. This nonprobability sampling technique can be considered as the best of all nonprobability samples because it includes all subjects that are available that makes the sample a better representation of the entire population.

Sequential Sampling

Here the sample size is not fixed. The investigator initially selects small sample and tries out to make inferences; if not able to draw results, he or she then adds more subjects until clear-cut inferences can be draw. For example, a researcher is studying association between smoking and lung cancer. Initially research takes a smallest sample and tries to draw inferences. If unable to draw any inferences he or she continues to draw the sample until meaningful inferences are drawn.

Snowball Sampling

Snowball sampling is usually done when there is a very small population size. In this type of sampling, the researcher asks the initial subject to identify another potential subject who also meets the criteria of the research. The downside of using a snowball sample is that it is hardly representative of the population. It is a nonprobability sampling technique where existing study subjects recruit future subjects from among their acquaintances. Thus the sample group appears to grow like a rolling snowball. This sampling technique is often used in hidden populations which are difficult for researchers to access; example populations would be drug users or sex workers. As sample members are not selected from a sampling frame, snowball samples are subject to numerous biases. Snowball sampling is a method used to obtain research and knowledge, from extended associations, through previous acquaintances. 'Snowball sampling uses recommendations to find people with the specific range of skills that has been determined as being useful.' An individual or a group receives information from different places through a mutual intermediary. This is referred to metaphorically as snowball sampling because as more relationships are built through mutual association, more connections can be made through those new relationships and a plethora of information can be shared and collected, much like a snowball that rolls and increases in size as it collects more snow. Snowball sampling is a useful tool for building networks and increasing the number of participants. However, the success of this technique depends greatly on the initial contacts and connections made. Thus it is important to correlate with those that are popular and honorable to create more opportunities to grow, but also to create a credible and dependable reputation.

Advantages

- **Locate hidden populations:** It is possible for the surveyors to include people in the survey that they would not have known.
- **Locating people of a specific population:** There are no lists or other obvious sources for locating members of the population (e.g., the homeless, users of illegal drugs).
- **Low cost:** As the subject is used to locate the hidden population, the researcher do not have invest money and time for the sampling process. Snowball sampling method does not require a complex planning and the staff used is considerably smaller in comparison to other sampling methods.

Disadvantages

- ❖ **Community bias:** The first participants will have strong impact on the sample. Snowball sampling is inexact, and can produce varied and inaccurate results. The method is heavily reliant on the skill of the individual conducting the actual sampling, and that individual's ability to vertically network and find an appropriate sample. To be successful requires previous contacts within the target areas, and the ability to keep the information flow going throughout the target group.
- ❖ **Not random:** Snowball sampling contradicts many of the assumptions supporting conventional notions of random selection and representativeness. However, social systems are beyond researcher's ability to recruit randomly. Snowball sampling is inevitable in social systems.
- ❖ **Vague overall sampling size:** There is no way to know the total size of the overall population.
- ❖ **Wrong anchoring:** Another disadvantage of snowball sampling is the lack of definite knowledge as to whether or not the sample is an accurate reading of the target population. By targeting only a few select people, it is not always indicative of the actual trends within the result group.
- ❖ **Lack of control over the sampling method:** As the subjects locate the hidden population, the research has very little control over the sampling method, which becomes mainly dependent on the original subject. This is because it is a chain sampling in which the original and subsequent subjects add the sampling pool using a method outside of the researcher's control.

SUMMARY

- ❖ A population is the entire aggregation of cases in which researcher is interested. It is a complete set of elements (persons or objects) that possess some common characteristics defined by the eligibility criteria established by the researcher.
- ❖ Before selection of population the researcher selects some predetermine criteria based on which the population will be selected. The exact criteria by which it could be decided whether an individual would or would not be classified as a member of the population is known as inclusion criteria.
- ❖ A sample is 'a smaller (but hopefully representative) collection of units from a population used to determine truths about that population'. A sample is simply a subset of the population. The concept of sample arises from the inability of the researchers to test all the individuals in a given population.
- ❖ Sampling is the process of selecting units from a population of interest so that by studying the sample we may fairly generalize our results back to the population from which they were chosen. It is a process of selecting subjects who are representative of population events, behaviors or other elements with which to conduct study.
- ❖ There are some principles of sampling technique which must be followed during selection of sample. Good sample should be complete, free from bias and errors, representative of the population and appropriate according to the study. There are also some basic steps followed during selection of sample.
- ❖ The purposes of sampling in research are economical, convenient to use, increase efficiency, greater accuracy and precision of data and better organization of research findings. There are various advantages and limitations of research.

- Sampling technique is the process of selection of sample for conducting a study. There are mainly two types of sampling technique like probability sampling technique and non-probability sampling technique.
- Probability sampling is based on the theory of probability. It is also known as random probability. The primary characteristics of probability sampling is the random selection of elements from the population.
- Probability sampling techniques are further classified in following subtypes, such as simple random sampling, systematic random sampling, stratified random sampling, cluster sampling, multistage sampling, multiphase sampling and sequential sampling.
- Nonprobability sampling is a sampling technique where the samples are gathered in a process that does not give all the individuals in the population equal chances of being selected because it does not involve random selection.

QUESTIONS TO TEST YOUR KNOWLEDGE

Q1. Enumerate the concept of sample and sampling. Describe the principles of sampling. Write the importance and limitations of sampling. (2 + 2 + 5 + 6)

Q2. What do you mean by population? Write the types of population. Explain the eligibility criteria of population during selection. (3 + 3 + 4)

Q3. Explain the sampling process in detail. Differentiate between sampling error and sampling bias. (10 + 5)

Q4. Write the classification of sampling technique. Explain probability sampling technique in detail. (3 + 12)

Q5. Multiple choice questions:

I. When each member of a population has an equally likely chance of being selected, this is called:
- a. A nonrandom sampling method
- b. A quota sample
- c. A snowball sample
- d. Probability sampling method

II. Which of the following techniques yields a simple random sample?
- a. Choosing volunteers from a gathering to participate
- b. Listing the individuals by ethnic group and choosing a proportion from within each ethnic group at random.
- c. Numbering all the elements of a sampling frame and then using a random number table to pick cases from the table.
- d. Randomly selecting schools, and then sampling everyone within the school.

III. The process of drawing a sample from a population is known as:
- a. Sampling
- b. Census
- c. randomizing
- d. None of the above

IV. The nonrandom sampling type that involves the researcher begins the research with the few respondents who are known and available to him, subsequently, there respondents give other names.
- a. Convenience sampling
- b. Quota sampling
- c. Purposive sampling
- d. Snowball sampling

V. Sampling which provides for a known non zero chance of selection is:
- a. Nonprobability sampling
- b. Multiple choice
- c. Analysis
- d. Random sampling

VI. A listing of all the elements of the population from which a sample is to be chosen is:
- a. Sampling frame
- b. Sampling table
- c. Population frame
- d. Data sheet

VII. A numerical characteristics of a sample is:
   a. Data sheet
   b. Statistics
   c. Coding
   d. Checklist

VIII. When a researcher accepts the null hypothesis that is false, he commits what type of error?
   a. Type I
   b. Type II
   c. Type III
   d. Type IV

IX. Determining every kth element for sample in a population for the research is called which type of sampling?
   a. Simple random sampling
   b. Stratified random sampling
   c. Systematic sampling
   d. Cluster sampling

X. Sequential sampling is a subtype of which of the following sampling technique:
   a. Nonprobability sampling
   b. Simple random sampling
   c. Stratified random sampling
   d. Probability sampling

ANSWERS				
I. d	II. c	III. a	IV. d	V. d
VI. a	VII. b	VIII. b	IX. c	X. a

Chapter 9

Methods of Data Collection

Learning Objectives

After completion of this chapter, the students will be able to:
- Explain the concept, types of research data and their sources.
- Enumerate data collection plan their benefits, instruction for developing data collection plan and the steps of development.
- Describe, interview, questionnaire, observation, biophysiological methods and projective techniques as the methods used for data collection.
- Explain how vignette method, visual analogue scale and Q-sorts methods can be used for data collection.
- Enumerate different types of tools like observation schedule, interview guide, interview schedule, mailed questionnaire, rating scale, checklist.
- Describe different levels of measurement and scaling technique.
- Explain how to check the reliability and validity of the tools.

INTRODUCTION

Data collection is an important aspect of any type of research study. Inaccurate data collection can impact the results of a study and ultimately lead to invalid results. Depending on the nature of the information to be gathered, different instruments are used to conduct the assessment: forms for gathering data from official sources, such as police or school records; surveys/interviews to gather information from youth, community residents, and others; and focus groups to elicit free-flowing perspectives the task of data collection begins. After the research problem has been identified and, research design/plan chalked out.

DATA

In general data is the information in raw or unorganized form (such as alphabet, number or symbols) that refers to or represent, ideas, and object. Data is limitless and present everywhere in the Universe. The piece of information obtained in the course of a study is called data.

The data of a research study are the pieces of information obtained in the course of the investigation. The term data refers to any kind of information researchers obtain on the subjects, respondents or participants of the study. In research, data are collected and used to answer the research questions or objectives of the study. Examples of data are demographic information, such as age, sex, household size, civil status or religion. Social and economic information, such as educational attainment, health status, extent of participants in social organizations, occupation, income, housing condition and the like. Scores in exams, grades, etc.

TYPES OF RESEARCH DATA

The research data are classified in two ways (Fig. 9.1); based on the study findings and based on the source. Based on the study finding it is classified as quantitative or qualitative. Based on their source, data fall under two categories namely: Primary data and secondary data.

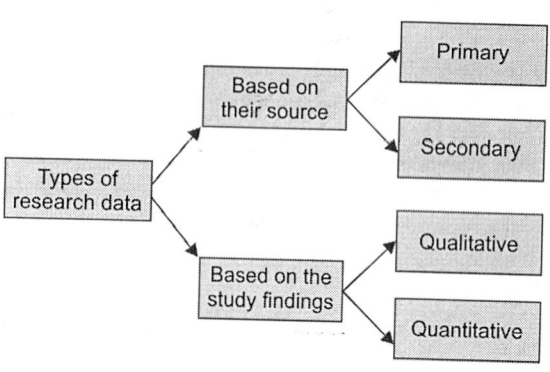

Fig. 9.1: Types of research data.

Qualitative and Quantitative Data

Qualitative Data

A study may be intended to generate precise quantitative findings or to produce qualitative descriptive information or both. Data that approximates or characterizes but does not measure the attributes, characteristics, properties, etc., of a thing or phenomenon is generally termed as qualitative data. Qualitative data describes whereas quantitative data defines. Qualitative data is a categorical measurement expressed not in terms of numbers, but rather by means of a natural language description. In statistics, it is often used interchangeably with 'categorical' data. Although we may have categories, the categories may have a structure to them. When there is not a natural ordering of the categories, we call these nominal categories, e.g., might be gender, race, religion, or sport.

When the categories may be ordered, these are called ordinal variables. Categorical variables that judge size (small, medium, large, etc.) are ordinal variables. Attitudes (strongly disagree, neutral, agree, strongly agree) are also ordinal variables, however we may not know which value is the best or worst of these issues. Note that the distance between these categories is not something we can measure.

Quantitative Data

Quantitative data are the informations which can be counted or expressed in numerical values. Data that can be quantified and verified, and is amenable to statistical manipulation is termed as quantitative data, e.g., age, grades, income, test score, number of children, level of satisfaction, amount of sales, length of service, etc. Quantitative data is a numerical measurement expressed not by means of a natural language description, but rather in terms of numbers quantitative data always are associated with a scale measure. Probably the most common scale type is the ratio-scale. Observations of this type are on a scale that has a meaningful zero value, but also have an equidistant measure (i.e., the difference between 10 and 20 is the same as the difference between 100 and 110). Some examples of quantitative data are height, weight, your shoe size and the length of your fingernails.

According to the data source there are two types of data.
1. **Primary data:** Data observed or collected directly from first-hand experience are called primary data. Primary data are collected from the research units, which may be individuals, objects, programs or institutions which provide the first-hand information. It is collected by the researcher directly from the respondents or situations. The source of your primary data is the population sample from which you collect the data.
2. **Secondary data:** Secondary data is the data that have been already collected by someone else and have been passed through the statistical process and readily available from other sources.

Such data are cheaper and more quickly obtainable than the primary data and also may be available when primary data cannot be obtained at all. Data can be collected either from internal or external secondary sources **(Table 9.1)**.

Table 9.1: Sources of data.

Primary sources	Internal sources (private documents)	Secondary sources	
		External sources (public documents)	
		Published records	Unpublished records
People, objects, programs, institutions, etc. (collected through interviews, questioning, observation, biochemical measurements and psychosocial measurement)	• Biographies • Diaries • Letters	• Journals and magazines • Newspapers • Government reports • Statistical abstracts • Census reports • Mass communication • Commission reports	• Unpublished thesis/dissertation • Official or patient records

DATA COLLECTION PLAN

Data collection is nothing more than planning for obtaining successful information for key quality characteristics. Data collection plan is mandatory to collect data in uniform and consistent pattern. The elements of data collection plan should be clear, unambiguous and operationally defined to get useful data.

Benefits of Data Collection Planning

- Well-developed data collection plan helps to gather accurate and bias-free information.
- It prevents errors and involvement of external variables in the data collection plan.
- It saves time and money.
- It gives direction for data collection.

Instruction for Developing Data Collection Plan

A formal data collection plan needs a lot of efforts, expert advice, guidance and experiences. The researcher should follow certain instruction while developing data collection plan.

- Data collection plan should be easy to follow for investigator as well as participant.
- Seek usefulness. Data which are useful for study should be collected rather than waiting for perfect data.
- Data collection process should be pretested with small size of similar sample.
- Cost of data collection should be less.
- Appropriate training should be given to the researcher.
- Instruction for data collection should be clear and unambiguous.
- Be objective while collecting data to avoid bias and errors.
- Data recording process should be easy to follow for data recorder.
- Record the data simultaneously to avoid any data loss.

Existing Data versus New Data

* One of the first decision that a researcher makes in regards to research data concern weather to use existing data or to collect new data.
* Existing records represent a very important source of data for nurse researchers. Researcher can use existing data available to them for exploration. The existing records may be hospital records, patient charts, physician order sheets, care plan statements, etc.

Historical researches also typically relay on available data, data for historical research are in the form of written records of—diaries, letters, newspapers, medical documents, reports, periodicals, etc.

DIMENSIONS OF DATA COLLECTION APPROACHES

If existing data are not available or not suitable for the research, the researcher must collect new data. Many methods of collecting new data are used for studies. Data collection methods have four important dimensions **(Fig. 9.2)**:
1. Structure
2. Quantifiability
3. Researcher obstructiveness
4. Objectivity

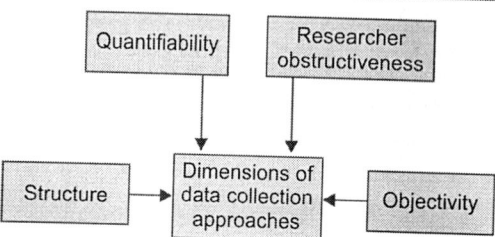

Fig. 9.2: Dimensions of data collection approaches.

Structure

Research data particularly in quantitative studies are often collected according to a structured plan that indicates what information is to be gathered and how to gather, e.g., most administered questionnaires are highly structured: they include a fixed set of questions that are generally answered in a specified sequences. In such structured methods, there is a little opportunity for participants to qualify their answer or to explain the underlying meaning of their response.

The structure methods are not suitable for in depth examination of a phenomenon. Structure methods often take considerable effort to develop and refine, but they yield data that are easy to analyze.

Quantifiability

Data that will subjected to statistical analysis must be gathered in such a way that they can be quantified. For statistical analysis, all variables must be quantitatively measured. Data that are to be analyzed quantitatively are typically collected in a close ended questionnaires. Structured data collection approaches generally yield data that are easily quantified.

Researcher Obstructiveness

Data collection methods differ in terms of the degree to which people are aware of their status as study participants. If study participants are fully aware of their role in a study, their behavior and responses may not be normal. When participants distort data, the entire value of research can be undermined. Study participants are most likely to distort their behavior and their responses to questions under certain circumstances.

Objectivity

It refers to the degree to which two independent researchers can arrive at similar 'scores' or make similar observations regarding the concepts of interest, i.e., make judgments regarding participants attributes or behavior that are not biased by personal feelings or beliefs. Some data collection approaches require more subjective judgment than others and some research problems require higher degree of objectivity than others.

DEVELOPING DATA COLLECTION PLAN

The decision that a researcher makes about the design of study are totally independent of his decision about which the data collection methods to use. The data collection plan should be accurate, trustworthy and meaningful data that are maximally effective in answering research questions. The data collection plan should contained the answers of the 6'W's of data collection.

6 'W's of Data Collection (Fig. 9.3)

1. WHAT data to be collected?
2. From WHOM data is to be collected?
3. WHO will collect data?
4. WHERE data will be collected?
5. WHEN the data will be collected?
6. HOW data will be collected?

WHAT Data will be Collected?

In this step decision is made about the type of data to be collected means what information will be obtained from the participants and what type of data, number of variables need for data, etc. For example, when physical growth of infant is the phenomenon under study, the data to measure about physical growth would be the body weight, height, chest and head circumferences.

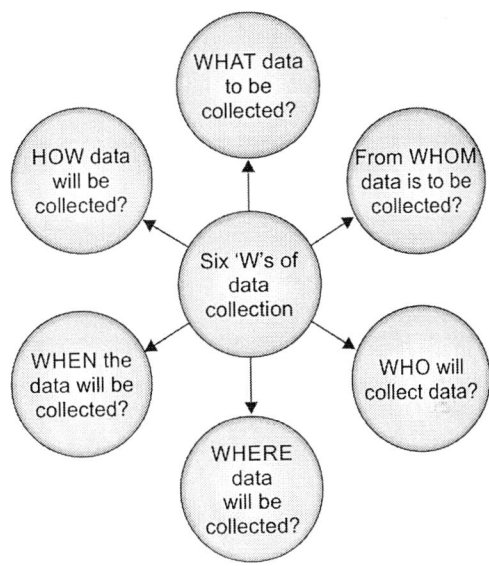

Fig. 9.3: Six 'W's of data collection.

From WHOM Data is to be Collected?

Information collected from different research studies generally depends upon various sources like primary source and secondary source. Primary data are directly collected from the research units, data provided by individuals, objects, programs or institutions. It is the first-hand information is collected by researcher directly from the respondents or the situations that is self-reports which is strong but secondary data are collected from either internal or external secondary sources which includes published or unpublished records. Published records include journal, magazines, newspapers, government reports, statistical abstracts, census, reports.

Unpublished records include official records, patient records, unpublished thesis, etc. Internal secondary sources also known as private documents may include the biographies, personal diaries, letters, memories, etc.

WHO will Collect Data?

Sometimes scientific investigation involve team of researchers for data collection. It concern with investigator who is going to collect data. If the researcher is going to collect the data it is easy. If more persons are, assumption must be made that the data are being collected in same manner training is needed for data collectors.

Selecting Research Personnel

Some consideration should be kept in mind when selecting research personnel are as follows:
- **Experiences:** Research staff should have prior experience with data collection.
- **Congruity with sample characteristics:** To the extent possible, data collectors should match the background of the study participants (especially in qualitative studies) with respect to such characteristics as racial or cultural background and gender.
- Unremarkable appearance should generally be avoided because participants may react to extremes and may alter their behavior or responses accordingly.
- **Personality:** It should be pleasant, sociable and nonjudgmental.
- **Availability to the participants:** Ideally the resource person will be available to the participant for the entire data collection period to avoid recruit and train new staffs.

Training Data Collectors

Depending on the prior experience of the research personnel, training will need to cover both general procedures of data collection and procedures specific to the study. All the personnel selected for data collection should have a manual which they can refer in between the data collection. The training manual should contain the detailed instructions relating to the administration of the specific data collection instruments.

WHERE Data will be Collected?

Determination of data collection setting is very important. Data setting should be explained to the person who is collecting data properly to avoid any confusion. A conducive comfortable environment may be provided to the participants. If the environment of the subjects is not comfortable then the answers that are provided may not be valid. If the environment of the subjects is not comfortable then the answers that are provided may not be valid. If questionnaires are being used for data collection, researcher might ask respondents to complete the questionnaire in same area.

If subjects are tired or temperature of room is not adequate then data collected may be improper.

WHEN will the data be Collected?

The determination of time is made about the month, date, time, etc., for how long data collection will take. The period for data collection may be varies from few days to years. So before data collection the length of data collection period and date will be determined.

HOW data will be Collected?

The data will be collected for the research by following some method and using some instruments which will be developed and validated before. The researchers or the persons who are ready to collect data should be ready with the tools and instruments and properly trained regarding data collection procedure.

STEPS OF DEVELOPING DATA COLLECTION PLAN (FIG. 9.4)

Identifying Data Needs

The researcher should begin by identifying types of data are needed to complete the study successfully. The researcher should give a thoughtful consideration to what data needs for accomplishing the following:

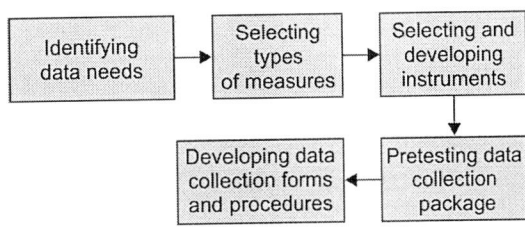

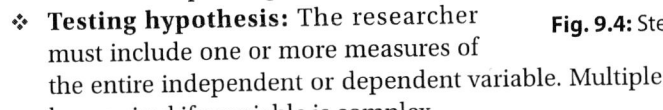

Fig. 9.4: Steps of developing data collection.

- **Testing hypothesis:** The researcher must include one or more measures of the entire independent or dependent variable. Multiple measures of some variables may be required if a variable is complex.
- **Describing the main characteristics of the sample:** The information should normally be gathered about major demographic characteristics of the sample and about relevant aspects of participant's health status. It is almost always advisable to gather information about the participant's age, gender, race, marital status, income, type of occupation, etc. if the sample includes health problems, data on the nature of that problem should also be gathered.
- **Controlling for important source of extraneous variables:** Thought should be given to gather the data on both external and intrinsic factors that should influence the outcome.
- **Analyzing potential bias:** The data that can help the researcher to identify potential biases should be collected. The researcher should know what potential source of bias might arise and then determine whether they can be measured.
- **Understanding subgroup effects:** It requires to answer the research questions not only for the entire sample but also for entire subgroup of participants.
- **Interpreting the results:** The researcher should try to anticipate alternative patterns of results and then determine what types of data would best help in interpreting those results.
- **Checking on the manipulation:** When a researcher manipulates the independent variable, if requires gathering information to determine if manipulation was actually achieved. Such a manipulation check provides a mechanism for interpreting negative results.
- **Obtaining administrative information:** It is necessary to gather various types of administrative information to help in management of the project. This includes participants identification numbers, date of attempted contacts, date of actual data collection, where and when the data is collected.

Selecting Types of Measures

After data needs have been identified, the next step is to select a method to gather information on each concept. Data collection is typically most time consuming process of a study. Because of this the researcher is likely to have to make a number of compromises about type and amount of data collection.

Selecting and Developing Instruments

Once the decisions have been made regarding the basic of data collection methods to be use, the researcher should select the instruments which are appropriate for data collection.

After potential data collection instruments have been identified, they should be carefully reviewed to determine their appropriateness for study.

The next factor is to consider is whether the instruments are likely to yield data of a sufficient high quality. There are six other criteria that often affect the researcher's decision in selecting the instruments are:

1. **Resources:** It constraints sometimes make it impossible to use the highest quality measures. There may be some direct cost associated with measure, but the biggest data collection cost often involve compensation to the people who are collecting data if you cannot do it single handled. In such situation, the length of instrument and time it takes to administer whether it can be used.
2. **Availability and familiarity:** In selecting measures, you may need to consider how readily available various tools are. Similarly, data collection strategy with which researcher is familiar are generally preferable to new measures.
3. **Norms and comparability:** Norms indicate normal values and distribution of values on the measure with respect to a specified population. It is advantageous to adopt a specific instrument because it was used in other similar studies and therefore offers a supplementary basis for putting the study findings in context.
4. **Population appropriateness:** The measure should be chosen with the characteristics of target population in mind. Characteristics of special important include age of participants, their intellectual ability, their culture, ethnic background, etc.
5. **Administration issue:** It is an important consideration often relates to the instrument's requirement for obtaining high quality data. Another administration issues concerns constraints on where the data must be collected.
6. **Reputation:** Instruments designs to measure the same construct often differ in the kinds of reputation they enjoy among specialists working in a field, even if they are comparable with regards to quality. Therefore, it may be useful to seek the advice of knowledgeable individuals, preferably people with personal direct experiences in using the instruments.

Based on such considerations one can conclude that existing instruments are not suitable for all research variables. In such situation one researcher will be faced with either adapting an existing instruments or developing a new one.

Pretesting Data Collection Package

Researchers who develop their own instrument typically subject it to rigorous pretesting so that it can be evaluated and refined. The researcher has to test the validity and reliability of the tools by consultation with experts and administration of same tool to different population in small scale and also for determining smoothness and effectiveness of data collection package and identifying any parts of data collection package that the participants find objectionable or offensive. After determining the validity or reliability of the tool if satisfactory result has not achieved it may be necessary to modify the instruments.

Developing Data Collection Forms and Procedures

After the instrument package has been finalize the final data collection plan with modification of tool has developed. The researcher should make a list of all things that will be needed during data collection. The plan must contain followings:

❖ Conditions that must be met for collecting data.
❖ Specific procedures for collecting the data.

- Standard information to provide participants who ask routine questions about the study.
- Procedures to follow in the event that a participant becomes distraught, disoriented or for any other reason cannot complete data collection.
- Finally procedures and forms may need to be developed for managing data as they are gathered from multiple sites or over an extended period.

METHODS AND TOOLS OF DATA COLLECTION

Data collection means gathering information to address those critical evaluation questions that a researcher has identified earlier in the evaluation process. The process by which the researcher collects the information needed to answer the research problem is data collection. In collecting the data, the researcher must decide which data to collect, when to collect the data, who will collect the data, how to collect the data.

There are various methods of data collection. The methods and tools are selected based on some study characteristics.

Selection of methods of data collection:
- The nature of phenomenon under study
- Type of research subjects
- The type of research study
- The purpose of research study
- Size of the study sample
- Distribution of the target population
- Time frame of the study
- Literacy level of the subjects
- Availability of resources and manpower
- Researcher's knowledge level and competence.

The different methods of data collection are described below.

INTERVIEW

Interviews are an attractive proposition for the project researcher. Interviews are something more than conversation. They involve a set of assumptions and understandings about the situation which are not normally associated with a casual conversation. Interviews are also referred as an oral questionnaire by some people, but it is indeed much more than that. Questionnaire involves indirect data collection, whereas interview data is collected directly from others in face-to-face contact research interview should be systematically arranged. It does not happen by chance. The interviews not done by secret recording of discussions as research data. The consent of the subject is taken for the purpose of interview. The words of the interviews can be treated as 'on the record' and 'for the record'. It should not be used for other purposes besides the research purpose.

The discussion therefore is not arbitrary or at the whim of one of the parties. The agenda for the discussion is set by the researcher. It is dedicated to investigating a given topic.

Definitions

- It is a method of data collection in which a person (interviewer) asks the question from another person (respondent); which is conducted either face-to-face or telephonically.

- An interview is a conversation between two or more people (interviewer and interviewee) where questions are asked by interviewer to obtain information from the interviewer.
- It may be defined as a two-way systematic conversation between an investigator and an informant, initiated for obtaining information relevant to a specific study. It involves not only conversations, but also learning from the respondent's gestures, facial expressions and pauses, his or her environment.

Characteristics of Interview

- The participants, the interviewer, and the respondent are strangers.
- The relationship between the participants is a transitory one.
- It is a mode of obtaining verbal answers to questions put verbally.
- The investigator records information furnished by the respondent in the interview.
- Interview is not a mere casual conversational exchange but a conversation with a specific purpose.
- The interview is not need be face-to-face, it can be conducted over telephone also.
- Although interview is usually a conversation between two person, it is not always limited to a single respondent.
- It is an interaction process between the interviewer and respondent.
- It is not a standardized process; it can be modified according to situation.

Benefits of Interview

- **Provide in-depth and detailed information:** When used in well-conceived schedule, interview can often a great deal of information (in detail). They allow more detailed questions to be asked.
- **Permits greater depth of response:** The interview permits greater depth of response, which is not possible through any other means. It also enables an interviewer to get information concerning feelings and attitude related to the phenomenon under research and also achieve a high response rate.
- **Data from different subjects:** Interview is advantageous for illiterate subjects who do not write as fluently as they speak. It is also appropriate when dealing with young children, language difficulty and limited, intelligence, who are unable to write their responses, like patients with eye patches or in tractions, etc., interview is very advantageous for them.
- **High response:** Interview method results in better, more elaborate response of questionnaires, people who would normally ignore questionnaire are willing to talk with the interviewer, which elicit interesting information, e.g., hospitalized patients.
- **Clarify misunderstandings:** When conducting an interview, a researcher can be sensitive to the subject's misunderstandings to the questions, and provide further clarification on the topic under discussion.
- **Ask questions at several levels:** A researcher can plan to ask questions at several levels and gather maximum information from the subjects.
- **Helps to gather other supplementary information:** The interview can gather other supplementary information, such as the economic level, living condition, etc.
- **Use of special devices:** The interviewer can use special scoring devices, visual material, etc., in order to improve the quality of interviewing.
- **Accuracy can be checked:** The accuracy and dependability of the answers given by the respondent can be checked by observation. Ambiguities can be clarified and incomplete answers followed up.

- **Flexible and adaptable:** Interviews are flexible and adaptable to individual situations. The requisite amount of control can be exercised over the interview situation.
- Respondents' own words are recorded. So it cannot be misinterpreted.
- Precise wording can be tailored to respondent and precise meaning of questions clarified.
- Interviewees are not influenced by others in the group.
- It can be combined with other tools in order to corroborate facts using a different approach.

Limitations of Interviews

The main limitations of interviews are:
- **They can be very time-consuming:** Setting up, interviewing, transcribing, analyzing, feedback, reporting.
- They can be costly.
  Different interviewers may understand and transcribe interviews in different ways.

Types of Interview

Interviews vary in purpose, nature and scope. They may be conducted for guidance, therapeutic or research purposes. They may be confined to one individual or extended to several people. Based on the construction of the tool it is of three types **(Fig. 9.5)**:
1. Structured interview
2. Unstructured interview
3. Semistructured interview

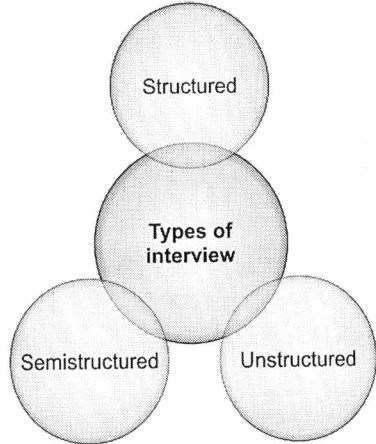

Fig. 9.5: Types of interview.

Structured Interview

Structured interview involves fight control over the format of questions and answers. It is like a questionnaire which is administered face-to-face with a respondent. The researcher has a predetermined list of questions. Each respondent is faced with identical questions. The choice of alternative answers is restricted to a predetermined list. This type of interview is rigidly standardized and formal. It is a means of data collection in which the interviewer has an interview schedule in which the questions are listed in the order in which they are to be answered. The aim of this approach is to ensure that each interview is presented with exactly the same questions in the same order. This ensures that answers can be reliably aggregated and that comparisons can be made with confidence between sample subgroups or between different survey periods. Structured interviews are a means of collecting data for a statistical survey. In this case, the data is collected by an interviewer rather than through a self-administered questionnaire. Interviewers read the questions exactly as they appear on the survey questionnaire. The choice of answers to the questions is often fixed (close-ended) in advance, these interviews are also known as standardized interviews. Structured interview consists of following characteristics:
- Interview schedule is formalized and has limited set of questions.
- The aim is to answer that each interview is presented with exactly the same questions in the same order.
- It increases the reliability and credibility of research data.
- It minimizes context effects, wherein answers given to survey questions depend on the nature of preceding questions.

Merits

Structured interviews are easy to replicate as a fixed set of closed questions are used, which are easy to quantify—this means it is easy to test for reliability. Data from one interview to the next one are easily comparable.

Structured interviews are fairly quick to conduct which means that many interviews can take place within a short amount of time. This means a large sample can be obtained resulting in the findings being representative and having the ability to be generalized to a large population. Recording and coding data does not pose any problem. Attention is not diverted to irrelevant and time consuming conversation.

Demerits

- Structure interviews are not flexible. This means new questions cannot be asked impromptu (i.e., during the interview) as an interview schedule must be followed. It tends to lose the spontaneity of natural conversation.
- The answers from structured interviews lack detail as only closed questions are asked which generates quantitative data. This means a researcher may not know why a person behaves in a certain way.
- The way in which the interview is structured may be such that the respondent's views are minimized and investigator's own biases regarding the problems under study are assessed.
- The scope of exploration of information of data is limited.

Unstructured Interview (Nondirective Interview)

The unstructured interviews are sometimes referred to as 'discovery interviews' and are more like a 'guided conversation' than a strict structured interview. They are sometimes called informal interviews. An interview schedule might not be used, and even if one is used, they will contain open-ended questions that can be asked in any order. The questions can be changed to meet the respondent's intelligence, understandings and beliefs. Hence, the interviewer encourages the respondents to talk freely about given topic with minimum prompting. In this, no preplanned schedule is used. These interviews are also known as nonstandardized interviews. Unstructured interview consists of the following characteristics:

- Interview schedule is not formalized and has open-ended questions, where there is opportunity to ask questions which are not planned before.
- The aim is to explore the information from the respondents.
- It increases the reliability and credibility of research data.
- It facilitates the natural unobstructed proceedings of the interview procedure.

Merits

- It is less prone to interviewer's bias.
- It provides greater opportunity to explore the problem in an unrestricted manner.
- It is useful for gathering information on sensitive topics, such as divorce, social discrimination, drug addiction, etc. Unstructured interviews are more flexible as questions can be adapted and changed depending on the respondents' answers. The interview can deviate from the interview schedule.
- Unstructured interviews generate qualitative data through the use of open questions. This allows the respondent to talk in some depth, choosing their own words. This helps the researcher develop a real sense of a person's understanding of a situation.

- They also have increased validity because it gives the interviewer the opportunity to probe for a deeper understanding, ask for clarification and allow the interviewee to steer the direction of the interview, etc.

Limitations

- It can be time consuming to conduct an unstructured interview and analyze the qualitative data (using methods such as thematic analysis).
- Employing and training interviewers is expensive, and not as cheap as collecting data via questionnaires. For example, certain skills may be needed by the interviewer. These include the ability to establish rapport and knowing when to probe.

Semistructured Interview

In semistructured interview, the interviewer also has a clear list of issues to be addressed and questions to be answered. There is some flexibility in the order of the topics. In this type of interviewee is given chance to develop his ideas and speak more widely on the issues raised by the researcher. The answers are open-ended and more emphasis is on the interviewee elaborating points of interest. It is a flexible method that allows new questions to be brought up during the interview, depending upon the situation during the interview. Semistructured interviews have the following characteristics:

- Interviewer prepares an interview guide, which is an informal list of topics and questions that the interviewer can ask in different ways from different participants.
- Interview guide helps the researcher to focus on the topics at hand without constraining them to a particular format.
- Explain the purpose of the interview.
- Address terms of confidentiality.
- Explain the format of the interview.
- Indicate how long the interview usually takes.
- Ask them if they have any questions.

Other Types of Interview

- Personal interview
- Telephone interview
- Depth interview
- Focus group interview
- Projective techniques

Personal Interview

It is a face-to-face way communication between the interviewer and the respondents. It is carried out in a planned manner and is referred to as 'structured interview'.

Telephone Interview

Here the information is collected from the respondent by asking him questions on telephone. The combination of telephone and computer has made this method even more popular.

Focus Group Interview

A focus group can be defined as a group of interacting individuals having some common interest or characteristics, brought together by a moderator, who uses the group and its interaction as a way to gain information about a specific or focused issue.

A focus group is typically consists of 7–10 people who are unfamiliar with each other. These participants are selected because they have certain characteristics in common that relate to the topic of the focused group. The moderator or interviewer creates a permissive and nurturing environment that encourages different perceptions and the points of view, without pressuring participants to vote, plan or reach consensus.

The group discussion is conducted several times with similar types of participants to identify trends and patterns in perceptions. Careful and systematic analysis of the discussion provide clues and insights as to how a product, service, or opportunity is perceived by the group.

Strengths

- It enables the researcher to examine the level of understanding a respondent has about a particular topic—usually in more depth than with a postal questionnaire.
- It can be used as a powerful form of formative assessment. That is, it can be used to explore how a respondent feels about a particular topic, before using a second method (such as observation or in-depth interviewing) to gather a greater depth of information. Structured interviews can also be used to identify respondents whose views you may want to explore in more detail (through the use of focused interviews, for example).
- All respondents are asked the same questions in the same way. This makes it easy to repeat ('replicate') the interview. In other words, this type of research method is easy to standardize.
- Provides a reliable source of quantitative data.
- The researcher is able to contact large numbers of people quickly, easily and efficiently.
- It is relatively quick and easy to create, code and interpret (especially if closed questions are used).
- There is a formal relationship between the researcher and the respondent with the latter knowing exactly what is required from them in the interview, e.g., a respondent is unable or unwilling to answer a question the researcher (because they are present at the interview) is aware of the reasons for a failure to answer all questions.
- The researcher does not have to worry about response rates, biased (self-selected) samples, incomplete questionnaires and the like.
- Group interviews generate qualitative data through the use of open questions. This allows the respondents to talk in some depth, choosing their own words. This helps the researcher develop a real sense of a person's understanding of a situation.
- They also have increased validity because some participants may feel more comfortable being with others as they are used to talking in groups in real life (i.e., it is more natural).

Limitations

- It can be time consuming if sample group is very large (this is because the researcher or their representative needs to be present during the delivery of the structured interview).
- The quality and usefulness of the information is highly dependent upon the quality of the questions asked. The interviewer cannot add or subtract questions.
- A substantial amount of preplanning is required.

- The format of questionnaire design makes it difficult for the researcher to examine complex issues and opinions. Even where open-ended questions are used, the depth of answers the respondent can provide tend to be more-limited than with almost any other method.
- There is limited scope for the respondent to answer questions in any detail or depth.
- There is the possibility that the presence of the researcher may influence the way a respondent answers various questions, thereby biasing the responses. For example, an aggressive interviewer may intimidate a respondent into giving answers that do not really reflect the respondent's beliefs. Similarly, a young male researcher asking a middle-aged woman how frequently she had sexual intercourse in the past month may be embarrassing for the respondent and make her unlikely to answer truthfully. This is known as the interview effect.
- A problem common to both postal questionnaires and structured interviews is the fact that by designing a 'list of questions', a researcher has effectively decided-in advance of collecting any data-the things they consider to be important and unimportant.
- The researcher must ensure that they keep all the interviewees details confidential and respect their privacy. This is difficult when using a group interview. For example, the researcher cannot guarantee that the other people in the group will keep information private.
- Group interviews are less reliable as they use open questions and may deviate from the interview schedule making them difficult to repeat.
- Group interviews may sometimes lack validity as participants may lie to impress the other group members. They may conform to peer pressure and give false answers.

Demerits

- The data obtained from one interview is not comparable to the data from the next.
- Time may be wasted in unproductive conversation.
- There is no order or sequence in this interview.
- This requires more skills on the part of the research.

Depth Interview

Depth interview is nondirective in nature where the respondent is given freedom to answer within the boundaries of the topic of the interview. An in-depth interview is a conversation with an individual conducted by trained staff that usually collects specific information about the person.

Characteristics of Depth Interview

- **It is a qualitative method:** In-depth interviews are most appropriate for situations in which one wants to ask open-ended questions that elicit depth of information from relatively few people.
    This allows the interviewer to deeply explore the respondent's feelings and perspectives on a subject. This results in rich background information that can shape further questions relevant to the topic.
- **Open-ended questions:** Questions beginning with 'why' or 'how', which gives freedom to answer the questions using their own word.
- **Semistructured format:** For example, the elections are approaching, an appropriate response would be, 'how do you feel about the candidates involved?'

- **Seek understanding and interpretation:** Active listening skills to reflect upon what the speaker is saying. The interviewer should try to interpret what is being said and should seek clarity and understanding throughout the interview.
- **Recording responses:** The responses are typically audio-recorded and complemented with written notes (i.e., field notes) by the interviewer. Written notes include observations of both verbal and nonverbal behaviors as they occur, and immediate personal reflections about the interview.

Projective Techniques Interviews

In projective techniques, the respondents are assessed to interpret the behavior of others and this way they indirectly reveal own behavior in the same situation.

A projective test is a personality test designed to let a person respond to ambiguous stimuli, presumably revealing hidden emotions and internal conflicts projected by the person into the test. This is sometimes contrasted with a so-called 'objective test' or 'self-report test' in which responses are analyzed according to presumed universal standard (for example, a multiple choice exam), and are limited to the content of the test. The responses to projective tests are content analyzed for meaning rather than being based on presuppositions about meaning, as is the case with objective tests.

Steps of Conducting an Interview

Generally an interview should go through the following five stages, which are as follows:

Rapport Building

Building and maintaining rapport are essential in conducting any type of interview. Without good rapport there is a lack of credibility and trust and without trust and credibility, true communication is impossible. An interviewer who does not have a firm grasp of these concepts will not obtain any truly relevant information. Interviewer should increase the receptiveness of the responders by making him believe that his opinion are very useful for research, and is going to be pleased than an ordeal.

Introduction

An introduction involves the interviewer identifying himself by giving him his name, purpose and sponsorship if any.

Probing

Probing is the technique of encouraging the respondents to answer completely, freely and relevantly.

Recording

The interviewer can either write the interview or after the interview. In certain cases, where the respondent allows for it, audio or visual aids can be used to record answers.
- It is essential to record responses as they take place.
- Good information can be taken by note taking.
- A tape recorder should be used to record the responses of respondent.
- Shorthand should be used to record responses.

Closing

After the interview, interviewer should thank the respondent and once again assure him about the worth of his answers and the confidentiality of the same.

After the interview is over, a polite leave of the respondent should be taken, thanking him or her with a friendly smile and saying 'goodbye'.

Carrying the Interview Forward

Interviewing is an art governed by certain scientific principles. Effort should be made to create friendly atmosphere of trust and confidence, so that respondents may feel at ease while talking to and discussing with the interviewer. The interviewer must ask questions properly and intelligently and must record the responses accurately and completely. The interviewers approach must be friendly, courteous, conversational and unbiased. The following points should be remembered during interview process.

After establishing rapport, following guidelines should be used:
- Start the interview.
- Ask only one question at a time.
- Repeat a question if necessary.
- Try to make sure that subject understands the questions.
- Listen carefully to the subject's answers.
- Observe the subject's facial expressions, gestures and tone of voice.
- Allow the subject sufficient time to answer the questions.
- Do not signs of surprise, shock or anger.
- Maintain a neutral attitude with respect to controversial issues during the interview.
- Take note of answers that seem to be vague or ambiguous.
- Ask additional questions to follow up clues or to obtain additional information.
- Do not hurry the interview. If silence is too prolonged, introduce a stimulus.

Advantages of Interview

- Useful to obtain information about people's feelings, perceptions and opinions.
- Allow more detailed questions to be answered.
- High response rate is achieved.
- Respondent's own words are recorded.
- Ambiguities can be clarified and incomplete answers are followed up.
- Interviews are not influenced by others in the group.
- Meaning of questions can be clarified.

Disadvantages of Interview

- There is greater flexibility under this method as the opportunity to restructure questions is always there, especially in case of unstructured interviews.
- Observation method can as well be applied to recording verbal answers to various questions.
- Personal information can as well be obtained easily under this method.
- Samples can be controlled more effectively as there arises no difficulty of the missing returns; nonresponse generally remains very low.
- Interviews are time consuming and costly affairs.
- Different interviewers may understand and translate interviews in different ways.

- There are high degree chances of interview's bias.
- Cultural assets may influence people's willingness to participate in an interview.

QUESTIONNAIRE

A questionnaire is a structured instrument consisting of a series of questions prepared by researcher that a research subject is asked to complete, to gather data from individuals about knowledge, attitude, beliefs and feelings.

A set of questions designed to generate the statistical information from a specific demographic needed to accomplish the research objectives is called as a questionnaire.

The instrument is called a questionnaire or sometimes a self-administered questionnaire (SAQ), when respondents complete the instrument themselves, usually in a paper and pencil format but occasionally directly onto a computer.

Characteristics of Good Research Questions (Fig. 9.6)

- **The question should be feasible:** It can be investigated without an undue amount of time, energy, or money.
- **The question should be clear:** Most people would agree as to what the key words in the question mean.
- **The question is significant:** The question should be worth investigating in terms of time needed, energy required, effect on or for subjects.
- **The question is ethical:** It will not involve physical or psychological harm or damage to human beings, or to the natural or social environment of which they are apart.
- **It should create interest:** Questionnaire should create interest among respondents simple, direct, conversational language should be used in questions.

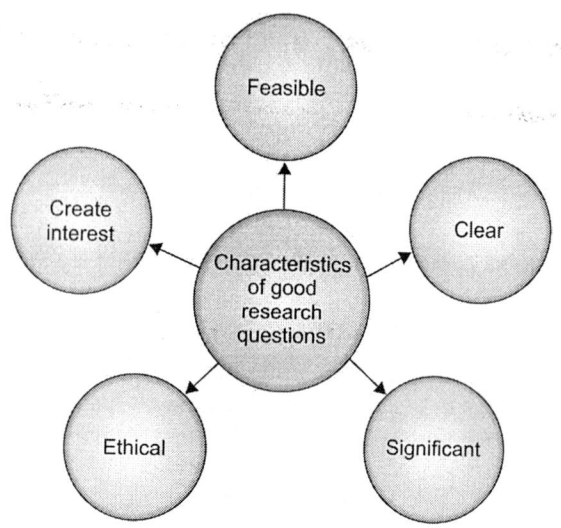

Fig. 9.6: Characteristics of good research question.

Types of Questions (Fig. 9.7)

Structured Questionnaires

Structured questionnaires are those questionnaires in which there are definite, concrete and predetermined questions. The questions are presented with exactly the same wording and in the same order to all respondents. The questions will be formulated before. There should be no alteration of questionnaires during data collection. Resort is taken to this sort of standardization to ensure that all respondents reply to the same set of questions. Structured questionnaires may also have fixed alternative questions in which responses of the informants are limited to the stated alternatives. Thus a highly structured questionnaire is one in which all questions and answers are specified and comments in the respondent's own words are held to the minimum.

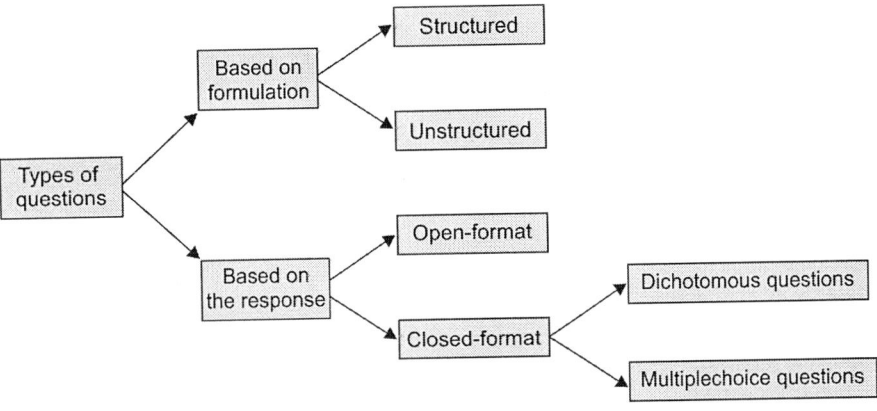

Fig. 9.7: Types of questions.

Unstructured Questionnaires

When the characteristics of structured questionnaires are not present in a questionnaire we can called it as as unstructured or nonstructured questionnaires. In nonstructured questionnaries the questions can be changed based on the situations. In questionnaries it may be mentioned how to change and where to changes questionnaries but the questionnaries are always distributed in written form and cannot be asked like interview.

Open-format Questions

Open-ended questions are unstructured question in which possible answers are not suggested, and the respondent answers it in his or her own words. Such questions usually begin with a how, what, when, where, and why open-ended questions are those questions which provide opportunity to the respondents to express their opinions and answers in their own way. It provides qualitative instead of quantitative information. On open-ended questions are asked generally during exploratory research and where statistical validity is not a prime objective.

Characteristics

- There is no predetermined set of responses.
- An open question is likely to receive a long answer.
- They provide true, insightful and unexpected suggestions.
- They ask the respondent to think and reflect.

Advantages

- Wide range of responses and information can be obtained.
- Answers based on respondent's not researcher's frame of reference–consumer's terms.
- Lack of influence. Do not channel respondents thinking.
- Can help interpret closed-ended questions-why.
- Particularly useful as introduction to survey or topic.
- When it is important to measure the salience of an issue.
- When too many possible responses to be listed or unknown. It is free from the bias of the interviewer; answers are in respondents' own words.

Disadvantages

* It depends upon the ability and/or willingness of respondent to answer.
* Interviewer's ability to record answers quickly or summarize accurately and probe effectively.
* Interviewer's attitude influences response.
* Time consuming (interview sessions, tabulation, classification, assignment, validation).
* Difficulty in coding.
* Require respondents to be articulate.
* Respondents may miss important points.
* Nonresponse.

Closed-format Questions

The question that call for short check responses are known as restricted or closed form type. These questions limits respondents with a list of answer choices from which they must choose to answer the question. Commonly these types of questions are in the form of multiple choices, either with one answer or with check-all-that-apply or may be yes or no. They provide for marking a yes or no, a short response or checking an item from a list of responses. Here the respondent is not free to write of his own, he was to select from the selected from the supplied responses. These questions offer respondents a number of alternatives replies, from which the subjects must choose the one that most likely matches the appropriate answer.

Characteristics

* Facilitate easy statistical calculation of data.
* Provide easy preliminary analysis.
* Can be asked to different groups at different intervals.
* Facilitate efficient tracking of opinion.

Subtypes of Closed-format Questions

Dichotomous Questions

Fixed-alternative question that can only be answered in one of the two indicated ways, such as 'A' or 'B', Agree or Disagree, True or False, Yes or No. These require the respondent to make a choice between two.

Example: Have you ever been hospitalized?
a. Yes   b. No

Multiple Choice Questions

Multiple choice is a form of assessment in which respondents are asked to select the best possible answer (or answers) out of the **choices** from a list. These questions require respondents to make a choice between more than two response alternatives.

Example: Which of the following disease is sexually transmitted?
a. Diabetes mellitus
b. Hypothyroidism
c. Syphilis
d. Hypertension

Cafeteria Question

These are special type of multiple choice questions that ask respondents to select a response that most closely corresponds to their views. Here there will be no single correct response. It is depends upon the individuals own views.

Example: What do you think about hormone replacement therapy?
a. It is dangerous, should be avoided
b. One should be cautious while using it
c. I am uncertain about my views
d. It is beneficial, should be promoted

Rank-order Questions

These questions ask respondents to rank their responses from most favorable to least favorable. Here also there is no single correct answer. This is depends upon the participants views. This type of questions cannot be applicable to assess the knowledge of the individual. By this questions we can assess the individual's, interest, perception thinking, etc.

Example: What according to you is most important for your life? Rank from most favorable to least favorable.
a. Money   b. Education   c. Family   d. Health

Contingency Questions

Contingency questions are also not fully structured questions, because here according to the answer of first part of the questions we will move to the next part of the questions. A question that is asked further only if the respondents gives a particular response to previous question.

Example: Are you having any reproductive health problems?
a. No
b. Yes
    If yes what are that ?...............

Rating Questions (Table 9.2)

These questions ask respondent to judge something along an ordered dimension. Respondent is asked to rate a particular issue on a scale that ranges from poor to good. We can call it also rating scale which may provide a number of choices. Here per each option there is marks which will be added lastly in analysis and interpretation.

Example: How you rank the education quality in India?

Table 9.2: Rating of education quality.

Excellent	Good	Average	Poor	Very poor
5	4	3	2	1

Important Question (Table 9.3)

In this, respondents are asked to rate the importance of a particular issue, on a rating scale of 1–5. This helps to know the things/issue that are important to a respondent. This is also one type of rating scale.

Example: Exercising every day is ....for the health.

Table 9.3: Example of important question.

5	4	3	2	1
Extremely important	Very important	Somewhat important	Not very important	Not at all important

Likert Questions (Table 9.4)

Likert questions helps to know how strongly the respondent agrees with a particular statement. It helps to assess how respondent feels towards a certain issue/services. The scoring process is depends upon the types of statements. In negative types of statements the scoring process will be altered. For example, in a study assessing the attitude of adolescence, here for the statement. 'Junk food should be avoided by the adolescents'.

Table 9.4: Example of Likert question.

5	4	3	2	1
Strongly agree	Agree	Uncertain	Disagree	Strongly disagree

For negative statement
'Junk food should not be avoided by the adolescents'

1	2	3	4	5
Strongly agree	Agree	Uncertain	Disagree	Strongly disagree

Bipolar Questions

Questions that have two extreme answers. Respondent has to mark his/her response between two opposite ends of the scale.

Example: What is your balance of preference here?
I like going for walks [ ] [ ] [ ] [ ] [ ] I like watching movie.

Matrix Questions (Table 9.5)

Include multiple questions and identical response categories are assigned. Questions are placed one under another.

Response categories are place along the top and a list of questions down the side.

Table 9.5: Example of matrix question.

	Mon	Tue	Wed	Thu	Fri	Sat	Sun
Gym							
Aerobics							
Eating (Dinner outside)							

Guidelines for Designing a Good Questionnaire

- The questions must be developed exactly in accordance with the study objectives.
- The questionnaire should begin with the instructions for the respondents to provide the response. Each question must be very clear to avoid any sort of misunderstanding.
- The drafting of the questionnaire should be concise, precise and brief.
- Language of the questionnaire should be according to the respondents knowledge about a particular knowledge.
- Questions outside the respondents experience should not be asked.
- In asking questions about past events, too much reliance should not be placed on the respondents memory.
- Questions which are likely to lead to bias in the respondents should be avoided.
- Questions should be very clear and simple.
- Avoid questions with difficult concepts, which are not easily understandable for respondents.
- Controversial and ambiguous questions should be avoided.
- The structure of the questionnaire should be according to the form in which the responses are to be recorded.
- Cross check the respondent by asking same questions in two different ways.
- A mailed questionnaire should be accompanied by introduction to the study, purpose and directions to fill the questionnaire.
- Answer to question is not influenced by previous question.
- It should be as short as possible but should be comprehensive.
- It should be attractive.
- Directions should be clear and complete.
- It should be represented in good psychological order proceeding from general to more specific responses.
- Double negatives in questions, annoying or embarrassing questions should be avoided and putting two questions in one question also should be avoided.
- It should be designed to collect information in such a way that which can be make easy subsequently as data for analysis.
- The questionnaire should also be used appropriately. Over all the questions should be easily understood, should be simple, i.e., should convey only one thought at a time, should be concrete and should conform as much as possible to the respondent's way of thinking.
- Words such as 'often', 'occasionally', 'usually', 'regularly', 'frequently', 'many', should be used with caution. If these words have to be used, their meaning should be explained properly.

Question Construction

- Use statement which can be interpreted in same way by all subjects.
- Use statements where persons that have different opinions will give different answers.
- Avoid asking double-barrelled questions which contain two distinct ideas or concepts.
- Avoid leading, loaded, ambiguous and long questions.
- Use positive statement.
- Use clear and comprehensible wording.
- Use correct spelling, grammar and punctuation.

Methods of Questionnaire Administration

A questionnaire can be sent and returned by post or e-mail, completed on the web, or handed directly to the respondent who completes it on the spot and hands it back.

Postal

The questionnaires can be sent through post to the target group or the study subject and the study subject can fill up the questionnaires and make it return back to the investigator. This process is economic but time consuming, not labor intensive and anonymity can maintain.

Electronic

Electronics makes the survey easy. Usually through mailing self-completed questionnaires can be distributed to a large target group of people. The main advantages of this method is that large numbers of questionnaires can be sent out at fairly low cost. Questions that are difficult to ask on the telephone or in face-to-face interviews can be asked in a postal questionnaire or through mail. For example, personally sensitive information (about income, sexual orientation, drinking behavior) are best asked about in a way that saves the respondent the embarrassment of facing a stranger and reporting something they may feel awkward about. This method is low cost, not labor intensive and anonymity can maintain. Directly in the website the data can be collected.

Handed Directly to the Respondent

Sometime the researcher will visit to the target population and directly distribute the questionnaires though direct survey. This method is time consuming. It will be difficult to conduct the study if the participants are staying far away from the researcher and not available in a particular place.

Advantages of Questionnaires

- Questionnaire are cost effective
- Easy to collect and analyze data
- Requires less time and energy to administered
- Offer the possibility of anonymity
- Reduce bias
- Used for large sample size
- Less intrusive than face-to-face interview
- Respondents have adequate time to give well throughout answers.
- Respondents, who are not easily approachable, can also be reached conveniently.
- Large samples can be made use of and thus the results can be made more dependable and reliable.

Disadvantages

- Not suitable for all, e.g., children, blind, illiterate
- Low response rate if it will be sent
- Sent by mail may be filled by someone other than the intended person
- It can be used only when respondents are educated and cooperating.
- The control over questionnaire may be lost once it is sent.
- Provide only superficial information
- Probing of response is not possible
- Chances of misinterpretation
- People can lie and answer the question vaguely.

There is also the possibility of ambiguous replies or omission of replies altogether to certain questions; interpretation of omissions is difficult.

Difference between Questionnaires and Schedules

Both questionnaire and schedule are popularly used methods of collecting data in research studies.

There is much resemblance in the nature of these two methods and this fact has made many people to remark that from a practical point of view, the two methods can be taken to be the same. But from the technical point of view there is difference between the two. The important points of difference are discussed in **Table 9.6**.

Table 9.6: Difference between questionnaire and schedule.

Questionnaires	Interview schedules
The questionnaire is generally sent through mail or e-mail to informants to be answered	The interviewer has to visit the place with interview schedule to collect the data
Questionnaire is relatively cheap and economical	To collect data through schedules is relatively more expensive
Non-response is usually high in case of questionnaire as many people do not respond and may return the questionnaire without answering all questions	In interview schedules nonresponse is generally very low because these are filled by researcher/enumerators who are visiting to the field and will try to get answers of all questions
Bias due to nonresponse often remains indeterminate	There may be the danger of interviewer bias and cheating if they are not properly trained
In case of questionnaire, if it will be send through mail; it is not always clear as to who replies. If the person replies also he/she may follow the material and reply. So actual knowledge of the person cannot be assessed	In case of interview schedule the identity of respondent is known. So actual knowledge of the person can be assessed
The questionnaire method is likely to be very slow as it is generally send through mail or e-mail	In case of interview schedules the information is collected well in time as the enumerator is going to field and collecting data
Personal contact is generally not possible in case of the questionnaire method as questionnaires are sent to respondents by post who also in turn return the same by post	In case of schedules direct personal contact is established with respondents
Questionnaire method can be used only when respondents are literate and cooperative	Interview schedule can be used for illiterate persons also
Wider and more representative distribution of sample is possible under the questionnaire method	In respect of schedules there usually remains the difficulty in sending enumerators over a relatively wider area
The success of questionnaire method lies more on the quality of the questionnaire itself	In case of interview schedules it depends upon the honesty and competence of the enumerators
In order to attract the attention of respondents, the physical appearance of questionnaire must be quite attractive	The physical appearance of interview schedule does not require it as it is filled by the enumerators

OBSERVATION

Observation offers the researcher a distinct way of collecting data. It does not rely on what people say they do, or what they say they think. It is more direct than that. Instead, it draws on the direct evidence of the eye to witness events first hand. It is a more natural way of gathering data. Whenever direct observation is possible it is the preferable method to use. Here the researcher gathering data by watching behavior, events or physical characteristics in their natural setting. Moreover observation is a method of data collection that can be used together either information or characteristics and conditions of individual both verbal and nonverbal communication, etc.

Meaning of Observation

Observation means viewing or seeing. We go on observing something or other while we are awake. Most of such observations are just casual and have no specific purpose. But observation as a method of data collection is different from such casual viewing. It is a technique that involves systematically selecting, watching and recording behavior and characteristics of living beings, objects or phenomena.

Definition

Observation is a technique for collecting all the data or acquiring information through occurrences that can be observed through senses with or without mechanical devices.

It is a two part process to collect data for study that includes an observer (someone who is observing) and the observed (there is something to observe).

Gorman and Clayton define observation studies as those that 'involve the systematic recording of observable phenomena or behavior in a natural setting'.

An observation with the following characteristics will be scientific observation.
- Observation is systematic.
- It is specific.
- It is objective.
- It is quantitative.
- The record of observation should be made immediately.
- Expert observer should observe the situation.
- It is result can be checked and verified.

Characteristics of Observational Method

Observation as a method of data collection has certain characteristics.
- **It is both a physical and a mental activity:** The observation eye 'catches' many things which are sighted, but attention is focused on data which are necessary for study.
- **Observation is selective:** A researcher does not observe anything and everything, but select the range of things to be observed on the basis of the nature, scope and objectives of his study.
- **Observation is purposive and not casual:** It is made for the specific purpose of which is relevant to the study.
- **It captures the natural behavior:** In observation the researcher capture the natural behavior of the participant which is required for the study.

Classifications of Observational Method

Observation can be classified in a number of ways:
- **Overt observation:** When everyone knows they are being observed. When we are observing a group of people in their workplace by taking their concern.
- **Covert observation:** When the participants do not know that they are being observed. For example, observing the behavior of children when they are playing.

- **Participant observation:** In participant observation, the observer becomes more or less involvement with the groups under observation and shares the situation as a visiting stranger, an attentive listener, an eager learner or as a complete participant observer. During observation he/she is registering, recording and interpreting behavior of the group. In seeking to explore the natural scene, the qualitative researcher aims to be as unobtrusive as possible, so that neither research presence nor methods disturb the situation. This is why participant observation is one of the favored approaches. Here, the researcher adopts a recognized role within the institution or group. He/she becomes a part of the phenomenon or group which observed and he or she acts as both an observer and a participant. For example, a study of tribal customs by an anthropologist can be undertaken by taking part in tribal activities like folk dance. The person who is observed should not be aware of the researcher's purpose. Then only their behavior will be 'natural.' In this method unstructured tools are used to collect the data such as logbooks, field notes, field diary and tape or video recording, etc.

Advantages

- It blends in with natural activity.
- It gives the researcher access to the same places, people and events as the subjects.
- It gives access to documents relevant to the role, including confidential reports and records.
- It facilitates the use of mechanical aids, such as tape recorders and cameras.
- It provides personal first-hand experience of the role and thus heightens understanding of it.
- It makes a worthwhile contribution to the life of the institution.

Disadvantages

- It might be more difficult to observe the situation as a stranger especially if one is a member of the institution before starting the research. Indeed there is a danger of 'going native' - an over-identification with people's views so that one's perspective as a researcher is submerged beneath them. One must work hard to achieve 'analytic distance' from the role, to set aside taken-for-granted assumptions and to see oneself in the role. The cultivation of reflectivity, and keeping personal diaries, have helped here.
- It adds to the demands on the researcher. Qualitative research in any form is demanding, typically presenting a mass of confusing and intricate data. Participation adds to this, taking up valuable time and adding to one's responsibilities.
- There is a possibility of conflict between one's role as a participant and one's role as a researcher.
- There is ethical problems as we are not taking their permission.

Nonparticipant Observation

In nonparticipant observation, the observer observes through one way screens and hidden microphones. The observer remains a look to the group. He keeps his observation as inconspicuous as possible. In this method, the observer stands apart and does not participate in the phenomenon observed. The purpose of nonparticipant observation is to observe the behavior in a natural setting. The subject will not shift his behavior or he will not be conscious that someone is observing his behavior. Naturally, there is no emotional involvement on the part of the observer. This method calls for skill in recording observations in an unnoticed manner.

Example: Use of recording devices to examine the details of how people talk and behave together.

Advantages

- This mode is less taxing, and is a defense against 'going native'.
- No conflict between the role of participant and researcher.

Disadvantages

- It lacks the benefits of participation.
- There are also practical and ethical problems.
- It does not provide sufficient data within limited time period.
- Sometimes unforeseen factors may interfere with the observational task.

Direct Observation

This means observation of an event personally by the observer when it takes place. This method is flexible and allows the observer to see and record all aspects of events and behavior as they occur. He is also free to shift places, change the focus of the observation. For example, observer is physically present to monitor.

Indirect Observation

This does not involve the physical presence of the observer, and the recording is done by mechanical, photographic or electronic devices. For example, recording customer and employee movements by a special motion picture camera mounted in a department of large store.

Controlled Observation

Controlled observation is carried out either in the laboratory or in the field. It is typified by clear and explicit decisions on what, how, and when to observe. It is primarily used for inferring causality, and testing casual hypothesis.

Uncontrolled Observation

This does not involve over extrinsic and intrinsic variables. It is primarily used for descriptive research. Participant observation is a typical uncontrolled one.

Structured Observation

Researcher in advance prepares a structured or semistructured tool to observe the phenomenon under study. He/she observes only specific attributes or behavior in accordance with planned observation guidelines. The structured observation helps researcher to be in the track which can be carried out by using, checklist and rating scale, etc.

Strengths of Structured Observation

- It is relatively free of observer bias. It can establish frequencies, and is strong on objective measures which involve low inference on the part of the observer.
- Reliability can be strong. Where teams of researchers have used this approach, 80% reliability has been established among them.
- Generalizability. Once you have devised your instrument, large samples can be covered.

- It is precise. There is no 'hanging around' or 'muddling through'.
- It provides a structure for the research.

Weaknesses

- There is a measure of unreliability. Qualitative material might be misrepresented through the use of measurement techniques.
- Much of the interaction is missed.
- It usually ignores the temporal and spatial context in which the data is collected.
- It is not good for generating fresh insights.
- The prespecification of categories predetermines what is to be discovered and allows only partial description.
- It ignores process, flux, development, and change.

Unstructured Observation

Unstructured observation where observation made with minimally structured or researcher imposed categories is used for complete and no specific observation of phenomenon. This unstructured observation was carried out by using unstructured tools, such as logbooks and field notes anecdotes, field diary and video recording, etc.

Uses of Observation Method

Uses: Observation as a method of data collection is used in following situation:
- **To understand an ongoing process or situation:** Through observation a process or situation can be monitor or evaluated as it occur as a particular time.
  Example: A researcher wants to assess the existing ward management practice in public and private hospital. In this situation observation only could be a best method of data collection.
- **To gather data on individual behavior interaction between people:** Observation allow researcher to watch people's behavior and interaction directly or watch for the results of behavior or interactions.
  Example: How nurses respond to the agitated patient in emergency situation.
- **To know about physical setting:** Observing the place or environment where something take place and help increase understanding for the event, activity, or situation that the researcher is evaluating.
  Example: A researcher can observe whether a classroom or training facility is conductive to learning.
- **Data collection where other methods are not possible:** If respondents are unwilling or unable to provide data through questionnaires or interview, observation is a method that requires little forms the individuals for whom we need data.
  Example: A researcher conducting the study of the deaf and dumps illiterate children residing in a rehabilitation center in the situation the researcher has only observation method to observe their nonverbal gestures and behavior to assess their satisfaction.

Steps of Effective Observation

As a research tool effective observation needs effective:
- Planning
- Execution

- Recording
- Interpretation

Planning for Observation

- **Determine the focus:** Thinking about the evaluating question you want answered through observation and select a few areas of focus for your data collection.
  Example: You may want to know how well HIV awareness curriculum is being implemented in the classroom. Your focus area might be interaction between students and teachers, teacher's knowledge, skill, behavior, and in teaching this particular.
- **Design a system for data collection:** Once you have to focus your evaluation, thinking about the specific ideas for which you want to collect data and then determine how you will collect the information you need. There are three primary ways of collecting observation data. These three methods can also be combine to meet our data collection needs.
  - **Recording sheet and checklist:** It is the most standardized ways of data collection observation data that include both questions and responses.
    These forms are typically used for collecting data that can be easily describe in advance.
    Example: Topics that might be covered in HIV prevention lesson.
  - **Observation guide:** List the interaction, process or behavior to be observed with space to record open-ended narrative data.
  - **Field note:** Field note are the least standardized way of data collecting observation data and do not include present question or response.
    Field notes are open-ended narrative data that can be written or recorded into tape recorder.
- **Select the sites:** Select the adequate number of sites to ensure that they are representative of larger population, and will provide an understanding of the situation you are observing.
- **Select the observer:** You may choose to be the only observer or you may want to include other in conducting observation.
- **Train the observers:** It is critical that the observers are well-trained in your data collection process to ensure high quality and consistent data.
- The level of training will be different, based on the complexity of data collection and the individual capacity of the observers.
- **Time your observations appropriately:** Programs and process typically follow a sequence of events. It is critical that we schedule our observation. So we can observe the component of the activity that will answer our evaluation question. This requires advance planning.

Execution

A good observation plan lends to success only when followed with skill and expert execution. Expert execution needs:
- Proper arrangement of special conditions for the subject.
- Assuming the proper physical position for observing.
- Focusing attention on the specific activities or units of behavior under observation.
- Observing discreetly the length and number of periods and internals decided upon.
- Handling well the recording instruments to be used utilizing the training received in terms of expertness.

Recording

The two common procedures for recording observations are:
1. Simultaneous
2. Soon after the observation

Which methods should be used by the observer depend on the nature of the group and the type of behavior to be observed. Both methods have their merits and limitations. The simultaneous form of recording may distract the subjects while after observation the observer may fill the record with the complete and exact information, but if the observation is long and time consuming the observer may fill up the record in between. Therefore, for a systematic collection of data the various devices of recording should be used. They are like checklist, rating scale and score card, etc. But in qualitative study sometimes the observer record the whole data through tape recorder and then decide which aspect he/she will include in his/her data.

Interpretation

Interpretation can be done directly by the observer at the time of his observation. Where several observers are involved, the problem of confusion is there. Therefore, in such instances, the observer merely records his observations and leaves the matter of interpretation to an export that is more likely to provide a unified frame of reference. It must of course, be recognized that the interpreter's frame of reference is fundamental to any interpretation and it might be advisable to insist on agreement between interpreters of different background.

Advantages of Observation Method

- Data collected directly so they permit measurement of actual behavior rather than reports of intended or preferred behavior.
- There is no reporting bias, and potential bias caused by the interviewer and the interviewing process is eliminated or reduced.
- Certain types of data can be collected only by observation.
- If the observed phenomenon occurs frequently or is of short duration, observational methods may be cheaper and faster than survey methods.
- Sometime substantial amount of data can be collected in a relatively short time span.

Disadvantages

- The reasons for the observed behavior may not be determined since little is known about the underlying motives, beliefs, attitudes, and preferences.
- Establishing validity is difficult.
- Subjectivity is also there.
- It is a slow and laborious process.
- Selective perception (bias in the researcher's perception) can bias the data.
- In some cases, the use of observational methods may be unethical, as in observing people without their knowledge or consent.
- It is costly both in terms of time and money.

Observation Tools and Recording Devices

While using this observation method, the researcher should keep in mind things like: What should be observed? How the observations should be recorded? or how the accuracy of observation can be ensured?

To collect data in observation method there are some tools the researcher can use for proper observation which are as follows:
- Observation guides
- Recording sheets or checklist
- Field observation log
- Mechanical devices

Observation Guides

These are printed forms that provide space for recording observations. They are particularly useful when several observers are involved or when you wish to obtain comparable information from several sites/observation points or observations of many people. The more structured the guide, the easier it will be to tally the results.

Recording Sheets or Checklist

These forms are used to record observations as in yes/no option (present/not present) or on a rating scale to indicate extent or quality of something. Checklists are used when there are specific, observable items, actions or attributes to be observed. Checklist is a selected list of words, phrases, sentences and paragraphs following which an observer records a check mark to denote a presence or absence of whatever is being observed. It calls for a simple yes/no judgments. The main purpose is to call attention to various aspects of an object or situation, to see that nothing of importance is overlooked.

Field Observation Log

This may take the form of a diary or cards. Each item of observation is recorded under appropriate subheading.

At the time of observation, rough noting may be made, and at the end of the day, fully log may be made. The card system is flexible and facilitates arrangement and rearrangement of items in any desired order.

Mechanical Devices

These may include cameras, tape recorders, videotape and electronic devices. The camera makes a record that can be analyzed later and may be used to illustrate your evaluation report.

BIOPHYSIOLOGICAL METHODS

Biophysiological method involves the collection of biophysiological data from subjects by using the specialized equipment to determine physical and biological status of subjects, e.g., blood pressure measurement by using special equipment, such as sphygmomanometer and stethoscope.

Purposes

- To study basic physiological process.
- To study physiological outcome of nursing care.
- To evaluate nursing intervention.
- To study correlation of physiological functioning in patients with health problems.

Basic Physiology with Relevance for Nursing Care

- Ways that nursing actions or medical interventions affect patient health outcomes.
- Evaluation of specific nursing procedures or interventions testing a hypothesis.
- Improving measurement and recording of biophysiologic data collected by RN.
- Correlation of physiologic function in patient with health problems.

Use of Biophysiologic Measures in Nursing Research

- Study of biophysiologic processes.
- Effect of nursing intervention on human physiological process.
- Correlate physiologic functioning with health outcomes.

Types

It is classified into two categories:
1. **In vivo:** Performed directly to measure processes occurring internally within living organisms through medical or surgical instruments. In vivo, instruments are available to measure all bodily functions, and technologic advances continue to improve the ability to measure biophysiologic phenomena more accurately, and conveniently, e.g., TPR, BP monitoring. It may use complex instrumentation system with computers, X-ray, MRI, CT scan and may be simple—thermometer, pulse oximeter, stethoscope.
2. **In vitro:** By using this method data are gathered from participants by extracting some biophysiologic material from them and subjecting it to laboratory analysis. It is done outside the organism, in vitro measures include chemical measures (e.g., the measurement of hormone, sugar, or potassium levels); microbiologic measures (e.g., bacterial counts and identification); and cytologic or histologic measures (e.g., tissue biopsies).

Advantages

- Relatively more accurate and errorless, precise and sensitive.
- More objective in nature.
- Participant unlikely to be able to distort measurement.
- Provide valid measures for target variables.
- Easy access to the most of the instruments used for biophysiological measurement.
- Instruments used are valid and reliable.
- May biophysiologic measures are not expensive.

Disadvantages

- Some of the instruments are very expensive. The use of biophysiological measurement instruments may cause fear and it requires significant amount of training knowledge, and experience.
- The results produced by the biophysiological measurements instruments may be affected by the environment and calibration, for example, auxiliary temperature recording in a room with or without air conditioning may have different readings.
- Instrument may cause fear and anxiety among participants, e.g. the collection of blood sample.

- Interferences that create artifacts in biophysiologic measures.
- High degree of interaction among the major biophysiological systems of human being.
- Biophysiological measurements may have traumatic impact on the subjects.
- The use of some of the biophysiological methods may have harmful effect on the participants such as repeated exposure to X-ray increase the health risk for study subjects.

PROJECTIVE TECHNIQUES

Projective techniques, originally developed for use in psychology, can be used in an evaluation to provide a prompt for interviews. These techniques are based on the phenomenon of projection and are indirect and unstructured methods of investigation which have been developed by the psychologists and use projection of respondents for inferring about underline motives, urges or intentions which cannot be secure through direct questioning as the respondent either resists to reveal them or is unable to figure out himself. These techniques are useful in giving respondents opportunities to express their attitudes without personal embarrassment. In these techniques, relatively indefinite and unstructured stimuli are provided to the subject and he or she is asked to structured them in anyway they likes these techniques helps the respondents to project his or her own attitudes and feelings unconsciously on the subject under study. Thus projective techniques play a important role in motivational researches or in attitude surveys. Participants project their unconscious beliefs into other people or objects. Projective techniques have been categorized in terms of the response types required of subjects. The first category is association. The subjects are presented with a stimulus and they respond by indicating the first word, image or thought elicited by the stimulus (Burns and Lennon, 1993).

Important Projective Techniques

- Word association test
- Sentence completion test
- Construction test
- Expression techniques

Word Association Test

It is a simple technique devised by Galton in 1879. In the case of word association, the subjects are asked to read a list of words and to indicate the first word that comes to mind. He is given a clue or hint and asked to respond to the first thing that comes to mind. The association can take the shape of a picture or a word. There can be many interpretations of the same thing. A list of words is given to the respondent and the researcher do not know in which word they are most interested. The interviewer records the responses which reveal the inner feeling of the respondents. The frequency with which any word is given a response and the amount of time that elapses, before the response is given are important for the researcher. In word association respondents are presented with a list of words one at a time and asked to respond to each with the first word that comes to mind, e.g., out of 50 respondents 20 people associate the word 'fair' with 'complexion'.

Sentence Completion Test

In this the respondents are asked to complete an incomplete sentence or story. The completion will reflect their attitude and state of mind. In sentence completion or unfinished sentences, the respondents are given incomplete sentences and asked to complete them. Generally, they are asked to use the first word or phrase that comes to mind.

Examples
- My father seldom……………………
- Most people do not know that I am afraid of……………
- When I was a child, I……………………
- When encountering frustration, I usually……………

Rotters incomplete sentence blank (RISB): This includes list of 40 incomplete sentences and there is no specific time limit for the respondent and psychologist. The respondent makes such sentences that manifest his unconscious desires, thinking, frustrations, emotions, anxiety, mental state, etc.

Assessment for completing sentence: Five types of attitudes are kept in mind while assessing the personalities from resultant complete sentence.
1. Attitude towards family
2. Social attitude
3. Emotional attitude
4. Sexual attitude
5. Character traits

Construction Test

This is more or less like completion test. In this method, construction, the subject is asked to construct a story or a picture from a stimulus concept (Burns and Lennon, 1993). The construction procedure requires more complex and controlled intellectual activity on the part of the subject, for example, the subjects will be handed a picture or a series of pictures and asked to write a story about it. The initial structure is limited and not detailed like the completion test, e.g., two cartoons are given and a dialogue is to written.

Expression Techniques

In this the people are asked to express the feeling or attitude of other people. Here the subject is required to organize and incorporate a particular stimulus into a self-expressive process, such as role playing, psychodrama, dance, etc. In my view, some of the narrative interviews commonly used in qualitative research nowadays also fall into this category.

Drawing Techniques

This is also a projective technique in which a well-known early example is the Machover Draw-a- Person test (D-A-P Machover, 1949). In this test the individual is provided with paper and pencil and is told to 'draw a person'. He or she is asked to draw a person of the opposite sex or of a different gender. The drawing is usually followed by a series of question to elicit specific information about age, schooling, occupation. The results are based on a psychodynamic interpretation of the details of the drawing, such as the size, shape and complexity of the facial features, clothing and background of the figure. As with other projective tests, the approach has very little demonstrated validity and there is evidence that therapists may attribute pathology to individuals who are merely poor artists. A similar class of techniques is kinetic family drawing.

Autobiographical memories: Analyzing memories especially those of early life, in order to understand recurrent or intractable conflicts in later life. In Bruhn's cognitive–perceptual theory, autobiographical memories are central to the understanding of personality. The early memories procedure (EMP Bruhn, 1989) is a self-administered paper-and-pencil instrument that samples 21 autobiographical memories from the entire life span, not just childhood.

The first part calls for six general or spontaneous memories delimited primarily by specific time frames (the five earliest memories and a particularly important life time memory).

The second part comprises 15 specific or directed memories that explore a diverse set of events and areas that may be clinically relevant (e.g., a traumatic memory, one's first punishment memory or one's happiest memory).

Thematic Apperception Test

Another popular projective test is the thematic apperception test (TAT) in which an individual views ambiguous scenes of people, and is asked to describe various aspects of the scene; for example, the subject may be asked to describe what led up to this scene, the emotions of the characters, and what might happen afterwards. A clinician will evaluate these descriptions, attempting to discover the conflicts, motivations and attitudes of the respondent. A researcher may use a specific scoring system that establishes consistent criteria of expressed thoughts and described behaviors associated with a specific trait, e.g., the need for achievement, which has a validated and reliable scoring system. In the answers, the respondent 'projects' their unconscious attitudes and motivations into the picture, which is why these are referred to as 'projective tests.'

Disadvantages of Projective Techniques

- Highly trained interviewers and skilled interpreters are needed.
- Interpreters bias can be there.
- It is a costly method.
- The respondent selected may not be representative of the entire population.
- Psychological technique to get answers without asking a direct question.
- Reduces threat of personal vulnerability.
- Consists of a stimulus and a response.

VIGNETTE METHOD

Vignettes are short scenarios or stories in written or pictorial form which participants can comment upon. It is a method for collecting data by presenting hypothetical situations, and asking research participants a set of directed questions to reveal their values and perceptions. Vignettes are usually developed by drawing from previous research or examples of situations which reflect the local context, creating a story that participants can relate to. Participants are typically asked to comment on how they think the character in the story would feel or act in the given situation, or what they would do themselves. The questions posed to respondents after the vignettes may be either open-ended (e.g., how would you describe this patients' level of confusion?) or closed-ended (e.g., rate how confused you think this patient is on a 7-point scale). These are simulations of real events which can be used in research studies to elicit subject's knowledge, attitudes or opinions according to what they state how they would behave in the hypothetical situation depicted. The vignette provides enough context and information for participants to have an understanding of the scenario being depicted, but needs to be vague in ways that compel participants to 'fill in' detail. Another difference from the story completion method is that instead of completing a story, participants respond to a series of open-ended questions about the story. They can be asked about how a character should ideally act and/or how would they realistically act.

Vignettes have primarily been used quantitatively to study attitudes, perceptions, beliefs and norms. Some pioneering researchers have used vignettes qualitatively, exploring topics as diverse as violence between children in residential care homes, drug injectors' perceptions of HIV risk and safer behavior and social work ethics. They can also be used as 'elicitation tools' in interviews and focus groups, to generate talk data for discussion of interviews or focus groups.

Advantages

- ❖ The ability to collect information simultaneously from large numbers of subjects, to manipulate a number of variables at once in a manner that would not be possible in observation studies.
- ❖ Absence of observer effect and avoidance of the ethical dilemmas commonly encountered during observation.
- ❖ Vignettes are ideally suited to understandings the perceptions and construction-type research questions.
- ❖ They can also be used for experience, accounts of practice and influencing factors-type research questions.
- ❖ They are useful for studying potentially sensitive topics.
- ❖ They can be useful if participants lack *personal* experience and knowledge about at topic.
- ❖ Difficulties include problems establishing reliability and validity, especially external validity.

VISUAL ANALOGUE SCALE OR VISUAL ANALOG SCALE

The visual analogue scale or visual analog scale (VAS) is a psychometric response scale which can be used to measure subjective experiences that cannot easily be directly measured. It is a testing technique for measuring subjective or behavioral phenomena (as pain or dietary consumption) in which a subject selects from a gradient of alternatives (as from 'no pain' to 'worst imaginable pain' or from 'every day' to 'never') arranged in linear fashion **(Fig. 9.8)**. It is often used in epidemiologic and clinical research to measure the intensity or frequency of various symptoms, such as pain, fatigue, and dyspnea. The VAS is a straight line, the end anchors of which are labeled as the extreme limits of the sensation or feeling being measured. Patient

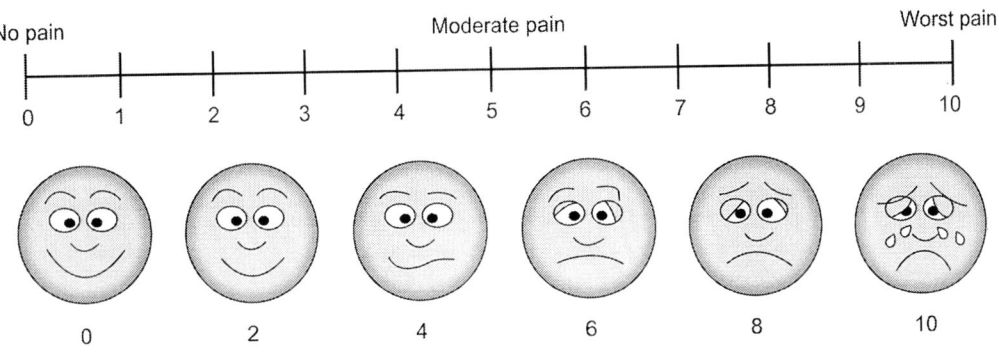

Fig. 9.8: Visual analogue scale for pain measurement.

has to mark on the continuum based on his/her pain or discomfort. The healthcare professional or investigator can help the patient in doing this. When responding to a VAS item, respondents specify their level of agreement to a statement by indicating a position along a continuous line between two end-points. Traditionally, a VAS line is 100 mm in length, which makes it easy to derive a score from 0 to 100 by simply measuring the distance from one end of the scale to the mark on the line which is modified for using research purpose.

Advantages of VAS

- Described permit researchers to efficiently quantify subtle gradations in the strength or intensity of individual characteristics.
- Can be administered either verbally or in writing and thus can be used with most people.
- Can be used to measured such characteristics or symptoms which cannot be measured by other methods.
- No training is required other than the ability to use a ruler to measure distance to determine a score.

Limitations

- They are of less value for comparing across a group of individuals at one time point.
- It could be argued that a VAS is trying to produce interval/ratio data out of subjective values that are at best ordinal.
- Scales are susceptible to several common problems, however, many of which are referred to as response set biases. The most important biases include the following:
  - *Social desirability response set bias:* A tendency to misrepresent attitudes or traits by giving answers that is consistent with prevailing social views.
  - *Extreme response set bias:* A tendency to consistently express extreme attitudes or feelings (e.g., strongly agree), leading to distortions because extreme responses may be unrelated to the trait being measured.
  - *Acquiescence response set bias:* A tendency to agree with statements regardless of their content by some people (*yea-sayers*). The opposite tendency for other people (*nay-sayers*) to disagree with statements independently of the question content is less common.

These biases can be reduced through such strategies as *counterbalancing* positively and negatively worded statements, developing sensitively worded questions, creating a permissive, nonjudgmental atmosphere, and guaranteeing the confidentiality of responses.

Q-sorts

In a Q-sort, participants are presented with a set of cards on which words or statements are written. Participants are asked to sort the cards along a specified bipolar dimension, such as agree or disagree. Typically, there are between 50 and 100 cards to be sorted into 9 or 11 piles, with the number of cards to be placed in each pile predetermined by the researcher. The sorting instructions and objects to be sorted in a Q-sort can vary. For example, patients could be asked to rate nursing behaviors on a most-to-least helpful continuum, or trauma patients could be asked to rate aspects of their treatment on a most-to-least distressing continuum. Q-sorts are versatile and can be applied to a wide variety of problems. Requiring people to place a predetermined number of cards in each pile eliminates many response biases that can occur in Likert scales. On the other hand, it is difficult and time-consuming to administer Q-sorts to a large sample of people. Some critics argue that the forced distribution of cards according to researchers' specifications is artificial and excludes information about how participants would ordinarily distribute their responses.

DEVELOPMENT OF TOOLS

Depending on the nature of the information to be gathered, different instruments are used to conduct the research. The tools of data collection translate the research objectives into specific questions/items, the responses to which will provide the data required to achieve the research objectives. In order to achieve this purpose, each question/item must convey to the respondent the idea or group of ideas required by the research objectives, and each item must obtain a response which can be analyzed for fulfilling the research objectives. Information gathered through the tools provides descriptions of characteristics of individuals, institutions or other phenomena under study. It is useful for measuring the various variables pertaining to the study. The variables and their interrelationships are analyzed for testing the hypothesis or for exploring the content areas set by the research objectives. A research instrument or tool is a device used to measure the concept of interest in a research project that a researcher uses to collect data. The selection of suitable instruments or tools is of vital importance for successful research. Different tools are suitable for collecting various kinds of information for various purposes. The research worker may use one or more of the tools in combination for his purpose. Research students should therefore familiarize themselves with the varieties of tools with their nature, merits and limitations. They should also know how to construct and use them effectively. The systematic way and procedure by which a complex or scientific task is accomplished is known as the technique. Techniques are the practical method, skill or art applied to a particulate task. So, as a researcher we should aware of both the tools and techniques of research. Depending on the nature of the information to be gathered, different instruments are used to conduct the assessment: forms for gathering data from official sources, such as records; surveys/interviews to gather information from youth, community residents, and others; and focus groups to elicit free-flowing perspectives. The major tools of research can be classified broadly into the following categories.

Principles of Construction of Research Tool

- Content of research tool should be based on aims and need of research problem.
- The questioning words must be concise comprehensive and unambiguous.
- Keep in mind the sequence and order of question, i.e., psychological order.
- One question should not influence the other.
- Tool must not be too long or too short. It should complete within 25–30 minutes.
- Should be attractive in appearance.

Types of Tools

The various methods of data gathering involve the use of appropriate recording forms. These are called tools or instruments of data collection. They consist of **(Fig. 9.9)**:

- Observation schedule
- Interview guide
- Interview schedule
- Mailed questionnaire
- Rating scale

* Checklist
* Document schedule/data sheet

Each of the above tools is used for a specific method of data gathering: Observation schedule for observation method, interview schedule and interview guide for interviewing, questionnaire for mail survey and so on.

Functions

* The tools of data collection translate the research objectives into specific questions/items, the responses to which will provide the data required to achieve the research objectives. In order to achieve this purpose, each question/item must convey to the respondent the idea or group of ideas required by the research objectives, and each item must obtain a response which can be analyzed for fulfilling the research objectives.

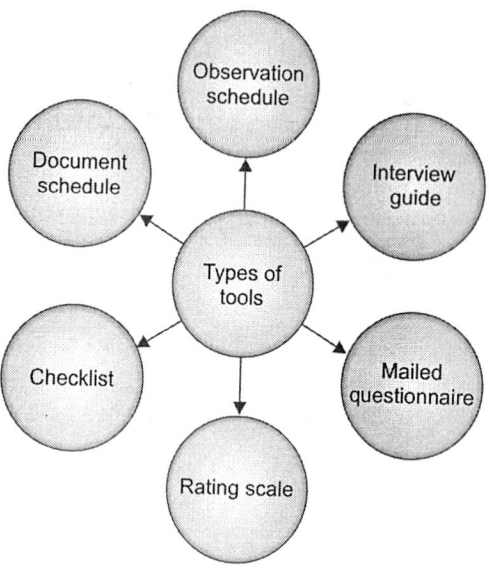

Fig.9.9: Types of tools.

* Information gathered through the tools provides descriptions of characteristics of individuals, institutions or other phenomena under study. It is useful for measuring the various variables pertaining to the study. The variables and their interrelationships are analyzed for testing the hypothesis or for exploring the content areas set by the research objectives.

Observation Schedule

* This is a form on which observations of an object or a phenomenon are recorded. The items to be observed are determined with reference to the nature and objectives of the study. They are grouped into appropriate categories and listed in the schedule in the order in which the observer would observe them.
* The schedule must be as devised as to provide the required verifiable and quantifiable data and to avoid selective bias and misinterpretation of observed items. The units of observation must be simple, and meticulously worded so as to facilitate precise and uniform recording.

Interview Guide

* This is used for nondirective and depth interviews. It does not contain a complete list of items on which information has to be elicited from a respondent. It just contains only the broad topics or areas to be covered in the interview.
* Interview guide serves as a suggestive reference or prompter during interview. It aids in focussing attention on salient points relating to the study and in securing comparable data in different interviews by the same or different interviewers.
* Interview schedule and mailed questionnaire both these tools are widely used in surveys.
* Both are complete lists of questions on which information is elicited from the respondents. The basic difference between them lies in recording responses. While the interviewer fills out a schedule, the respondent completes a questionnaire.

Rating Scale (Table 9.7)

A rating scale is a set of categories designed to elicit information about a quantitative or a qualitative attribute. It is a recording form used for measuring individual's attitudes, aspirations and other psychological and behavioral aspects, and group behavior. Rating scale is one of the enquiry form. Form is a term applied to expression or judgment regarding some situation, object or character. Opinions are usually expressed on a scale of values. Rating scale is one of the enquiry form. Form is a term applied to expression or judgment regarding some situation, object or character. Opinions are usually expressed on a scale of values.

Rating techniques are devices by which such judgments may be quantified. Rating scale is a very useful device in assessing quality, especially when quality is difficult to measure objectively. For example, 'How good was the care provided by a nurse?' Is a question which can hardly be answered objectively. Rating scales record judgment or opinions and indicates the degree or amount of different degrees of quality which are arranged along a line is the scale. For example, how good was the nursing care?

Table 9.7: Rating scale on nursing care.

Excellent	Very good	Good	Average	Below average	Poor	Very poor

This is the most commonly used instrument for making appraisals. It has a large variety of forms and uses. Typically, they direct attention to a number of aspects or traits of the thing to be rated and provide a scale for assigning values to each of the aspects selected. They try to measure the nature or degree of certain aspects or characteristics of a person or phenomenon through the use of a series of numbers, qualitative terms or verbal descriptions.

Scaling emerged from the social sciences in an attempt to measure or order attributes with respect to quantitative attributes or traits. Scaling provides a mechanism for measuring abstract concepts. The various types of scales used in research fall into two broad categories, (i) comparative and (ii) noncomparative.

Comparative Scales

A comparative scale is an ordinal or rank order scale that can also be referred to as a nonmetric scale. Respondents evaluate two or more objects at one time and objects are directly compared with one another as part of the measuring process. In comparative scaling, the respondent is asked to compare one product or service against another.

The researcher provides a point of comparison for respondents to provide answers. There are four types of comparative rating design:
1. **Paired comparison:** Description-paired comparison scales ask a respondent to pick one of two objects from a set based upon a given criterion. Rating personality characteristics was the man to man technique devised during World War I. This technique calls for a panel of raters to rate every individual in comparison to a standard person. This is known as the paired comparison approach.
2. **Rank order scales:** Rank order scales are used in comparative scales where respondents were asked to rate an item in comparison with another item or a group of items on a common

criterion. In this scale of measurement the researcher uses ranking questions as these are construed to be a form of opinion questions in which respondent is asked to rank.

3. **Constant sum:** This technique requires the respondent to divide a given number of points, typically 100, among two or more attributes based on their importance. Constant sum scales are used more often than paired comparisons because the long list of paired items is avoided.
4. **Noncomparative rating scale:** With noncomparative scaling respondents need only evaluate a single product. Noncomparative scaling is frequently referred to as monadic scaling and this is the more widely used type of scale in nursing research studies.

Graphic Rating Scales (Uncommon)

Respondents select a point on a graphic continuum anchored at the extremes. Respondents rate the objects by placing a mark at the appropriate position on a line that runs from one extreme of the criterion variable to the other. The form of the continuous scale may vary considerably. The ends of the continuum are sometimes labeled with opposite values. Respondents are required to make a mark at any point on the scale that they find appropriate. Sometimes, there are numbers along the markings of the line too. At other times, there are no markings at all on the line.

Multi-item Scales

With an itemized scale or multi-item scales respondents are provided with a scale having numbers and/or brief descriptions associated with each category and are asked to select one of the limited number of categories, ordered in terms of scale position. Examples of the itemized rating scale is a nurse researcher conducting by intervening a new intervention and assess the satisfaction of patient on that. The patient can answer they are highly satisfied, moderately satisfied, poorly satisfied or not satisfied at all. These are applied when it is difficult to measure people's attitude based on only one attribute, e.g., ask a person whether he/she is satisfied with Indian Railway. 'Overall I am satisfied.' 'But there are many factors with which I am dissatisfied.' In such cases it is impossible to capture the complete picture with one overall question. A number of scales have to be developed that can measure a respondent's attitude towards several issues from most favorable to most unfavorable.

Likert Scale

A Likert scale consists of several declarative items that express a view point on a topic. Respondents are asked to indicate the degree to which they agree or disagree with the opinion expressed by the statement. The Likert scale usually contains five degrees (but at times 3–7 may also be used). Likert scales are developed using item analysis approach. A particular item is evaluated on the basis of how well it discriminates between those whose total score is high and whose score is low. Likert-type or frequency scales use fixed choice response formats and are designed to measure attitudes or opinions. The original idea for the Likert scale is found in Rensis Likert's 1932 article in archive of psychology titled 'A Technique for the Measurement of Attitudes.' It is a psychometric scale commonly involved in research that employs questionnaires. It is the most widely used approach to scaling responses in survey research. Likert scales are a noncomparative scaling technique and are one-dimensional in nature. When responding to a Likert questionnaire item respondents specify their level of agreement or disagreement on a symmetric agree-disagree scale for a series of statements believe that ecological questions are the most important issues facing human beings today. Strongly agree/agree/do not know/disagree/strongly disagree—each of the five (or seven) responses would have a numerical value which would be used to measure the attitude under investigation. Choose a particular scale (3 point, 5 point, 7 point, etc.) and use it as your standard to cut down on potential confusion and fatigue. This will also allow for comparisons within and between your data sets. We can use it to get an overall measurement of a particular topic, opinion, or experience and also collect specific data on contributing factors.

This scale consists of a series of statements where the respondent provides answers in the form of agreement or disagreement. The respondent selects a numerical score for each statement to indicate the degree of agreement or otherwise. Each such score is finally added up to measure the respondents, attitude.

Staple Scales

It is an attitude measure that places a single adjective or an attitude describing an object in the center of an even number of numerical values. Generally, it is constructed on a scale of 10 ranging from -5 to +5, without a neutral point (zero). It is similar to semantic scale, except for it is single polar. This scale is useful for the researchers to understand the positive and negative intensity of attitudes of respondents. Likert scale questions use a scale, working with quantitative data, it is easy to draw conclusions, reports, results and graphs from the responses. Likert scale questions use psychometric testing to measure beliefs, attitudes and opinion and it is very easy and quick type of survey and it can be sent out through all modes of communication, including even text messages.

* People are not forced to express an either-or opinion, rather it allows them to be neutral.
* Participants may not be completely honest-which may be intentional or unintentional.
* Previous questions will have influenced responses to any further questions that have been asked.
* They are unidimensional, because they only give a certain amount of choices.

Guttman Scaling

Guttman scaling is a hierarchical scaling technique that ranks items such that individuals who agree with an item will also agree with items of a lower rank, e.g., Katz Index of activities of daily living (Katz et al. 1963).

Semantic Scales

This type of scale makes extensive use of words rather than numbers. Respondents describe their feelings about the products or brands on scales with semantic labels. When bipolar adjectives are used at the end points of the scales, these are termed semantic differential scales. The semantic scale and the semantic differential scale are illustrated in **Figure 9.10**. A semantic scale is a combination of more than one continuum. It usually contains an odd number of radio buttons with labels at opposite ends. Max differential scales are often used in trade-off analysis such as conjoint.

Max differential scale can be used in new product features research or even market segmentation research to get accurate orderings of the most important product features. Discriminate among feature strengths more effectively than derived importance methodologies. Like other trade-off analyzes, the analysis derives utilities for each of the most important product features which can be used to derive optimal products, using market segmentation to put respondents into groups with similar preference structures, or to prioritize strategic product goals.

You can have your respondents perform forced-choice nature of the tasks, and disentangle the relative feature importance in cases where average Likert-style ratings might all have very similar ratings.

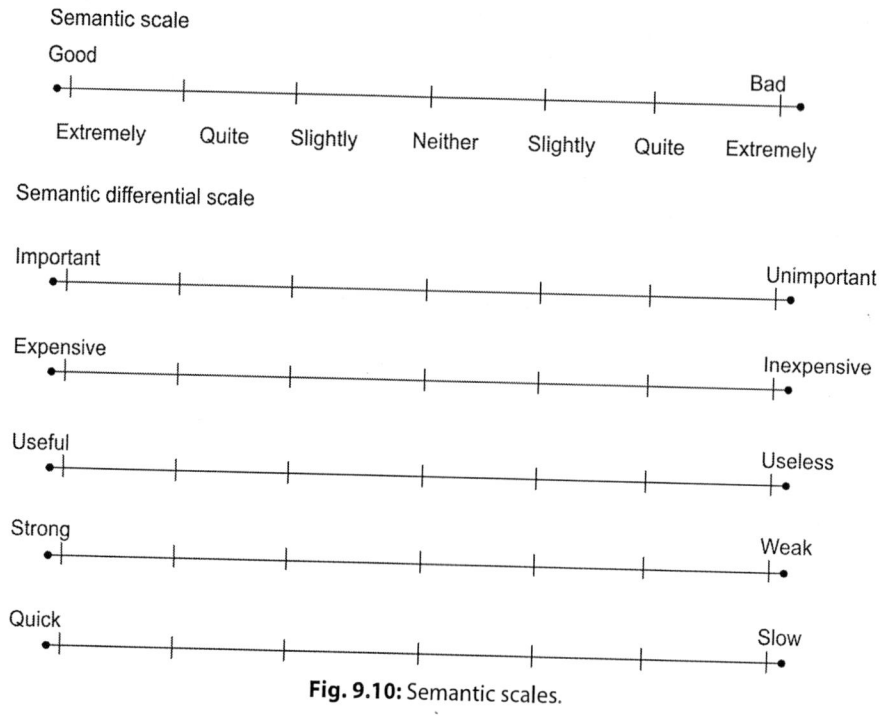

Fig. 9.10: Semantic scales.

Useful Hints on Construction of Rating Scale

A rating scale includes three factors like:
1. The subjects or the phenomena to be rated.
2. The continuum along which they will be rated.
3. The judges who will do the rating. All taken three factors should be carefully taken care by a researcher when he/she construct the rating scale.
    - The subjects or phenomena to be rated are usually a limited number of aspects of a thing or of a traits of a person. Only the most significant aspects for the purpose of the study should be chosen. The usual may to get judgment is on five to seven point scales as we have already discussed.
    - The rating scale is always composed of two parts:
        a. An instruction which names the subject and defines the continuum
        b. A scale which defines the points to be used in rating.
    - Anyone can serve as a rater where nontechnical opinions, likes and dislikes and matters of easy observation are to be rated. But only well-informed and experienced persons should be selected for rating where technical competence is required. Therefore, a researcher should select experts in the field as rater or a person who form a sample of the population in which the scale will subsequently be applied. Pooled judgments increase the reliability of any rating scale. So employ several judges, depending on the rating situation to obtain desirable reliability.

Checklist

This is the simplest of all the devices. It consists of a prepared list of items pertinent to an object or a particular task. The presence or absence of each item may be indicated by checking 'yes' or 'no' or multipoint scale. The use of a checklist ensures a more complete consideration of all aspects of the object, act or task. Checklists contain terms, which the respondent understands, and which more briefly and succinctly express his views than answers to open-ended question. It is a crude device, but careful pretest construction can make it at the best when used to test specific hypothesis. It may be used as an independent tool or as a part of a schedule/questionnaire.

Document Schedule/Data Sheet

This is a list of items of information to be obtained from documents, records and other materials. In order to secure measurable data, the items included in the schedule are limited to those that can be uniformly secured from a large number of case histories or other records.

CONSTRUCTION OF SCHEDULES AND QUESTIONNAIRES

Schedule versus Questionnaire

Schedules and questionnaires are the most common instruments of data collection. These two types of tools have much in common. Both of them contain a set of questions logically related to a problem under study; both aim at eliciting responses from the respondents; in both cases the content, response structure, the wordings of questions, question sequence, etc., are the same for all respondents. Then why should they be denoted by the different terms: 'schedule' and 'questionnaires'? This is because the methods for which they are used are different. While a schedule is used as a tool for interviewing, a questionnaire is used for mailing. A questionnaire is a form prepared and distributed to secure responses to certain questions. It is a device for securing answers to questions by using a form which the respondent fills by himself. It is a systematic compilation of questions that are submitted to a sampling of population from which information is desired. Questionnaire rely on written information supplied directly by people in response to questions. The information from questionnaires tends to fall into two broad categories—'facts' and 'opinions'. It is worth stressing that, in practice, questionnaires are very likely to include questions about both facts and opinions. The successful use of questionnaire depends on devoting the right balance of effort to the planning stage, rather than rushing too early into administering the questionnaire. Therefore, the researcher should have a clear plan of action in mind and costs, production, organization, time schedule and permission should be taken care in the beginning. When designing a questionnaire, the characteristics of a good questionnaire should be kept in mind. Structure schedule construction is same as questionnaire but the way of data collection is different. This difference in usage gives rise to a subtle difference between these two recording forms. That is, the interviewer in a face-to-face interviewing fills a schedule, whereas the respondent himself fills in a questionnaire. Hence the need for using two different terms. Tool is referred to as a schedule when it is used for interviewing; and it is called a questionnaire when it is sent to a respondent for completion and return. The process of construction of a schedule and a questionnaire is almost same, except some minor differences in mechanics. This process is not a matter of simply listing questions that comes to researchers mind. It is a rational process involving much time, effort and thought. It consists of the following major steps: As an interview schedule or a mailed questionnaire is an instrument for gathering data for a specific study, its construction should flow logically from the data required for the given study.

Determination of the Respondents' Level

Who are our respondents? Are they persons with specialized knowledge relating to the problem under study? Or are they lay people? What is their level of knowledge and understanding? The choice of words and concepts depends upon the level of the respondents' knowledge. After determining the data required for the study, first, a broad outline of the instrument may be drafted, listing the various broad categories of data. Second, the sequence of these groupings must be decided. Third, the questions to be asked under each group heading must be listed. All conceivable items relevant to the 'data need' should be compiled.

- **Evaluation of the draft instrument:** In consultation with other qualified persons, the researcher must rigorously examine each question in the draft instrument.
- **Pretesting:** The revised draft must be pretested in order to identify the weaknesses of the instrument and to make the required further revisions to rectify them.
- **Specification of procedures/instructions:** After the instruction is finalized after pretests, the procedures or instructions, relating to its use must be specified.
- **Designing the format:** The format should be suited to the needs of the research. The instrument should be divided into different sections relating to the different aspects of the problem.

Levels of Measurement and Scaling Technique

Measurement can be defined as a standardized process of assigning numbers or other symbols to certain characteristics of the objects of interest. There are four levels of measurement: (i) nominal, (ii) ordinal, (iii) interval and (iv) ratio. The four levels differ in how closely each matches the characteristics of the abstract number system scaling describes the procedures of assigning of numbers or symbols (i.e., quantitative measures) to subjective abstract concepts (or properties of objects). This can be done in two ways viz.: (i) Making a judgment about some characteristic of an individual and then placing him directly on a scale that has been defined in terms of that characteristic scaling involves creating a continuum upon which measured objects are located. (ii) Constructing questionnaires in such a way that the score of individual's responses assigns him a place on a scale. These scale-point positions are so related to each other that when the first point happens to be the highest point, the second point indicates a higher degree in terms of a given characteristic as compared to the third point and the third point indicates a higher degree as compared to the fourth and so on.

Nominal Scale

Nominal scales are defined as those that use only label; that is, they possess only the characteristic of description. The response does not include any level of intensity nominal variables (sometimes also called categorical) involve placing participants into separate categories, such as diagnostic or political groups, so are said to have the property of identity. Use a nominal question when the potential answers are categories and the participant must fit into only one category.

- Serve as tags for identifying objects.
- One-to-one correspondence.

- Do not reflect the amount of the characteristic.
- Counting is the only permissible operation.
- Limited number of statistics based on frequency counts.
- For example, percentages and mode.

ORDINAL SCALE

An ordinal scale is obtained by ranking objects or arranging the in order with regard to some common variables the question is simply whether each object has more or less than some other object. Ordinal variables have both the property of identity and magnitude, which is to say that they involve some notion of order or rank between the categories (e.g., highest to lowest, largest to smallest), but no strong sense that the distance between two adjacent points on a scale is equal to the distance between two other adjacent points. It permits the researcher to rank order the respondents or their responses the researcher can rank order the responses into hierarchical pattern this scale does not allow a researcher to determine the absolute difference in any of the ordinal relationship. A Likert scale is a type of ordinal scale and may also use names with an order such as: 'bad', 'medium' and 'good' or 'very satisfied', 'satisfied', 'neutral', 'unsatisfied', 'very unsatisfied. Another example is military rank; they have an order, but no well-defined numerical difference between ranks or result of a horse race, which says only which horses arrived first, second, or third but include no information about race.

INTERVAL SCALE

Interval scales are those in which the distance between each descriptor is known it demonstrates absolute differences between each scale point in an interval scale the numbers used to rank the objects also represent equal increments of the attribute being measured. Interval variables have the properties of identity, magnitude and equal intervals between points. A common example of an interval scale is the Fahrenheit scale of temperature. In the Fahrenheit temperature scale the distance between 10° and 20° is the same as the distance between 35° and 45°. However, since interval scales do not have an absolute zero point, the ratio of two scores will not be meaningful: it would not be appropriate to say that 40° is twice as hot as 20°. Other examples include IQ tests, neuroticism scores, attitude measures, personality measures, self-reported depression level, ability to solve problems. Such scales are normally constructed by adding together a number of separate questionnaire items that indicate a concept.

RATIO SCALE

Ratio scales are the ones in which true zero origin exists—such as actual number of purchases in a certain time period, rupees spent, miles traveled, etc. This characteristic allow us to construct ratios when comparing the results of measurement a ratio scale tends to be most sophisticated scale in the sense that it allows the researcher not only to identify the absolute differences between each scale point but also to make absolute comparisons between the responses. Ratio scales have all the properties of interval scales as well as a true zero point. Therefore, all mathematical operations are appropriate, including taking the ratio of two numbers. For example, someone who earns ₹ 3,000, earns twice as much as someone who earns ₹ 1,500. Data from ratio scales are also sometimes called *score data*. Examples include height, weight, age, annual income, number of responses, time duration, reaction time, heart rate, child's rate of hitting.

Scaling Technique

Alternatively, we can say that while measuring attitudes and opinions, we face the problem of their valid measurement. In research we quite often face measurement problem, especially when the concepts to be measured are complex and abstract and we do not possess the standardized measurement tools. This brings us to the study of scaling techniques. As such we should study some procedures which may enable us to measure abstract concepts more accurately. Scaling describes the procedures of assigning of numbers or symbols (i.e., quantitative measures) to subjective abstract concepts (or properties of objects). This can be done in two ways viz., making a judgment about some characteristics of an individual and then placing him directly on a scale that has been defined in terms of that characteristic. Scaling involves creating a continuum upon which measured objects are located and constructing questionnaires in such a way that the score of individual's responses assigns him a place on a scale.

Definition

Scaling has been defined as a procedure for the assignment of numbers (or other symbols) to a property of objects in order to impart some of the characteristics of numbers to the properties in question. Numbers for measuring the distinctions of degree in the attitudes/opinions are, thus, assigned to individuals corresponding to their scale-positions.

Reliability

Reliability is the consistency of the measurement instrument. The consistency of measurement instrument means the degree to which an instrument measures the same way each time. It is used under the same condition with the same subjects reliability is synonymous with the consistency of a test, survey, observation, or other measuring devices. Imagine your weight on a scale was 140 pounds, if your weight on the same scale changes to 180 pounds an hour later and 100 pounds an hour after then the tool is not reliable. It shows inconsistency of this scale, any research relying on it would certainly be unreliable. That weight machine cannot be allowed to conduct research.

Definitions

- ❖ Reliability is the consistency of measurement of an instrument.
- ❖ Reliability is the degree to which an instrument measures the same way each time it is used under the same condition with the same subjects.
- ❖ Reliability also refers to the dependability, consistency, and stability of a test.

Types of Reliability

Stability Reliability

The tool is thought to be stable in providing result in all repeated administration. This is used when the concept is to be measured over a period of time. Stability reliability of the tools can be tested through test-retest method.

Test-retest Method

Test-retest reliability refers to the test's consistency among different administrations. To determine the coefficient for this type of reliability, the same test is given to a group of subjects on at least two separate occasions. If the test is reliable, the scores that each student receives on the first administration should be similar to the scores on the second. We would expect the relationship between the first and second administration to be a high positive correlation. So it is a measure of reliability obtained by administering the same test twice over a period of time to a group of individuals. The scores from time 1 and time 2 can then be correlated in order to evaluate the test for stability over time.

One major concern with test-retest reliability is what has been termed the memory effect. This is especially true when the two administrations are close together in time. For example, imagine taking a short ten question test on vocabulary and then ten minutes later being asked to complete the same test. Most of us will remember our responses and when we begin to answer again, we may just answer the way we did on the first test rather than reading through the questions carefully. This can create an artificially high reliability coefficient as subjects respond from their memory rather than the test itself. When a pretest and post-test for an experiment is the same, the memory effect can play a role in the results.

Equivalence Reliability

In this type of reliability testing the tool will be rated either two researchers or one researcher in different samples and found the same percentage of agreement of an observed behavior. To observe the equivalence reliability in the tools the method of reliability testing are parallel form and rater method.

Parallel Forms Reliability

Parallel forms reliability is a measure of reliability obtained by administering different versions of an assessment tool (both versions must contain items that probe the same construct, skill, knowledge base, etc.) to the same group of individuals. The scores from the two versions can then be correlated in order to evaluate the consistency of results across alternate versions. It is one way to assure that memory effects do not occur is to use a different pre- and post-test. In order for these two tests to be used in this manner, however, they must be parallel or equal in what they measure. To determine parallel forms reliability, a reliability coefficient is calculated on the scores of the two measures taken by the same group of subjects. Once again, we would expect a high and positive correlation is we are to say the two forms are parallel. *For example*, if a researcher wanted to evaluate the reliability of a critical thinking assessment, you might create a large set of items that all pertain to critical thinking and then randomly split the questions up into two sets, which would represent the parallel forms.

Inter-rater Reliability

Whenever observations of behavior are used as data in research, we want to assure that these observations are reliable. One way to determine this is to have two or more observers rate the same subjects and then correlate their observations. If, for example, rater A observed a child act out aggressively eight times, we would want rater B to observe the same amount of aggressive acts. If rater B witnessed 16 aggressive acts, then we know at least one of these two raters is incorrect. If there ratings are positively correlated, however, we can be reasonably sure that they are measuring the same construct of aggression. It does not, however, assure that they are measuring it correctly, only that they are both measuring it the same. So, inter-rater reliability is a measure of reliability used to assess the degree to which different judges or raters agree in their assessment decisions. Inter-rater reliability is useful because human observers will not necessarily interpret answers the same way; raters may disagree as to how well certain responses or material demonstrate knowledge of the construct or skill being assessed. *Example:* Inter-rater reliability might be employed when different judges are evaluating the degree to which art portfolios meet certain standards. Inter-rater reliability is especially useful when judgments can be considered relatively subjective. Thus, the use of this type of reliability would probably be more likely when evaluating artwork as opposed to math problems.

Homogeneity or Internal Consistency

In this type the tool is concerned with sample of items used to measure the variable of interest. Internal consistency reliability is a measure of reliability used to evaluate the degree to which different test items that probe the same construct produce similar results. The methods of reliability tastings are:

- **Average inter-item correlation** is a subtype of internal consistency reliability. It is obtained by taking all of the items on a test that probe the same construct (e.g., reading comprehension), determining the correlation coefficient for each *pair* of items, and finally taking the average of all of these correlation coefficients. This final step yields the average inter-item correlation.
- **Split-half reliability** is another subtype of internal consistency reliability. The process of obtaining split-half reliability is begun by 'splitting in half' all items of a test that are intended to probe the same area of knowledge in order to form two 'sets' of items. The entire test is administered to a group of individuals, the total score for each 'set' is computed, and finally the split-half reliability is obtained by determining the correlation between the two total 'set' scores.

Validity

The word 'valid' is derived from the Latin 'validus' meaning 'strong'. The validity is a measurement tool (e.g., a test in education) is considered to be the degree to which the tool measures what it claims to measure. In the area of scientific research design and experimentation validity refers to whether a study is able to scientifically answer the question it is intended to answer. In clinical fields, the assessment of validity of a diagnosis and various diagnostic tests are extremely important. As diagnosis augments treatments, medications and the patient life, it is extremely important to known that when running diagnostic tests that clinicians are truly testing what they intend to test.

In psychometrics; validity has a particular application known as test validity 'the degree to which evidence and theory support the interpretations of test scores.'

Validity is important because it can help to determine what types of tests to use and help to make sure researchers are using methods that are not only ethical, and cost-effective but also a method that truly measures the idea or construct in question. It is the extent to which an instrument measures what it is supposed to measure and performs as it is designed to perform. Validity is generally measured in degrees. As a process, validation involves collecting and analyzing data to assess the accuracy of an instrument. There are numerous statistical tests and measures to assess the validity of quantitative instruments, which generally involves pilot testing. The remainder of this discussion focuses on external validity and content validity. Some of the constructs include motivation, depression, anger, and practically any human emotion or trait. If we have a difficult time defining the construct, we are going to have an even more difficult time measuring it. Construct validity is the term given to a test that measures a construct accurately and there are different types of construct validity that we should be concerned with.

Three of these, concurrent validity, content validity, and predictive validity are discussed below.

Definitions

- According to Treece and Treece, 'validity refers to an instrument or test actually testing what is supposed to be testing.'
- According to Polit and Hungler, 'validity refers to the degree to which an instrument measures what it supposed to measuring.'

Types of Validity

- Construct validity
  - Convergent validity
  - Divergent validity
- Content validity
- Face validity
- Criterion validity
  - Concurrent validity
  - Predictive validity
- Experimental validity
  - Internal validity
  - External validity
- Relationship to internal validity
- Statistical conclusion validity
- Diagnostic validity

Construct Validity

Construct validity is based on the extent to which a test measures a theoretical construct or trait. (i.e., practical tests developed from a theory) do actually measure what the theory says they do. For example, to what extent is an questionnaire actually measuring intelligence? It involves attempting to validate a baby of theory underlying the measure and testing hypothesized relationship. Evidence of construct validity can be provided by comparing the results obtained with the results obtained using other tests, other (related) characteristics of the individual or factors in the individual's environment which would be expected to affect test performance. Construct validity is usually measured using a correlation coefficient–when the correlation is high, the tool can be considered valid.

The major focus of construct validity is on the abstract concept that is being measured and its relationship to other concepts. Construct validation is a cyclical process that unites psychometric procedures with theory development. Constructs are specified and then interrelated with other in empirical testing. Empirical testing confirms of fails to confirm the relationship that would be predicted among concepts. It is complex process, often involves several studies. Two strategies for assessing construct validity include convergent and divergent approaches.

Convergent Validity

It refers to a search for other measures of the construct when two or more tools that theoretically measure the same construct are identified, they are both administered to the same subject. A correlational analysis is performed. If the measures are positively correlated, convergent validity is said to be supported.

Divergent Validity

It searchers further instruments that measure the opposite of the construct. It refers to the ability to differentiate the construct from others that may be similar. If the divergent measure is negatively related to the other measures, validity of the measure is strengthened.

A specific method of assessing convergent and divergent validity is that multitrait-multimethod approach (Campbell and Fiske 1959e). For example, anxiety could be measured by:
- Administering the state: Trait anxiety inventory
- Recording blood pressure reading
- Asking subjects about Indian feeling
- Observing the subject's behavior

Content Validity

Content validity is concerned with a test's ability to include or represent all of the content of a particular construct. It is concerned with scope of coverage of the content area to be measured. *Content validity* refers to the appropriateness of the content of an instrument. In other words, do the measures (questions, observation logs, etc.) accurately assess what you want to know? This is particularly important with achievement tests. More often it is applied in tests of knowledge measurement. It is mostly used in measuring complex psychological tests of a person. It is a case of expert judgment about the content area included in the research instrument measure a particular phenomenon. Judgment of the content viability may be subjective and are based on previous researchers and exports opinion about the adequacy, appropriateness and completeness of the content of instrument. Generally, this viability is ensured through the judgments of experts about the content.

Face Validity

Face validity involves an overall look of an instrument regarding its appropriateness to measure a particular attribute or phenomenon. Face validity ascertains that the measure appears to be assessing the intended construct under study. Though face validity is not considered a very important and essential type of validity for an instrument. However, it may be taken in consideration while assessing for other aspects of validity refers to the value or the outlook of an instrument. Face validity says whether a tool appears to others to be measuring what it says it does. Face validity is a simple form of content validity—the researcher can asks a few people to check the tool covers all areas.

For example: A Likert scale designed to measure the attitude of the nurses towards the patients admitted with HIV/AIDS, a researcher may judge the face value of this instrument by its appearance, that is it looked good or not; covers all areas or not but it provides no guarantee about the appropriateness and completeness of a research instrument with regards to its content, construct and measurement score.

Criterion Validity

It is used to predict future or current performance—it correlates test results with another criterion of interest. Concurrent or predictive validity are both measures of criterion validity. This type of validity is a relationship between measurements of the instrument with some other external criteria. For example, a tool is developed to measure the professionalism among nurses; to assess the criteria validity nurses were separately asked about the number of research papers they published and number of professional conferences they have attended. Later a correlation coefficient is calculated to assess the criterion validity. This tool is considered strong with criterion validity if a positive correlation exists between score of the tool measuring professionalism and the number of research articles published and professional conferences attended by the nurses. The instrument is valid if its measurements strongly respond to the score of some other valid criteria. The problem with criterion-related validity is finding a reliable and valid external criterion mostly we are to rely on a less than perfect criterion because the rating found by empirical and supervisory methods may be computed mathematically, which can correlate score if instrument with scores of criterion variable. Here the range of coefficient ≥ 0.70 is desirable. Criterion-related validity may be differentiated by predictive and concurrent validity.

Predictive Validity

It is the degree of forecasting judgment; for example, some personality tests on academic futures of students can be predictive of behavior patterns it is the differentiation between performances on some future criterion and instruments ability. An instrument may have predictive validity when its score significantly correlates with some future criteria. For example, does a tool developed to measure the risk of pressure sores in children in hospital in fact identify the children at risk?

Concurrent Validity

It is the degree of the measures in present. It relates to the present specific behavior and characteristics; hence the difference between predictive and concurrent validity refers to timing pattern of obtaining measurements of a criterion. Concurrent validity uses an already existing and well-accepted measure against which the new measure can be compared, e.g., if a researcher developing a new pain assessment tool you would compare the ratings obtained from the new tools with those obtained using a previously validated tool.

Experimental Validity

The validity of the design of experimental research studies is a fundamental part of the scientific method, and a concern of research ethics. Without a valid design, valid scientific conclusions cannot be drawn. If a study is valid then it truly represents what it was intended to represent. Experimental validity refers to the manner in which variables that influence both the results of the research and the generalizability to the population at large. It is broken down into two groups: (1) Internal validity and (2) External validity.

Internal Validity

Internal validity is an inductive estimate of the degree to which conclusion about causal relationship can be made (e.g., cause and effect), based on the measures used, the research setting, and the whole research design. Good experimental techniques in which the effect of an independent variable on a dependent variable is studied under highly controlled conditions, usually allow for higher degrees of internal validity than, single case designs. Eight kinds of confounding variable can interfere with internal validity (with the attempt to isolate causal relationship):
1. History, the specific events occurring between the first and second measurements in addition to the experimental variables.
2. Maturation, process within the participants as a function of the passage of time (not specific to particular events), e.g., growing older, hungrier, more tired and so on.

3. Testing, the effect of taking a test upon the scores of a second testing.
4. Instrumentation, changes in calibration of a measurement tool or changes in the observers or scores may produce changes in the obtained measurements.
5. Statistical regression: Operating where groups have been selected on the basis of their extreme scores.
6. Selection, biases resulting from differential selection of respondents for the comparison grasp.
7. Experimental morality; or different loss of respondents from the comparison groups.
8. Selection-maturation interaction, e.g., in multiple-group quasi-experimental designs.

External Validity

External validity concerns the extent to which the (internally valid) results of a study can be held to be true for other cases. For example, to different people, places or times. In other words, it is about whether findings can be validity generalized. If the same research study was conducted in those other cases, would it get the same results?

A major factor in this is whether the study sample (e.g., the research participants) are representative of the general population along relevant dimensions. Other factors jeopardizing external validity are:

❖ Reactive or interaction effect of testing, a pretest might increase the score on a post-test.
❖ Interaction effects of selection biases and the experimental variable.
❖ Reactive effects of experimental arrangement which would preclude generalization about the effect of the experimental variable upon persons being exposed to it nonexperimental settings.
❖ Multiple-treatment interference, where effects of earlier treatments are not erasable.

Relationship to Internal Validity

On first glance, internal and external validity seem to contradict each other to get an experimental design you have to control for all interfering variables. That is why you conduct your experiment in a laboratory setting. While gaining internal validity (excluding interfering variables by keeping them constant) you lose ecological or external validity because you establish an artificial laboratory setting on the other hand with observational research you cannot control for interfering variables (low internal validity), but you can measure in the natural (ecological) environment, at the place where behavior normally occurs. However, in doing so, you sacrifice internal validity.

The apparent contradiction of internal validity and external validity is, however, only superficial. The question of whether results from a particular study generalize to other people, places or times arises only when one follows an intuitivist research strategy, if the goal of a study is to deductively test a theory, one is only concerned with factors which might undermine the rigor of the study, i.e., threats to internal validity.

Statistical Conclusion Validity

Statistical conclusion validity is the degree to which conclusions about the relationship among variables based on the data are correct or 'reasonable'. This began an being solely about whether the statistical conclusion about the relationship of the variables was correct, but now there is a movement towards moving to 'reasonable' conclusions that use quantitative statistical and qualitative data. Statistical conclusion validity involves ensuring the use of adequate sampling procedures, appropriate statistical tests and reliable measurement procedures. As this type of validity is concerned solely with the relationship that is found among variables the relationship may be solely a correlation.

Diagnostic Validity

In clinical fields such as medicine, the validity of a diagnostic tests or screening tests may be assessed.

In regard to tests, the validity issues may be examined in the same way as for psychometric tests as outlined above, but there are often particular applications and priorities. In laboratory work the medical validity of a scientific finding has been defined as the degree of achieving the objective: namely of answering the question which the physician asks.

An important requirement in clinical diagnosis and testing is sensitivity and specificity a test needs to be sensitive enough to detect the relevant problem if it is present and therefore avoid too many false-positive results.

In psychiatry there is particular issue with assessing the validity of the diagnostic categories themselves. In these context:
- Content validity may refer to symptoms and diagnostic criteria.
- Concurrent validity may be defined by various correlates or markers and perhaps also treatment response.
- Predictive validity may refer mainly to diagnostic stability overtime.
- Discriminant validity may involve delimitation from other disorders.

SUMMARY

- The data of a research study are the pieces of information obtained in the course of the investigation. The term data refers to any kind of information researchers obtain on the subjects, respondents or participants of the study.
- The research data are classified in two ways; based on the study findings and based on the source. Based on the study finding it is classified as quantitative or qualitative. Based on their source, data fall under two categories namely primary data and secondary data
- Many methods of collecting new data are used for studies. Data collection methods have four important dimensions that's are structure, quantifiability, researcher obstructiveness and objectivity. The data collection plan should contained the answers of the 6'w's of data collection, that's are what, whom, who, where, when and how.
- There are a lots of methods like interviews, observations, questionnaires, biophysiological method, projective techniques, etc., are used to collect data.
- Based on the construction of the tool it is classified as structured interview, unstructured interview and semistructured interview. Some other types of interviews are personal interview, telephone interview, depth interview, projective techniques and focus group interviews.
- A questionnaire is a structured instrument consisting of a series of questions prepared by researcher that a research subject is asked to complete, to gather data from individuals about knowledge, attitude, beliefs and feelings.
- The questionaries' can be classified as structured/unstructured and open-ended/close-ended. A questionnaire can be sent and returned by post or e-mail, completed on the web, or handed directly to the respondent who completes it on the spot and hands it back.

- Observation offers the researcher a distinct way of collecting data. It does not rely on what people say they do, or what they say they think. It is more direct than that. Instead, it draws on the direct evidence of the eye to witness events first hand. It is a more natural way of gathering data.
- Biophysiological method involves the collection of biophysiological data from subjects by using the specialized equipment to determine physical and biological status of subjects, e.g., blood pressure measurement by using special equipments, such as sphygmomanometer and stethoscope.
- These techniques are based on the phenomenon of projection and are indirect and unstructured methods of investigation which have been developed by the psychologists and use projection of respondents for inferring about underline motives, urges or intentions which cannot be secure through direct questioning.
- Vignettes are short scenarios or stories in written or pictorial form which participants can comment upon. It is a method for collecting data by presenting hypothetical situations, and asking research participants a set of directed questions to reveal their values and perceptions.
- The visual analogue scale or visual analog scale (VAS) is a psychometric response scale which can be used to measure subjective experiences that cannot easily be directly measured. It is a testing technique for measuring subjective or behavioral phenomena.
- Depending on the nature of the information to be gathered, different instruments are used to conduct the research. These are observation schedule, interview guide, interview schedule, mailed questionnaire rating scale, checklist and document schedule, etc. Before administering the tool the validity and reliability of the tools must be tested.
- Reliability is the consistency of the measurement instrument. The consistency of measurement instrument means the degree to which an instrument measures the same way each time. There are different types of reliability. The word 'valid' is derived from the Latin 'validus' meaning 'strong. 'validity refers to the degree to which an instrument measures what it supposed to measuring

QUESTIONS TO TEST YOUR KNOWLEDGE

Q1. Define data. Write its classifications. Enumerate different source for collecting data.

(2 + 4 + 4)

Q2. What do you mean by data collection plan? As a nurse researcher explain how you will develop data collection plan.

(3 + 12)

Q3. Enlist different methods of data collection. Explain details about interview method.

(3 + 12)

Q4. Describe different types of questions for collecting data and explain the guidelines for designing a good questionnaire.

(9 + 6)

Q5. Enumerate different types tools for collecting the data.

(15)

Q6. What do you mean by observation method? Enumerate the characteristics and classification of observational method.

(3 + 4 + 8)

Q7. Write short notes on the following:
   a. Biophysiological method of data collection
   b. Visual analogous scale
   c. Q-sorts

d. Rating scale
e. Reliability
f. Types of validity

Q8. Multiple choice questions: (1 × 20)

I. A qualitative research question:
   a. Is generally an open-ended question
   b. Is generally a closed-ended question
   c. Is both closed and open-ended question
   d. Consists only dichotomous question

II. The type of closed-ended question that offers two answer choices that are usually opposites or contrasting thoughts is called:
   a. Dichotomous
   b. Trichotomous
   c. Multiple response
   d. Multiple choice

III. When two raters rate the same tool may or may not at same time that is considered as:
   a. Parallel forms reliability
   b. Inter-rater reliability
   c. Intra-rater reliability
   d. Homogeneity

IV. Construct validity is usually measured using a:
   a. Correlation coefficient
   b. Particular construct
   c. Particular content
   d. Good instrument

V. A study is "reliable", it states that that:
   a. The methods are specified clearly enough for the research to be replicated.
   b. The tools and measures devised for concepts are stable on different occasions.
   c. The findings can be generalized to whole
   d. The study was conducted by a reputable researcher.

VI. The degree of forecasting judgment is:
   a. Concurrent validity
   b. Predictive validity
   c. Criterion validity
   d. Internal validity

VII. Schedule is used as a:
   a. Questionnaire
   b. Tool
   c. Method
   d. Technique

VIII. Which of these is not a method of data collection?
   a. Questionnaires
   b. Interviews
   c. Experiment
   d. Observations

IX. Subjects are presented with a straight line that is anchored on each end with words or phrases that represent the extremes of some phenomenon is called:
   a. Rating scale
   b. Visual analogue scale
   c. Likert scale
   d. Checklist

X. The degree to which an instrument covers the scope and range of information that is sought is called:
   a. Concurrent validity
   b. Construct validity
   c. Content validity
   d. Criterion validity

XI. _____ is the ability of an instrument to measure the construct that it is intended to measure.
   a. Concurrent validity
   b. Construct validity
   c. Content validity
   d. Criterion validity

XII. A type of criterion validity in which a determination is made of the instrument's ability to obtain a measurement of subjects' behavior that is comparable to some other criterion used to indicate that behaviour is called:
   a. Concurrent validity
   b. Construct validity
   c. Content validity
   d. Criterion validity

XIII. The degree to which two forms of an instrument obtain the same results or two or more observers obtain the same results when using a single instrument to measure a variable is called as:
   a. Parallel forms reliability
   b. Stability reliability
   c. Equivalence reliability
   d. Homogeneity

XIV. The lowest level of measurement of data is:
   a. Nominal level
   b. Ordinal level
   c. Ratio level
   d. Rating level

XV. A type of validity used to identify clusters of related items on an instrument or scale is called:
   a. Parallel forms reliability
   b. Stability reliability
   c. Equivalence reliability
   d. Factor analysis

XVI. The degree to which two or more independent judges are in agreement about ratings or observations of events or behaviors.
   a. Inter-rater reliability
   b. Intra-rater reliability
   c. Parallel forms reliability
   d. Stability reliability

XVII. Questions that are relevant for some respondents and not for others are:
   a. Open-ended questions
   b. Close ended questions
   c. Contingency questions
   d. Delphi technique

XVIII. A data collection method that uses several rounds of questions to seek a consensus on a particular topic from a group of experts on the topic:
   a. Q-sort method
   b. Delphi technique
   c. Focus group discussion
   d. Unstructured interview

XIX. Questions that allow respondents to answer in their own words is:
   a. Close-ended questions
   b. Multiple choice questions
   c. Open-ended questions
   d. Rank order questions

XX. A data-collection method in which subjects are asked to sort statements into categories according to their attitudes toward, or rating of, the statements is called as:
   a. Q-sort method
   b. Delphi technique
   c. Focus group discussion
   d. Unstructured interview

ANSWERS

I. a	II. a	III. b	IV. a	V. b
VI. b	VII. b	VIII. c	IX. b	X. c
XI. b	XII. a	XIII. c	XIV. a	XV. d
XVI. a	XVII. c	XVIII. b	XIX. c	XX. a

Chapter 10

Analysis of Data and Application of Biostatistics in Nursing Research

Learning Objectives

After completion of this chapter, the students will be able to:
- Explain the concept of analysis of quantitative and qualitative data.
- Enumerate the steps of quantitative data analysis.
- Explain about tabulation it's general principles, parts of table, types of the tables and how the data can be put in the forms of tabulation.
- Describe regarding graphical presentation of data, different types of diagram and graphs and how to construct diagrams/graphs.
- Enumerate measures of central tendency like different types of mean, median, mode and there calculation in different types of series with examples.
- Describe different types of measures of dispersion like the range, mean deviation, quartile deviation variance, standard deviation and able to calculate the values.
- Find out relationship between values of two or more variables by calculating correlation coefficient and through regression analysis.
- Difference between correlation and linear regression.
- Find out significant relationship between two or more variables though inferential analysis like t-test, ANOVA, MANCOVA, Chi-square test, etc.
- Enumerate the approaches, process and steps of qualitative data analysis.
- Identify problems in qualitative data analysis.

INTRODUCTION

The data, after collection, has to be processed and analyzed in accordance with the outline laid down for the purpose at the time of developing the research plan. It is the most important phase of the research process, which involves the computation of the certain measures along with searching for patterns of relationship that exists among data groups. Data collection is followed by the analysis and interpretation of data, where collected data are analyzed and interpreted in accordance with study objectives. The term analysis refers to the computation of certain measures along with searching for patterns of relationship that exist among data-groups which includes compilation, editing, coding, classification, and presentation of data. Analysis and interpretation of qualitative and quantitative data follow different paths, which are discussed in this chapter distinctly in detail.

The purpose of analyzing the data collected in a study is to describe the data in meaningful terms as the data collected does not answer the research questions or test research hypothesis. The data used is to be systematically analyzed so that trends and patterns of relationships can be detected.

DEFINITIONS

❖ Analysis is the process of organizing and synthesizing the data so as to answer research questions and test hypothesis.
❖ Analysis referred as a method of organizing data in such a way that research questions can be answered and hypothesis can be tested.
❖ Analysis is the process of breaking a complex topic into smaller parts to gain better understanding of it.

It is also defined as 'the process of systematically applying statistical and logical techniques to describe, summarize and compare data'.

ANALYSIS OF QUANTITATIVE DATA

Analysis of quantitative data deals with information collected during research study, which can be quantified, and statistical calculations can be computed. Quantitative data is presented in a numerical format, collected in a standardized manner (e.g., surveys, closed-ended interviews, tests) and analyzed using descriptive and inferential statistical techniques.

Steps of Quantitative Data Analysis

Data analysis process includes the following four steps (**Fig 10.1**):

Data Preparation (Cleaning and Organizing Data for Analysis)

Data preparation involves checking or logging the data which can be done just after data collection, checking the data for accuracy by comparing with original raw data, entering the data into the computer, transforming the data, and developing and documenting a database structure that integrates the various measures. Data preparation involved the following steps:

❖ **Compilation:** Compilation process includes gathering together all the collected data in manner that a process of analysis can be initiated. While compiling the data, care is to be taken to arrange all the data in an order so that editing and coding process can be implemented with case.

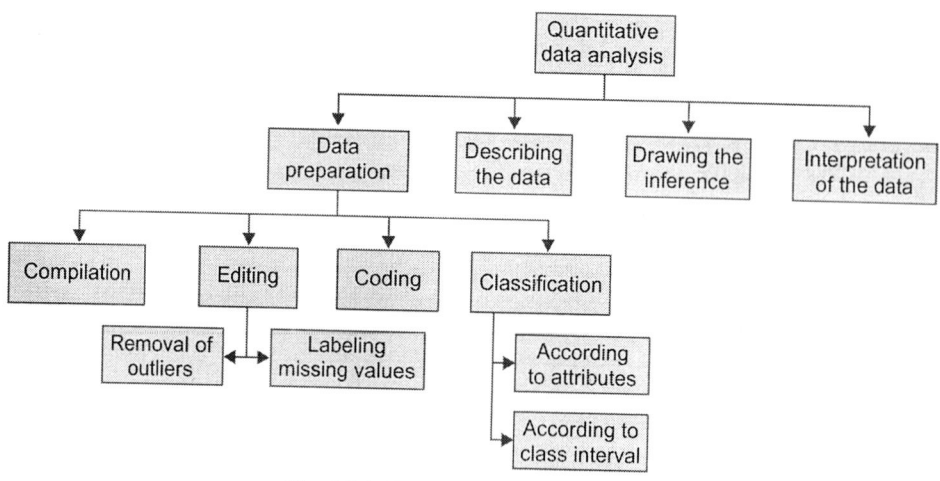

Fig. 10.1: Quantitative data analysis.

- **Editing:** Editing implies the checking of the gathered data for accuracy, utility, and completeness. It involves a careful scrutiny of the completed questionnaires and/or schedules. Editing is done to assure that the data are accurate, consistent with other facts gathered, uniformly entered, as completed as possible and have been well arranged to facilitate coding and tabulation. If the raw data are erroneous or inconsistent, these deficiencies will be carried through all subsequent stages of processing and will greatly distort the result of any enquiry. Editing of data is nothing but a process of examining the collected raw data. During editing the editor/researcher must see that none of the questions has been skipped, all the answers have been recorded, and all the replies are internally consistent with each other. During editing the researcher has to do followings:
  - **Removal of outliers:** Invalid, impossible, or extreme values may be removed from the dataset. Outliers might also be marked for exclusion for the purpose of certain analyzes.
  - **Labeling missing values:** It may be necessary to label each missing value with the reason it is considered missing in order to guarantee accurate bases for analysis. In a survey, missing values correspond to skipped questions or unendorsed options. A discussion between analyst and client should take place in determining how missing values should be handled.

  Editors must keep in view several points while performing their work:
  - They should be familiar with instructions given to the interviewers and coders as well as with the editing instructions supplied to them for the purpose.
  - While crossing out an original data/entry for one reason or another, they should just draw a single line on it so that the same may remain legible.
  - They must make entries (if any) on the form in some distinctive color and that too in a standardized form.
  - They should initial all answers which they change or supply.
  - Editor's initials and the date of editing should be placed on each completed form or schedule.

- **Coding:** It is important for analysis as numerous replies can be reduced to a small number of classes through coding. The original data is transformed into symbols compatible with manual or computer-assisted analysis. Coding refers to the process of assigning numerals or other symbols to answers so that responses can be put into a limited number of categories or classes. Such classes should be appropriate to the research problem under consideration. Coding can be carried out before or after the actual data is collected. Code is an abbreviation, a symbol, a number, or an alphabet, which is assigned by the researcher to every schedule item and response category.

  For coding some important criteria should be considered, such as categories should be exhaustive, so that all the responses can be classified in one or other category; codes should be mutually exclusive, which means one code should be specific to only one kind of information and not overlapping criteria of other codes. Separate categories can be created for recording 'no response' and 'no-knowledge response'.

  Coding decisions may be taken at the designing stage of a research tool, which is helpful for computer tabulation. In case of manual coding some standard methods may be used, such as coding in the margin with a colored pencil or transcribe the data instrument to a coding sheet. Care must be taken to avoid errors in the coding method.

- **Classification:** The classification of data is necessary, as many researches result in large volumes of raw data which must be reduced to homogeneous groups. In the process of classification, we divide and arrange the entire data into different categories, classifications, groups, or classes on the basis of common characteristics. The data can be classified based on their attributes or according to class-intervals. (a) Classification according to attributes: Descriptive characteristics refer to qualitative phenomenon which cannot be measured quantitatively; only their presence or absence in an individual item can be noticed. Data obtained this way on the basis of certain attributes are known as statistics of attributes and their classification is said to be classification according to attributes. At the end when the data are classified on the basis of common characteristics or qualities of individual which can either be descriptive (such as literacy, sex, honesty, etc.) or numerical (such as weight, height, income, etc.), this classification is termed as classification according to attributes. Such classification can be simple classification or manifold classification. In simple classification we consider only one attribute and divide the universe into two classes—one class consisting of items possessing the given attribute and the other class consisting of items which do not possess the given attribute. (b) Classification according to class-intervals: Unlike descriptive characteristics, the numerical characteristics refer to quantitative phenomenon which can be measured through some statistical units. Data relating to income, production, age, weight, etc., come under this category. Such data are known as statistics of variables and are classified on the basis of class intervals. For example, the family income or per-capita income of the family where it can represent within a range 1000 to 2000 or 2001 to 3000. Those people income falls on these range they will be grouped together. In this way the entire data may be divided into a number of groups or classes or what are usually called, 'class-intervals'. Class limits may generally be stated in any of the following forms:

Exclusive type class intervals: They are usually stated as follows:

10–20
20–30
30–40
40–50

The above intervals should be read as under:

10 and under 20
20 and under 30
30 and under 40
40 and under 50

Thus, under the exclusive type class intervals, the items whose values are equal to the upper limit of a class are grouped in the next higher class. For example, an item whose value is exactly 30 would be put in 30–40 class interval and not in 20–30 class interval.

Inclusive type class intervals: They are usually stated as follows:

11–20
21–30
31–40
41–50

In inclusive type class intervals the upper limit of a class interval is also included in the concerning class interval. Thus, an item whose value

❖ **Tabulation:** Tabulation is the recording of the classified data in accurate mathematical terms; for example, marking and counting the frequency tallied. In simple tabulation there is an orderly arrangement of data in columns and rows. The arrangement of the assembled data has to be done in concise and logical order. Tabulation is tedious process where raw data is to be summarized and displayed in compact form, which can be done manually or by computer.

Tabulation is essential because of the following reasons:
1. It conserves space and reduces explanatory and descriptive statement to a minimum.
2. It facilitates the process of comparison.
3. It facilitates the summation of items and the detection of errors and omissions.
4. It provides a basis for various statistical computations.

Describing the Data

Descriptive statistics are used to describe the basic features of data to provide simple summaries about the sample and the measures used in a study. They form the basis of virtually every quantitative analysis of data and concern the development of certain indices from the raw data. Descriptive statistics are used to present quantitative descriptions in a manageable form. They are used to describe the main features of a collection of data in quantitative terms. Percentages, means of central tendency and means of dispersion are the examples of descriptive statistics.

Drawing the Inference of the Data or Inferential Statistics

Inferential statistics helps in drawing inferences from the data, e.g., finding the differences, relationship and association between two more variables by the help of the parametric and nonparametric statistical tests. The most commonly used inferential statistical tests are Z-test, t-test, ANOVA, chi-square tests, etc. An inference is a conclusion or judgment based on evidence and made cautiously with great care.

Interpretation of the Data

The critical examination of the analyzed study results to draw inferences and conclusion. Interpretation of the research findings of a study involves a search for their meaning in relation to the research problems, objectives, conceptual framework and hypothesis. This is an activity of critical thinking, which is done carefully through brainstorming to infer the condensed and statistically computed data.

Strategies for the Effective Interpretations

- Interpretation must be made in light of research problem, objectives, conceptual framework, hypotheses and assumptions.
- Critical examination of the each element of the study results before framing the interpretations.
- Careful consideration and recognition of the limitations of the research study so that inappropriate interpretations of the unstudied facts can be avoided.
- Each part, aspect and segment of the analyzed result must receive close attentions, so that misrepresentation can be avoided.

APPLICATION OF STATISTICS

Statistics is the study of the collection, analysis, interpretation, presentation, and organization of data. The role of statistics in research is to function as a tool in designing research, analyzing its data and drawing conclusions there from. Most research studies result in a large volume of raw data which must be suitably reduced so that the same can be read easily and can be used for further analysis. Statistical analysis helps researchers make sense of quantitative information.

Statistical procedures enable researchers to summarize, organize, evaluate, interpret, and communicate numeric information. Without statistics, quantitative data would be a chaotic mass of numbers.

Biostatistics is the branch of statistics responsible for the proper interpretation of scientific data generated in the biology, public health and other health sciences (i.e., the biomedical sciences).

DESCRIPTIVE STATISTICS

Descriptive statistics are brief descriptive coefficients that summarize a given data set, which can be either a representation of the entire or a sample of a population. Actually, when such indexes are calculated on data from a population, they are called parameters. A descriptive index from a sample is called a statistic. Research questions are about parameters, but researchers calculate statistics from the samples to estimate them, using inferential statistics to make inferences about the population. Descriptive statistics, in short, help describe and understand the features of a specific data set by giving short summaries about the sample and measures of the data. The descriptive statistics is calculated in the following forms:

- Measures to condense data
- Measures of central tendency
- Measures of dispersion
- Measures of relationship (correlation coefficient)

Measures to Condense Data

An appropriate presentation of data involves organization of data in such a manner that meaningful conclusions and inferences can drawn to answer the research question. Unsorted and ungrouped records do not allow us to draw clear conclusion. Measures to condense data include summarization of data, find out frequency distributions, find out percentage and graphic presentations of data. Quantitative data are generally condensed and presented through tables, charts, graphs and diagram.

Frequency Distribution

Frequency distribution in statistics provides the information of the number of occurrences (frequency) of distinct values distributed within a given period of time or interval, in a list, table, or graphical representation. The frequency of any value is the number of times that value appears in a data set. The frequency of any value is the number of times that value appears in a data set. Frequency distributions are the methods of organizing numeric data. A frequency distribution is a systematic arrangement of values from lowest to highest, together with a count of the number of times each value was obtained. The frequency distribution is classified into following types.

Types of Frequency Distribution

- Ungrouped frequency distribution
- Grouped frequency distribution
- Relative frequency distribution
- Cumulative frequency distribution
- Relative cumulative frequency distribution

Ungrouped Frequency Distribution

A frequency distribution can be shown on a **Table 10.1** or plotted on a chart which list only each data point and its frequency. Ungrouped frequency distribution consists of ungrouped data and is given as individual data points. The tables consist of two parts, i.e., observed values or measurements or any categorical variables and the frequency of cases at each value. Values are listed in numeric order in one column, and corresponding frequencies are listed in another. In frequency distributions, the categories or score values must be mutually exclusive and collectively exhaustive. The sum of numbers appearing in the frequency column must equal the sample size.

Table 10.1: Frequency distribution table with tally mark N=71.

Education of mothers	Tally mark	Frequency
No formal education	ⵉⵙ ⵉⵙ ⵉⵙ ⵉⵙ ⵉⵙ ⵉⵙ IIII IIII III	43
Primary	ⵉⵙ	5
Secondary	ⵉⵙ IIII IIII	14
Higher secondary	ⵉⵙ IIII	9
Graduation and above		

In **Table 10.1** education is a categorical variable and the total sample size is 71. The number of different categories are calculated by the researcher from the total sample and presented in the table by frequency as well as tally marks. This is a simple way to construct. First draw tally mark for each category when identified in the coding sheet. After four draw a cross mark to represent it as five. Then calculate the tally marks and write the frequency.

Grouped Frequency Distribution

To construct a grouped frequency distribution, the data are sorted and separated into groups called classes. Usually 5–20 classes are used, but in any case, make sure that you use enough classes to give a good description of the data. The number (frequency) of data belonging to each class is then recorded in a table of frequencies called a frequency table. This table describes the distribution of frequencies.

There are four rules for the classes in a grouped frequency distribution.
1. The classes must be mutually exclusive (non-overlapping). This means that there is no way that any of the data could fall into two different classes at once.
2. The classes must be continuous. This means that there can be no gaps in the classes. Even if there are no values in a particular class, you cannot omit that class unless it is the first or last class (in which case it should not have been included in the first place).
3. The classes must be exhaustive. This means that there must be a class for every data value in the data set so that every data value is included in the frequency distribution.
4. The classes must be of equal width, otherwise the frequency distribution would give a distorted view of the data. The class width is found by either subtracting the upper (or lower) class limit of one class from the upper (or lower) limit of the next class or by

subtracting the upper boundary from the lower boundary of any given class. Note that an exception is made for open-ended distributions that have no specific beginning or ending value. An example of the class limits for two such open-ended distributions are shown in **Table 10.2**.

Table 10.2: Frequency distribution table N=71.

Age of the mothers in year	Frequency
<21 years	15
21–25	17
26–30	20
31–35	17
>35 years	2

Relative Frequency Distribution

The frequency distribution is called relative frequency distribution when it is calculated in percentage. Generally in research the frequency distribution is calculated in percentage to give a clear idea about the data. When the sample size is too large and too small or whatever the sample size is the reviewer can analyze the result by seeing it if it will represents in percentage.

In this frequency distribution the researcher has to calculate percentage after calculating frequencies.

Cumulative Frequency Distribution

A cumulative frequency distribution is the sum of the class and all classes below it in a frequency distribution. Here for calculating the cumulative frequency the frequency of previous class interval will be added to the subsequent class intervals and the cumulative frequency can be plotted in the graph known as cumulative frequency curve or Ogive curve (**Table 10.3 and Fig. 10.2**).

Table 10.3: Cumulative frequency distribution table N= 174.

Knowledge score	Frequency	Cumulative frequency
1–4	0	0
5–8	6	6
9–12	21	27
13–16	20	47
17–20	20	67
21–24	4	71

Table 10.3 shows cumulative frequency distribution table.

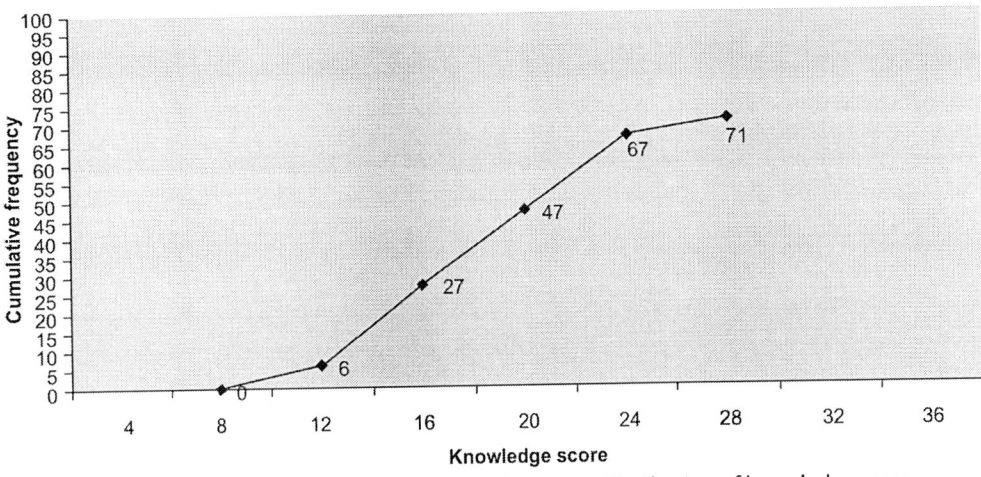

Fig. 10.2: Ogive curve showing cumulative frequency distribution of knowledge score.

Relative Cumulative Frequency Distribution

Relative cumulative frequencies (RCF) is calculated by dividing the cumulative frequency (CF) by total frequency and multiplying by 100 means the cumulative frequency percentage have to calculate. For relative cumulative frequency first we have to calculate frequency then cumulative frequency and cumulative frequency percentage. Like cumulative frequency distribution this relative cumulative frequency distribution can also be plotted on Ogive curve which is drawn below **(Table 10.4** and **Fig. 10.3)**.

Table 10.4: Cumulative frequency percentage distribution table.

Knowledge score	Frequency	Cumulative frequency	Cumulative frequency percentage
1–4	0	0	
5–8	6	6	8.44
9–12	21	27	37.5
13–16	20	47	66.2
17–20	20	67	94.36
21–24	4	71	100

Tabulation/Construction of Table

A table is a tabular representation of statistical data. Tabulation is the first step before data can be used for further statistical analysis and interpretation. The tabulation means the systematic presentation of the information contained in the data in rows and columns in accordance with some common features and characteristics. Rows are horizontal and columns are vertical arrangements.

General Principles of Tabulation

A table can be simple or complex depending upon the number or measurement of a single set or multiple set of items. Whether simple or complex there are certain general principles which

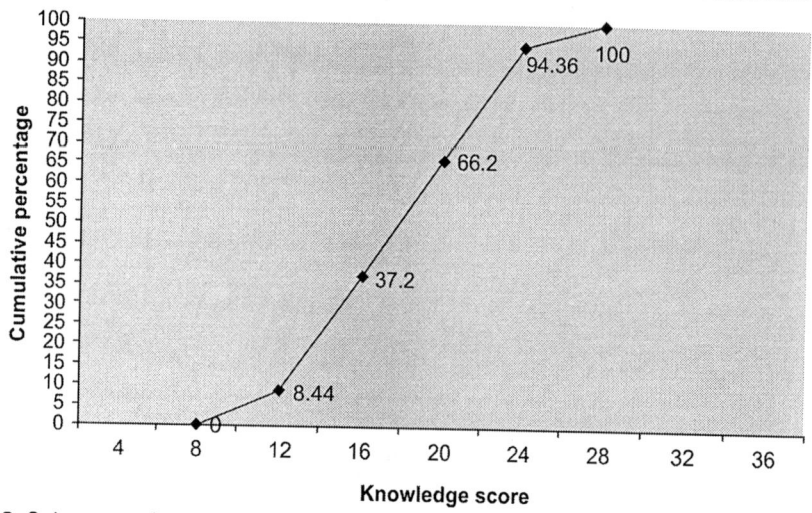

Fig 10.3: Ogive curve showing cumulative frequency percentage distribution of knowledge score.

must be kept in mind while designing table. Certain basic principles must be followed while presenting the data in the form of a statistical table; some of these are:
- The table should be precise, understandable, and self-explanatory.
- Every table should have title, which is placed at the top of the table. The title must describe the content clearly and precisely.
- Items should be arranged alphabetically or according to size, importance and casual relationship to facilitate comparison.
- Rows and columns are to be compared with one another, and should therefore have similar arrangement.
- The contents of the table, as a whole as well as item-wise in each column and row should be defined clearly and fully.
- The unit of measurement must be clearly stated.
- Percentage can be given in parenthesis or can be worked out to one decimal figure to draw the reader attention to the fact that the figure is a percentage and not an absolute number.
- Totals can be placed at the bottom of the columns.
- Explanatory cues can be placed directly beneath the table for any explanatory footnotes.
- Two or small tables are to be preferred to one large one.

Parts of Table

The various parts of table vary from problem-to-problem, depending upon the nature of the data and purpose of investigation. A good statistical table must contain:
- **Table number:** It should be placed at the top of the table.
- **Title:** Every table must have a suitable title. A title means brief and concise to describe about the content of the table. The content of table should be self-explanatory.
- **Subheads:** Subheadings is given just below the title in a prominent type usually enclosed in brackets for further description of the content of table.
- **Caption and stubs:** Captions are the headings or designate for vertical columns and stubs are the headings for horizontal rows.
- **Body of table:** Arrangement of the data according to description given in the form of captions and stubs compose the body of the table.
- **Footnotes:** When some characteristics or items of the table are not, or cannot be, adequately explained in the body of the table, footnotes are used to explain those items.

* **Source note:** It is used when secondary data is used, to mention the source from which these data are retrieved.

Types of the Table

Basically tables are of four types:
1. **Frequency distribution table:** These tables present the frequency and percentage distribution of the information collected, where an attribute is grouped number of classes, which may vary between three to eight classes. Too many or too few groups or classes may fail to reveal the salient features of the data. It should also be kept in mind that class or group intervals are kept constant. An example of a frequency distribution table **(Table 10.5)**.

Table 10.5: Sociodemographic variables of factory workers.

Sociodemographic variables of factory workers	N = 90	
	Frequency	Percentage
Age (in years)		
20–30	18	20
31–40	22	24.5
41–50	30	33.3
51–60	20	22.2
Gender		
Male	49	54.44
Female	41	45.56
Educational status		
Illiterate	18	20
Primary	22	24.5
High school	30	33.3
Higher secondary	20	22.2
Graduate and above	–	
Marital status		
Married	62	68.9
Unmarried	28	31.1
Habitat		
Urban	30	
Rural	40	
Religion		
Hindu	60	66.66
Muslims	15	16.67
Christian	15	16.67

2. **Contingency tables:** Tables that report on the frequency distribution of two nominal variables simultaneously and that include the totals are known as contingency tables. The categories considered should be mutually exclusive as well as exhaustive (i.e., observations cannot be beyond these categories). A contingency tables are also knows as cross-tables, which present the frequency distribution of two or more variables to establish the relationship or association between them. These tables could be 2 × 2, 2 × 3, and 3 × 3 depending on the number of variables on which the subjects are cross-classified. The number of subjects in a cell is called the cell frequency. These tables are generally used in chi-square test. Following is an example of a 2 × 2 contingency table **(Table 10.6)**.

Table 10.6: Presence of malnutrition according to their age.

Age in year	Malnutrition		Total f	χ² value
	Present	Absent		
0–2	391 (64.0)	32 (29.4)	423	45.87×
3–5	220 (36.0)	77 (70.6)	297	
Total	611	109	720	df = 1

3. *Multiple-response tables:* When classification of the cases is to be done into categories that are neither exclusive nor exhaustive, a multiple response table is used. For example, a patient can have two or more complaints, while say only the major ones may be listed. In such cases, the sum total of frequencies would exceed the total number of subjects and may lead to confusion. Therefore, the total number of subjects in cases of multiple responses is given as base, and from this we calculate the percentages. Example of a multiple-response table is presented in **Table 10.7**.

Table 10.7: Agewise distribution of health problems of geriatric people.

Age (in years)	HTN		DM		Insomnia		Obesity	
	Frequency	% age	Frequency	% age	Frequency	% age	Frequency	% age
60–70	60	50	55	45.83	40	33.33	38	31.66
Above 70	60	50	60	50	60	50	45	37.5

4. *Miscellaneous tables:* These tables are used present data other than frequency or percentage distributions, such mean, median, mode, range, standard deviation, and so on **(Table 10.8)**.

Table 10.8: Area wise distribution of mean, SD and mean % of knowledge score of mothers regarding prevention of malnutrition among under fives.

Sl. No.	Area	Max score	Mean	SD	Mean %
1.	Importance of nutrition among under fives	8	2.63	1.39	32.87
2.	Definition, cause and effect of malnutrition	4	1.00	0.78	25
3.	Antenatal care and breastfeeding	4	2.37	0.87	25
4.	Weaning	12	4.96	1.23	41.33
5.	Food hygiene	4	2.34	0.99	58.5
6.	Weight monitoring	5	2.41	0.88	48.2
7.	Prevention of common communicable disease	3	1.54	0.87	51.33
8.	Consequence of long-term untreated malnutrition	4	0.76	0.86	19

A table is called miscellaneous when the presentation of data cannot be classified under the frequency distribution table contingency table, or multiple response tables.

Graphs and Diagrams

Graphical Presentation of Data

The main reasons of using the diagrammatic and graphic representation of data are as follows:
- It is one of the most systematic and concise ways in which statistical results may be presented.
- They give overall view of entire data.
- The tabular appearance is easy to assimilate and more appealing than the same data or presented in text.
- The data becomes much easier to understand and memorize.
- It facilitates comparison of data represented in different columns and rows.

Constructing Diagrams/Graphs

While constructing a diagram or graph the following points should be considered:
- They must have a title, and an index.
- The proportion between width and height should be balanced.
- The selection of scale must appropriate.
- Footnotes may be included wherever they are needed.
- Principle of simplicity must be kept in mind.
- Neatness and cleanliness in construction of graph must be ensured.

Types of Diagram and Graph

The commonly used diagrams and graphs in the presentation of data of the research studies are bar diagram, pie chart, histogram, frequency polygon, line graphs, cumulative frequency curve, scattered diagrams, pictograms, map diagrams, etc.

Bar Diagram

Bar charts are used to create a visual display of the data from a table. The bars may be either horizontal or vertical. Bar charts are one of the easiest, graphically attractive and hence most commonly used methods of presenting all types of data. They are especially useful for representing various data series. The data series comprises the continuous variables while the values of the specific instances at which the value of the data series is measured represents the values of the discrete variables.

It is a convenient graphical device that is particularly useful for displaying nominal or ordinal data. It is an easy method adopted for visual comparison of the magnitude of different frequencies. Length of the bars drawn vertical or horizontal indicates the frequency of a character are called vertical bar charts (or column charts) if the bars are placed vertically. When the bars are placed horizontally, we get horizontal bar charts. There are three types of bar diagrams: (a) simple, (b) multiple, and (c) proportional bar diagram. Some points to be kept in mind while making a bar diagram are as follows:
- The width of bars should be uniform throughout the diagram.
- The gap between one bar and another should be uniform throughout.
- Bars may be vertical or horizontal.

Simple Bar Diagram

The simple bar chart is the 'simplest' bar chart which has one continuous variable charted along with one discrete variables used to display the data from a frequency distribution (one variable table). Each bar represents one value of the variable. It is classified on spatial, quantitative or temporal basis. In simple bar chart, we make bars of equal width but variable length, i.e., the magnitude of a quantity is represented by the height or length of the bars (**Fig. 10.4**).

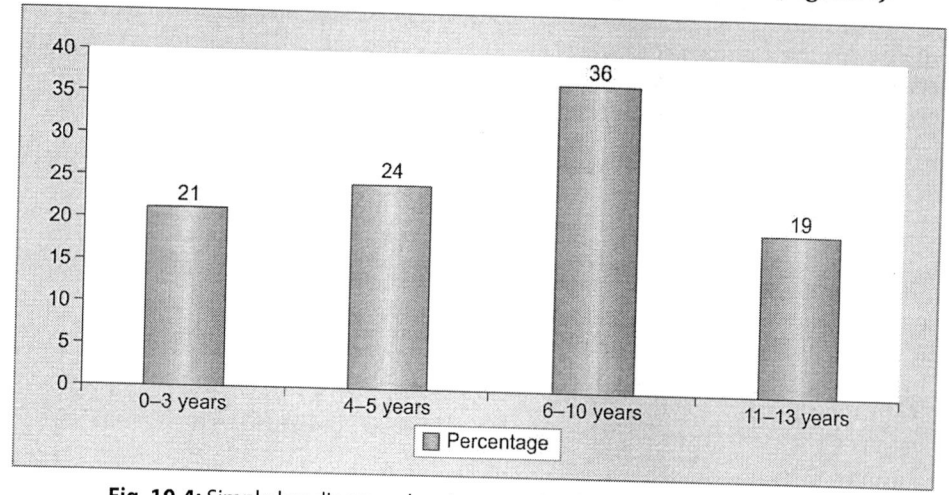

Fig. 10.4: Simple bar diagram showing agewise distribution of the children.

Multiple Bar Diagram

If two or more sets of continuous variables are to be shown on the same bar chart, we use what is called a composite or multiple bar diagram. **Figure 10.5** shows an example of the multiple bar diagram. This bar diagram depict the agewise and sexwise distribution of children. This bar diagram is quite convenient for comparing two or more sets of data.

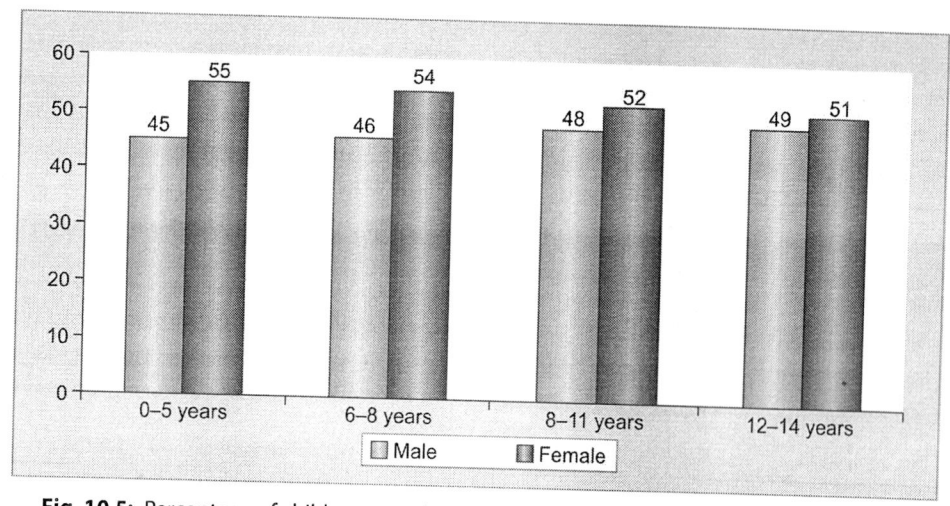

Fig. 10.5: Percentage of children according to their age and sex in a multiple bar diagram.

Proportion (Percentage) Bar Diagram

Proportion (percentage) bar diagram is a variant of bar diagram, in which all of the bars are pulled to the same height (100%) and show the components as percentages of the total rather than as actual values. This type of diagram is useful for comparing the contribution of different subgroups within the categories of the main variable (**Fig. 10.6**).

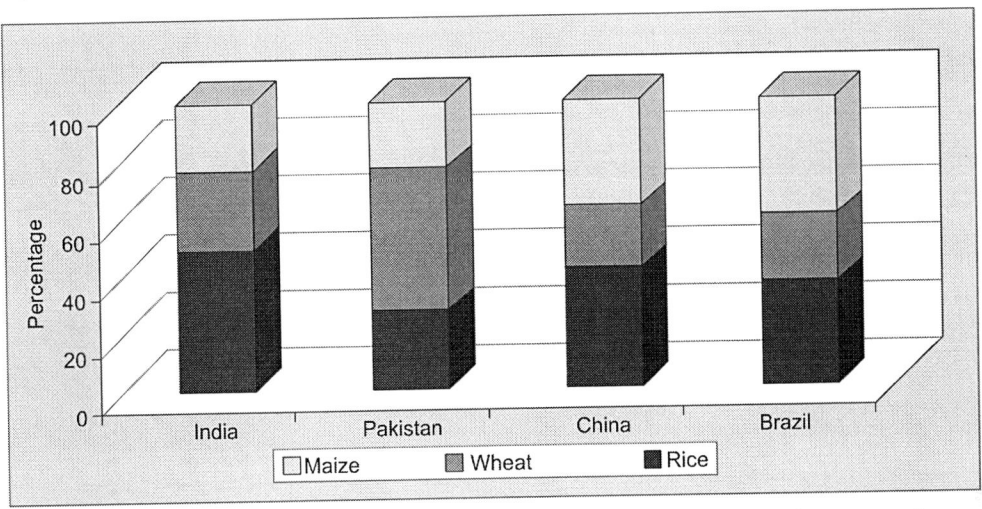

Fig. 10.6: Proportion (percentage) bar diagram on production of crops in different countries.

Pie Diagram or Sector Diagram (Fig. 10.7)

It is another useful pictorial device for presenting discrete data of qualitative characteristics, such as age group, gender, and occupational group in a population. The complete circle represents the entire data under consideration. Researcher must remember that only a percentage of data must be used to prepare a pie diagram. It gives comparative differences at a glance. The size of each angle is calculated by multiplying class percentage with 360 or a formula may be used, that is:

$$\text{Degree to be presented} = \frac{\text{Given \%}}{100} \times 360$$

Histogram

It is the most commonly used graphical representation of grouped frequency distribution. Variable characters of the different groups are indicated on the horizontal line (x-axis) and frequencies (number of observation) are indicated on the vertical line (y-axis). Frequency of each group forms a column or rectangle. Such a diagram is called 'histogram'. The area of rectangle is proportional to the frequency of the correspondence class interval and the total area of the histogram being proportional to the total frequency of all the class intervals. A histogram may be drawn by using the following steps:

* Set of vertical bars, the areas of which are proportional to frequencies represented.
* The difference of histogram from bar diagram is that bar diagram is one-dimensional and only length of bar has its significance while in histograms both length and width matters.
* When class intervals are equal, take frequency on y-axis, the variables on x-axis and construct adjacent rectangles.
* When the class intervals are unequal, a correction for unequal class intervals must be made.

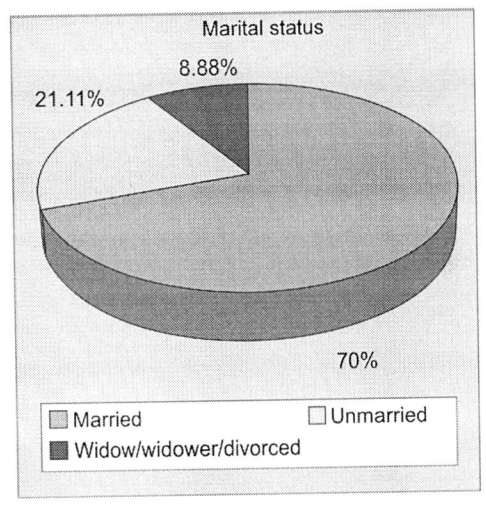

Fig. 10.7: Pie diagram showing percentagewise distribution of TB client according to their marital status.

In following **Table 10.9** frequency distribution is represented graphically in the form of histogram (**Fig .10.8**).

Table 10.9: Agewise distribution of male.

Age group (in years)	(15–20)	(20–25)	(25–30)	(30–35)	(35–40)
No. of males	15	20	40	60	50

Here, we will take classes boundaries along the horizontal axis and frequencies along with vertical axis.

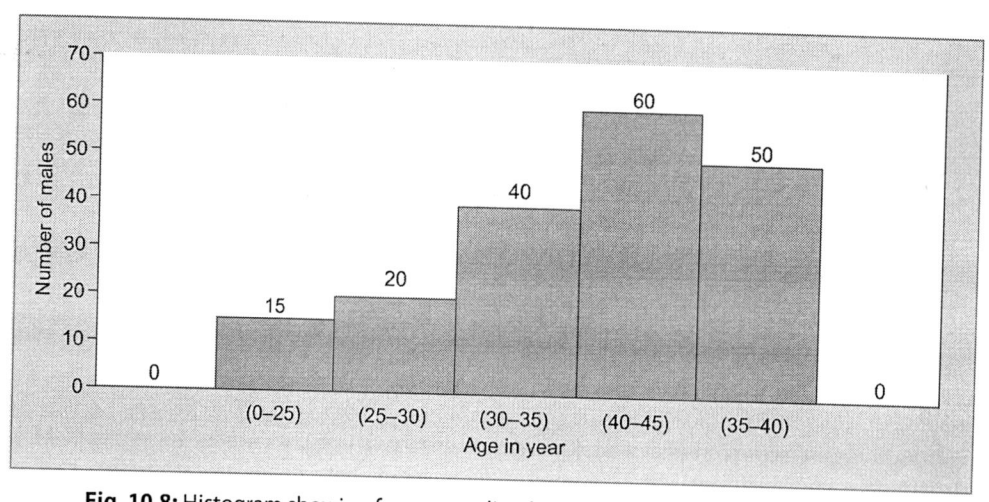

Fig. 10.8: Histogram showing frequency distribution of male according to their age.

Frequency Polygon

It is the curve obtained by joining the midpoints of the tops of the rectangles in a histogram by straight line. It gives a polygon, i.e., figure with many angles. In this, the two end points of the line drawn are joined to the horizontal axis at the midpoint of the empty class-intervals at both ends of the frequency distribution. Frequency polygons are simple and sketch an outline of data pattern more clearly than histograms. On same axis, one can plot frequency polygons of several distributions thereby making the comparisons possible. A histogram can be drawn by using following steps:

1. Draw the histogram of given data.
2. Join the midpoint of upper horizontal sides of each rectangle with adjacent one by a straight line.
3. Close the polygon at the both ends of distribution by extending them to baseline.
4. Hypothetical classes at the each end would have to be included each end with a frequency of zero.

The frequency polygon (**Fig. 10.9**) is drawn by considering following data.

Age group (in years)	(15–20)	(20–25)	(25–30)	(30–35)	(35–40)
No. of males	15	20	40	60	50

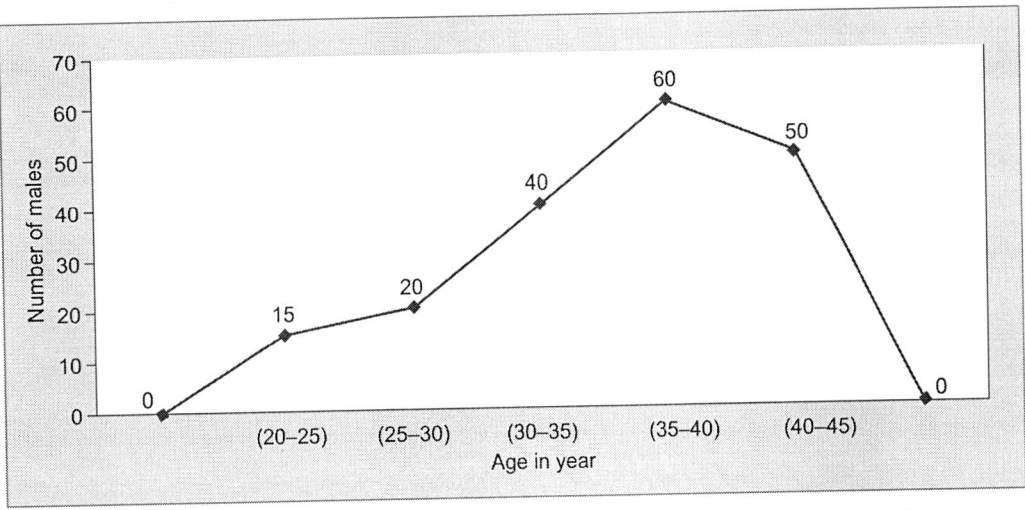

Fig. 10.9: Frequency polygon showing frequency distribution of male according to their age.

Line Graphs

In this, variables in the frequency polygon are depicting by line. It is mostly used where data is collected over a long period of time. On x-axis, values of independent variables are taken and values of dependent variables are taken on y-axis. Vertical axis may not start from zero, but at some point from where the frequency starts. With reference to x-axis and y-axis, the given data may be plotted and these consecutive points or data are then joined by straight lines (**Table 10.10** and **Fig. 10.10**).

Table 10.10: Timewise sale of cares in Delhi.

Year	2001	2002	2003	2004	2005	2006	2007
Sale of cares in Delhi (in thousands)	123	203	328	298	337	417	486
Sale of cares in Mumbai (in thousands)	456	402	387	347	342	307	298

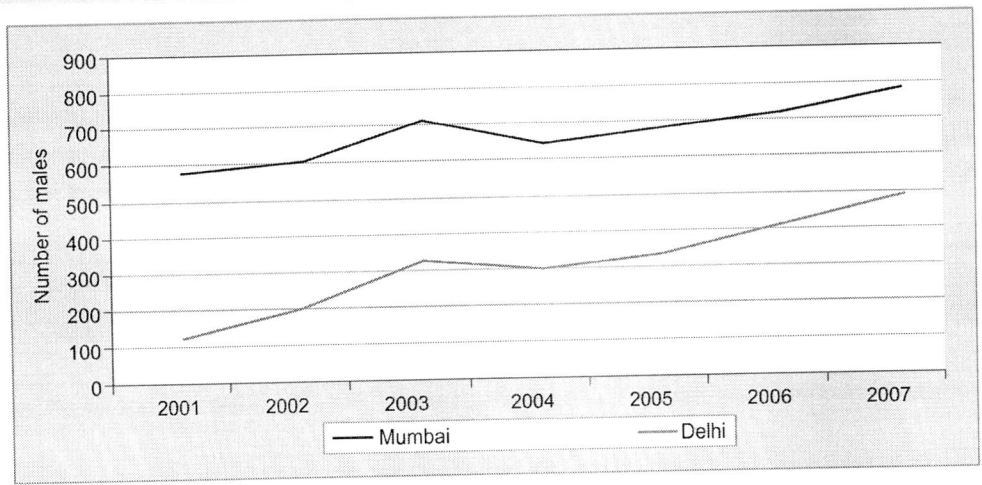

Fig. 10.10: Line graph showing comparison of the sale of cares between Mumbai and Delhi.

Cumulative Frequency Curve or Ogive

This graph represents the data of cumulative frequency distribution. For drawing Ogive, an ordinary frequency distribution table is converted into cumulative frequency table. The cumulative frequencies are then plotted corresponding to the midpoint of the class interval. The points corresponding to cumulative frequency at each upper limit of the classes are joined by a free-hand (S-shaped) curve. The diagram made is called Ogive curve **(Fig. 10.11)**. In **Figure 10.12** Ogive curve can also be drawn by plotting cumulative frequency percentage with class interval. **Table 10.11** shows cumulative frequency table.

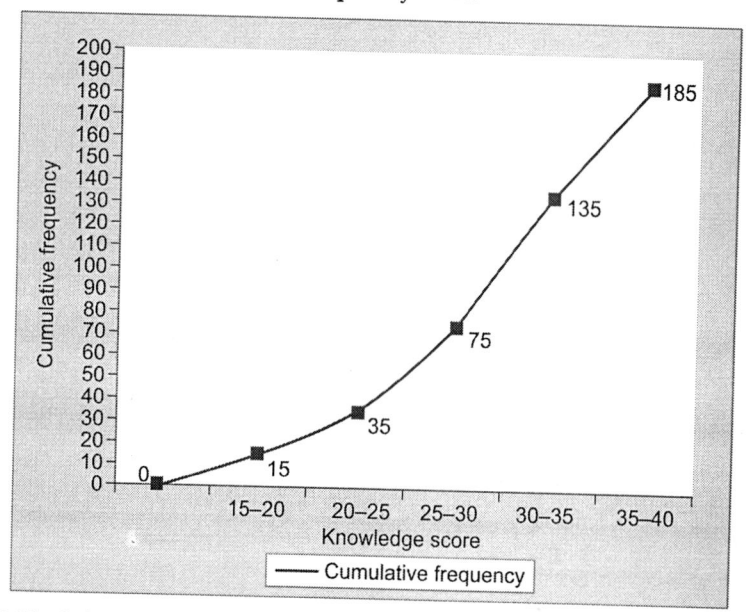

Fig. 10.11: Ogive curve showing cumulative frequency distribution of knowledge score.

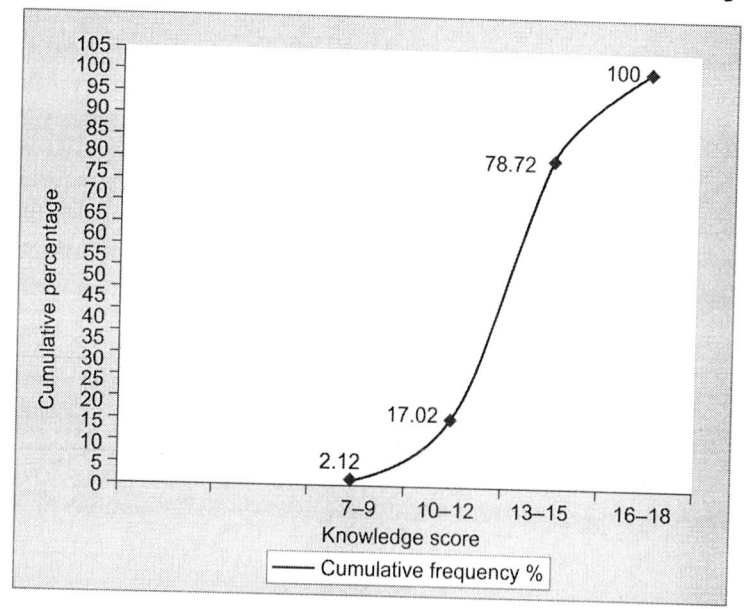

Fig. 10.12: Ogive curve showing cumulative frequency percentage distribution of knowledge score.

Table 10.11: Cumulative frequency table.

Age group (in years)	(15–20)	(20–25)	(25–30)	(30–35)	(35–40)
No. of males	15	20	40	60	50
Cumulative frequency	15	35	75	135	185

Scattered Diagrams

It is a graphic presentation, made to show the nature of correlation between two variable characters x and y on the same groups, such as height and weight in men aged 20 years. Therefore, it is also called correlation diagram. Example of a scattered or dotted diagrams is presented in **Figure 10.13**.

Pictograms or Picture Diagrams (Fig. 10.14)

This method is used to impress the frequency of the occurrence of events to common people such as attacks, deaths, number operations, admissions, accidents, and discharge in a population.

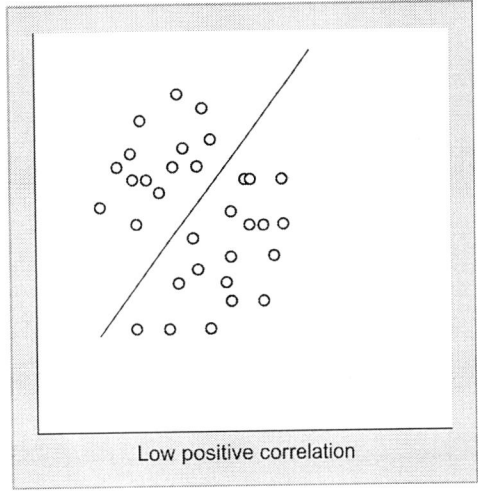

Fig. 10.13: Scatter diagram showing low positive correlation.

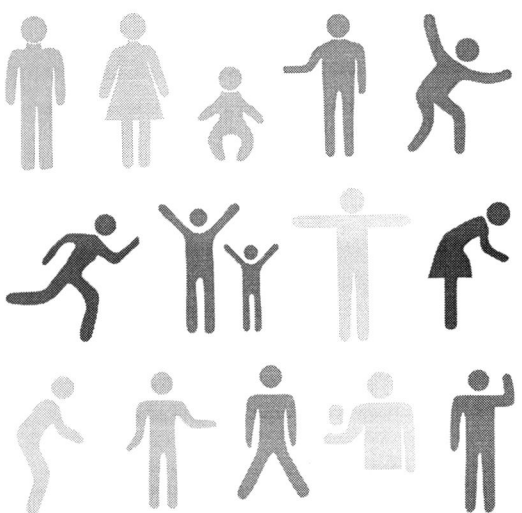

Fig. 10.14: Example of a pictogram.

Map Diagram or Spot Map

These maps are prepared to show geographical distribution of frequencies of characteristics, e.g., cases of an infectious disease. It is generally used in epidemiological investigation. The spot map can focuses on 'place' by showing where each of the known cases lives **(Fig. 10.15)**.

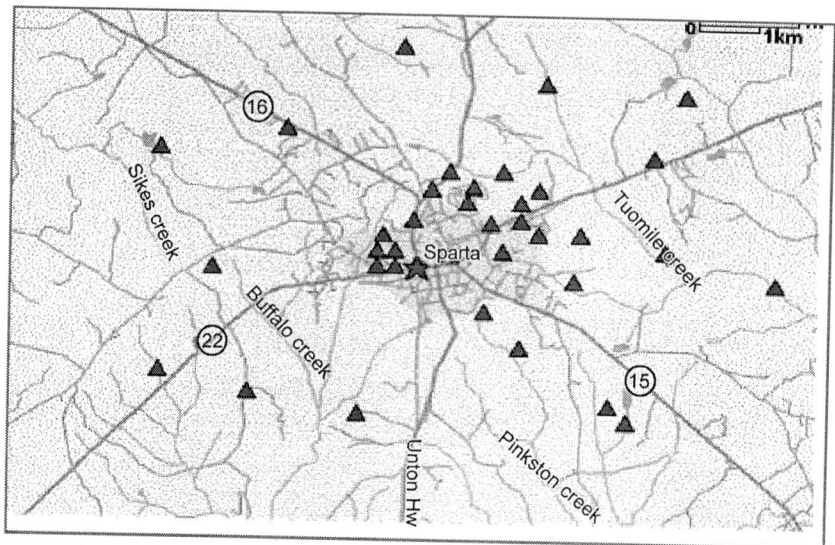

Fig. 10.15: The spot map showing the scattering of hepatitis at Sparta.

Limitations of Graphs

Some of the drawbacks of graphs may be as follows:
- Confusing (may be false or true).
- Present only quantitative aspect.
- Getting limited information on only one or two aspects or characteristics under study.
- They can present only approximate values.
- Easily misinterpreted.

Measures of Central Tendency

One of the most important objectives of statistical analysis is to get one single value that describe the characteristics of the entire mass of unwieldy data. Such a value is called central value or average. When a researcher collects the values of any characteristic, like hemoglobin percentage from a large population, he/she can see that the observation values cluster around a central value. This property of concentration of the value round a central value is known as central tendency. The central value around which there is a concentration is called the measure of central tendency. By calculating the measures of central tendency, we can find a single value to represent the whole data. It also helps us to compare the value of two or more groups.

Definition

- According to Ya-Chou, 'The average is sometimes described as a typical value in the sense that it is sometimes employed to represent the entire individual in a series of a variable'.
- According to Croxton and Cowden, 'An average value is a single value within the range of the data that is used to represent all of the value of series. Since an average is somewhere within the range of data, it is also called a measure of central value'.

Objectives of Central Value

- To get a single value that describes the characteristics of the entire group.
- To facilitate comparisons.

Requisites of Good Averaging

- Easy to understand
- Simple to compute
- Based on all the items
- Not be unduly affected by the extreme observations
- Rigidly defined
- Capable of further algebraic treatment
- Sampling stabilities

Important Measures of Central Tendency

- Arithmetic mean
- Median
- Mode
- Geometric mean
- Harmonic mean

Arithmetic Mean (AM)

The arithmetic mean (or mean or average) is the most commonly used and readily understood measure of central tendency. In statistics, the term average refers to any of the measures of central tendency. The arithmetic mean is defined as being equal to the sum of the numerical values of each and every observation divided by the total number of observations. It is represented by $\bar{x}$.

Arithmetic mean can be calculate in three different types of series:

Arithmetic Mean in Individual Series

The arithmetic mean of a variable is often denoted by a bar, for example, as in $\bar{x}$ (read x bar), which is the mean of the n values $x_1, x_2,..., x_n$. The process of computing mean in case of individual series (i.e., where frequencies are not given) is very simple. The various values of the variable will be added and divided by the number of items.

$$\bar{x} = \frac{x_1 + x_2 + x_3 \ldots \ldots x_n}{n}$$

$$\Rightarrow \bar{x} = \frac{1}{n}\sum_{i=1}^{n} x_i$$

Arithmetic Mean in Discrete Series

If $x_1, x_2,\ldots x_n$ are the n items and $f_1, f_2,\ldots f_n$ are the corresponding frequencies, then the mean is given by,

$$\bar{x} = \frac{f_1 x_1 + f_2 x_2 + f_3 x_3 \ldots \ldots + f_n x_n}{\sum f}$$

$$\text{Mean } (\bar{x}) = \frac{\sum_{i=1}^{n} f_i x_i}{\sum_{i=1}^{n} f_i}$$

Example: From the following data of the marks obtained by 60 students of a class **(Table 10.12)**.

Marks	20	30	40	50	60	70
No. of students	8	12	20	10	6	4

Table 10.12: Data of the marks obtained by 60 students.

Marks (x)	No. of students (f)	fx
20	8	160
30	12	360
40	20	800
50	10	500
60	6	360
70	4	280
	N = 60	$\sum fx = 2{,}460$

$$\Rightarrow \bar{x} = \frac{2{,}460}{60} = 41$$

Arithmetic Mean in Continuous Series

In the case of continuous series, we use the same formula as in discrete series. In this case, mid values will be taken as m.

Mid value = (lower limit + upper limit)/2

If $m_1, m_2, m_3, \ldots, m_n$ are 'n' midpoints of the classes and $f_1, f_2, f_3, \ldots, f_n$ be the corresponding frequencies then the arithmetic mean is defined as

$$\Rightarrow \bar{x} = \frac{\sum_{i=1}^{n} f_i m_i}{\sum_{i=1}^{n} f_i}$$

where, m_i is the midpoint of the 'i' th class.

Question 1: Find the mean of the following marks.

Class	0–10	10–20	20–30	30–40	40–50
F	4	6	13	6	1

Solution:

Table 10.13: The calculation of mean of a continuous class interval.

Class	f	m	fm
0–10	4	5	20
10–20	6	15	90
20–30	13	25	325
30–40	6	35	210
40–50	1	45	45
Total	30		690

$\Sigma fm = 690$ and $\Sigma f = 30$

The mean is given by

$$\bar{x} = \frac{f_1 m_1 + f_2 m_2 + f_3 m_3 \ldots + f n m n}{\Sigma f}$$

$= 690/30$

$= 23$

Mean = 23

Merits of Arithmetic Mean

- Arithmetic mean is most popular among averages used in statistical analysis.
- It is very simple to understand and easy to calculate.
- The calculation of AM is based on all the observations in the series.
- The AM is responsible for further algebraic treatment.
- It is strictly defined.
- It provides a good means of comparison.
- It has more sampling stability.

Demerits of Arithmetic Mean

- The AM is affected by the extreme values in a series.
- In case of a missing observation in a series it is not possible to calculate the AM.
- In case frequency distribution with open end classes the calculation of AM is theoretically impossible.
- The arithmetic mean is an unsuitable average for qualitative data.

Median

The median is the middle most or central value of the observations made on a variable when the values are arranged either in ascending order or descending order. As distinct from the arithmetic mean which is calculated from each and every item in the series, the median is what is called 'positional average'. The term position refers to the place of value in a series. The place of the median in a series is such that an equal number of items lie on either side of it, i.e., it splits the observations into two halves.

Calculation of Median in Individual Series

Step 1: Arrange the data in ascending or descending order of magnitude.

Step 2: If the number of observations is odd then median is the $\frac{n+1}{2}$ th observation in the arranged order.

Step 3: If the number of observations is even then the median is the mean of $\frac{n}{2}$ th and $\left(\frac{n}{2}+1\right)$ th observations in the arranged order.

Example: Let us find the median of following series
3, 13, 7, 5, 21, 23, 39, 23, 40, 23, 14, 12, 56, 23, 29

Step 1: First data has arranged in ascending order
3, 5, 7, 12, 13, 14, 21, 23, 23, 23, 23, 29, 39, 40, 56.

There are fifteen numbers. The middle number is the eighth number which is 23. The median value of this series is 23. But, with an even amount of numbers things are slightly different.

In that case we find the middle pair of numbers, and then find the value that is half way between them. This is easily done by adding them together and dividing by two.

Example: 29, 38, 39, 39, 40, 45, 54, 55, 56, 56, 57, 59, 60, 60.

Here for this series the total there are fourteen numbers and the series has arranged in ascending order. For this series the median is 54 + 55/2 = 54.5.

Calculation of Median in Discrete Series (Table 10.14)

Steps to calculate

- Arrange the data in ascending or descending order
- Find cumulative frequencies
- Apply the formula median is the $\frac{n+1}{2}$ th item, where $N = \Sigma f$
- Note the cumulative frequency either equal or just more than $\frac{n+1}{2}$ th item
- Locate the value of the variable corresponding to that cumulative frequency. This is the value of median:

Marks	20	30	40	50	60	70
No. of students	8	12	20	10	6	4

Table 10.14: The calculation of median in discrete series.

Marks (x)	No. of students (f)	cf
20	8	8
30	12	20
40	20	40
50	10	50
60	6	56
70	4	60
	N = 60	

N/2 = 60/2
= 30
Here, median is the corresponding terms of cumulative frequency 40 which is also 40. Hence, median is 40.

Computation of Median in Continuous Series

The median of a continuous series can be calculated by the below interpolation formula.
Median = (For continuous frequency distribution)

$$\text{Median} = L + \frac{N/2 - cf}{f} \times i$$

Where,
L = lower limit of the median class
f = frequency corresponding to the median class
N = total frequency
cf = cumulative frequency of the class preceding to the median class
i = size of median class

Merits

- The median is useful in case of frequency distribution with open-end classes.
- The median is recommended if distribution has unequal classes.
- Extreme values do not affect the median as strongly as they affect the mean.
- It is the most appropriate average in dealing with qualitative data.
- The value of median can be determined graphically whereas the value of mean cannot be determined graphically.
- It is easy to calculate and understand.

Demerits

- For calculating median it is necessary to arrange the data, whereas other averages do not need arrangement.
- Since it is a positional average its value is not determined by all the observations in the series.
- Median is not capable for further algebraic calculations.
- The sampling stability of the median is less as compared to mean.

Mode

The mode or the modal value is that value in a series of observations which occurs with the greatest frequency. The mode of a discrete probability distribution is the value x at which its probability mass function takes its maximum value. In other words, it is the value that is most likely to be sampled. The mode of a continuous probability distribution is the value x at which its probability density function has its maximum value, so the mode is at the peak. The mode of a sample is the element that occurs most often in the collection. For example, the mode of the sample [1, 3, 6, 6, 6, 7, 7, 12, 12, 17] is 6.

The mode of the series 3, 5, 8, 5, 4, 5, 9, 3 would be 5.
In certain cases there may not be a mode or there may be more than one mode.

Example:
1. 40, 44, 57, 78, 84 (no mode)
2. 3, 4, 5, 5, 4, 2, 1 (modes 4 and 5)
3. 8, 8, 8, 8, 8 (no mode)

A series of data which having one mode is called 'unimodal' and a series of data which having two modes is called 'bimodal'. It may also have several modes and be called 'multimodal'.

Calculation of Mode in Discrete Series

Simple Inspection Method

In a discrete series the value of the variable against which the frequency is the largest, would be the modal value.

Example:

Age	5	7	10	12	15	18
No. of boys	4	6	20	7	5	3

From the above data we can clearly say that mode is 10 because 10 has occurred maximum number of times, i.e., 20.

In discrete series, arithmetic mode can be determined by inspection and finding the variable which has the highest frequency associated with it. However, when there is very less difference between the maximum frequency and the frequency preceding it or succeeding it, then grouping table method is used.

Grouping and Analysis Table Method

This method is practically applied when the below problems occurs.
❖ When the difference between the maximum frequency and the frequency preceding it or succeeding it is very small.

Process

In order to find mode, a grouping table and an analysis table are to be prepared in the following manner.

Grouping Table

A grouping table consists of 6 columns.
❖ Arrange the values in ascending order and write down their corresponding frequencies in the column 1.
❖ In column 2 the frequencies are grouped into two's and added.
❖ In column 3 the frequencies are grouped into two's, leaving the first frequency and added.
❖ In column 4 the frequencies are grouped into three's, and added.
❖ In column 5 the frequencies are grouped into three's, leaving the first frequency and added.
❖ In column 6 the frequencies are grouped into three's, leaving the first and second frequencies and added.
❖ Now in each these columns mark the highest total with a circle.

Chapter 10: Analysis of Data and Application of Biostatistics in Nursing Research

Analysis Table

After preparing a grouping table, prepare an analysis table. While preparing this table take the column numbers as rows and the values of the variable as columns. Now for each column number see the highest total in the grouping table (which is marked with a circle) and mark the corresponding values of the variable to which the frequencies are related by using bars in the relevant boxes. Now the value of the variable (class) which gets the highest number of bars is the modal value (modal class).

Example: Find the mode of the following series.

Table 10.15: Calculation of mode in discrete series.

Size of the item	Frequency	Size of the item	Frequency
5	48	13	52
6	52	14	41
7	56	15	57
8	60	16	63
9	63	17	52
10	57	18	48
11	55	19	40
12	50	—	—

Solution:

Table 10.16: Location of mode by grouping.

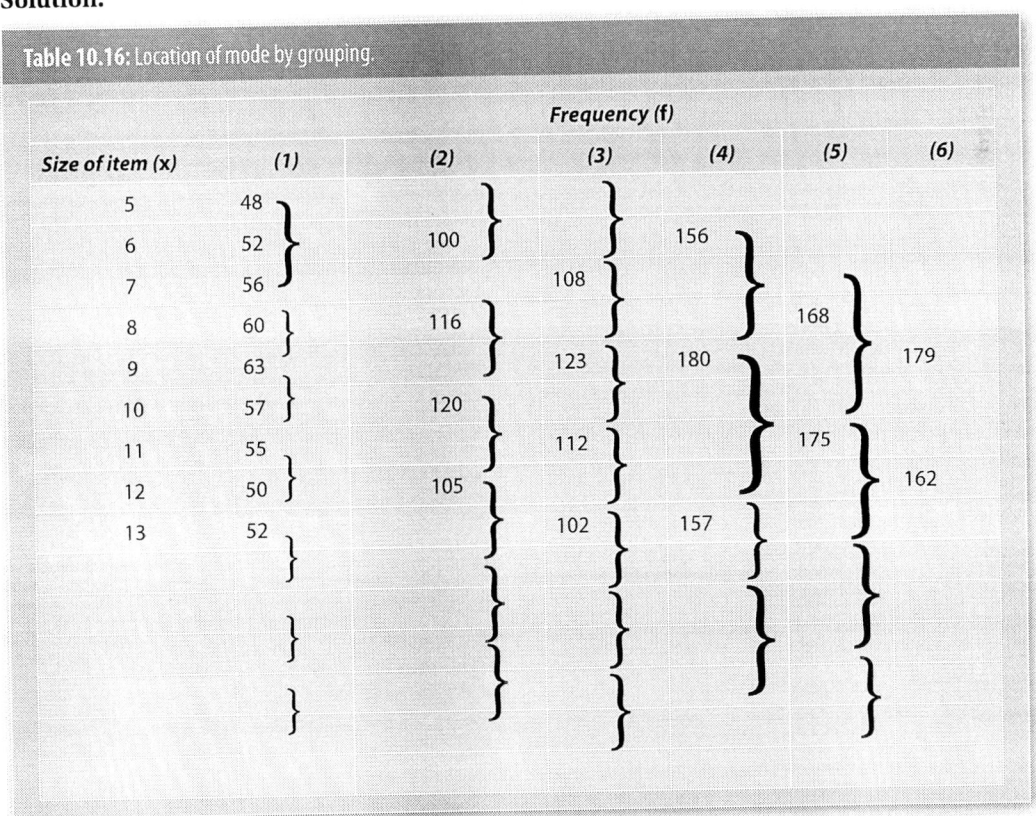

The frequencies in column 1 are first added in two's in column 2 and leaving first frequency and then add two in column 3. Then they are added in three's in columns 4, leaving first frequency and then add threes in column 5 and leaving first two frequencies add three's for column 6. The maximum frequency in each column is identified. It will be observed that mode changes with the change in grouping. Thus according to column 1 mode should be 9 or 16. To find out maximum concentration the data can be arranged in the shape table as follows **(Table 10.17)**:

Table 10.17: Analysis table.

Columns	Size of item containing maximum frequency							
1			9					16
2			9	10			15	16
3		8	9					
4		8	9	10				
5			9	10	11			
6	7	8	9					
	1	3	6	3	1		1	2

Number of times a size of the item occurs is considered as mode. Since the size 9 occurs the largest number of times it is the modal size or mode is 9.

If we look at the frequencies in the original table, we shall find that the frequency of 63, which is the maximum single frequency, is against two values, 9 and 16. The series thus appears to be bimodal but the process of grouping leads us to the conclusion that the concentration of items round 9 is more than the concentration round 16. Even if the frequency against 16 was 64 instead of 63 probably grouping would have disclosed that the concentration of items round about 9 is more, even though the individual frequency against 9 is only 63. It is thus never safe to rely only on the inspection of a series and to locate the mode at the point of maximum frequency. Mode is affected by the frequencies of the neighboring items also, and, therefore, grouping is essential, as it reveals the true point of maximum concentration.

Calculation of Mode in Continuous Series

In a continuous series, to find out the mode we need one step more than those used for discrete series. As explained in the discrete series, modal class is determined by inspection or by preparing grouping and analysis tables. Then we apply the following formula.

$$\text{Mode } (M_0) = l_1 + \frac{f_1 - f_0}{2f_1 - f_0 - f_2} \times i \quad \text{Or} \quad l_1 + \frac{\Delta_1}{\Delta_1 + \Delta_2} \times i$$

Where,

$\Delta_1 = f_1 - f_0$

$\Delta_2 = f_1 - f_2$

l_1 = lower limit of the modal class.
f_1 = frequency of the modal class.
f_0 = frequency of then class preceding to the modal class.
f_2 = frequency of the class succeeding to the modal class.
i = size of the class.

Example: The scores of 40 BSc Nursing students in research from 100 is given below. Find out the mode.

Table 10.18: Mode in a continuous series.

Marks	30–40	40–50	50–60	60–70	70–80	80–90
Students	4	5	8	9	9	5

Solution:

CI	f
30–40	4
40–50	5
50–60	8
60–70	11
70–80	7
80–90	5

By inspection it was confirm that the modal class is 60–70.

$$Mo = l_1 + \frac{f_1 - f_0}{2f_1 - f_0 - f_2} \times i$$

$$60 + \frac{11 - 8}{22 - 8 - 7} = 60 + \frac{3}{7} = 60.42$$

∴ Mode of the modal class is 60.42.

Note:
- While applying the above formula for calculating mode, it is necessary to see that the class intervals are uniform throughout. If they are unequal they should first made equal on the assumption that the frequencies are equally distributed throughout.
- In case of bimodal distribution the mode cannot be found.

Finding Mode in Case of Bimodal Distribution

In a bimodal distribution the value of mode cannot be determined by the help of the above formulae. In this case the mode can be determined by using the empirical relation given below.

Mode = 3 Median – 2 Mean

And the mode which is obtained by using the above relation is called 'Empirical mode'.

Merits

- It is easy to calculate and simple to understand.
- It is not affected by the extreme values.
- The value of mode can be determined graphically.
- Its value can be determined in case of open-end class interval.
- The mode is the most representative of the distribution.

Demerits

- It is not suitable for further mathematical treatments.
- The value of mode cannot always be determined.
- The value of mode is not based on each and every items of the series.
- The mode is strictly defined.
- It is difficult to calculate when one of the observations is zero or the sum of the observations is zero.

Empirical Relation between Mean, Median and Mode

The relationship between mean, median and mode depends upon the nature of the distribution. A distribution may be symmetrical or asymmetrical.

In asymmetrical distribution the mean, median and mode are equal
i.e., **Mean(AM) = Median(M) = Mode(Mo)**

In a highly asymmetrical distribution it is not possible to find a relationship among the averages. But in a moderately asymmetric distribution the difference between the mean and mode is three times the difference between the mean and median.

i.e., **Mean − Mode = 3 (Mean − Median)**
Mean − mode = 3 mean − 3 median
− Mode = 2 mean − 3 median
Mode = 3 median − 2 mean

Geometric Mean

A geometric mean (GM), unlike an arithmetic mean, tends to dampen the effect of very high or low values, which might bias the mean if a straight average (arithmetic mean) were calculated. This is helpful when analyzing bacteria concentrations, because levels may vary anywhere from 10 to 10,000 fold over a given period.

The nth root of the product of n numbers. The average of the logarithmic values of a data set, converted back to a base 10 number. Geometric mean is often used to evaluate data covering several orders of magnitude, and sometimes for evaluating ratios, percentage changes, or other data sets bounded by zero.

The easiest way to think of the geometric mean is that it is **the average of the logarithmic values, converted back to a base 10 number**.

However, the actual formula and definition of the geometric mean is that it is the nth root of the product of n numbers, or

Geometric Mean = nth root of $(x_1)(x_2)...(x_n)$

Where x_1, x_2, etc., represent the individual data points, and n is the total number of data points used in the calculation.

Calculation of GM in Individual Series

If $x_1, x_2, x_3, ..., x_n$ be n observations studied on a variable x, then the GM of the observations is defined as:

$$GM = (x_1 x_2 x_3........x_n)^{1/n}$$

Let us take an example
Find the GM of 2, 16, 32, 64
= $(2 \times 16 \times 32 \times 64)^{1/4}$

$2 = 2^1$
$16 = 2^4$
$32 = 2^5$
$64 = 2^6$
$(2 \times 16 \times 32 \times 64)^{1/4}$
$= (2^1 \times 2^4 \times 2^5 \times 2^6)^{1/4} = (2^{16})^{1/4} = 2^4$
$= 16$

Applying log both sides $\log GM = \dfrac{1}{n} \log(x_1, x_2 \ldots x_n)$

$= \dfrac{1}{n}[\log x_1 + \log x_2 + \ldots + \log x_n]$

$= \dfrac{1}{n}\sum_{i=1}^{n} \log x_i$

$\Rightarrow GM = antilog\left(\dfrac{1}{n}\sum_{i=1}^{n} \log x_i\right)$

Calculation of GM in Discrete Series

If $x_1, x_2, x_3, \ldots, x_n$ be n observations of a variable x with frequencies respective $f_1, f_2, f_3, \ldots, f_n$ then the GM is defined as:

$$GM = \left(x_1^{f_1} x_2^{f_2} x_3^{f_3} \ldots x_n^{f_n}\right)^{1/N} \qquad (i)$$

Where, $N = \sum_{i=1}^{n} f_i$ i.e. total frequency

Applying log both sides in the equation (i), we get

$GM = antilog\left(\dfrac{1}{N}\sum_{i=1}^{n} f_i \log x_i\right)$

Calculation of GM in Continuous Series

In continuous series the GM is calculated by replacing the value of x_i by the midpoints of the class, i.e., m, (median).

$GM = antilog\left(\dfrac{1}{N}\sum_{i=1}^{n} f_i \log m_i\right)$

Where, m_i is the mid value of the i th class interval.

Harmonic Mean

The harmonic mean (HM) is defined as the reciprocal of the arithmetic mean of the reciprocal of the individual observations.

Calculation of HM in Individual Series

If $x_1, x_2, x_3, \ldots, x_n$ be 'n' observations of a variable x then harmonic mean is defined as:

$$HM = \dfrac{n}{\dfrac{1}{x_1} + \dfrac{1}{x_2} + \ldots + \dfrac{1}{x_n}}$$

$$\Rightarrow HM = \dfrac{n}{\sum\limits_{i=1}^{n} \dfrac{1}{x_i}}$$

Calculation of HM in Discrete Series

If $x_1, x_2, x_3, \ldots, x_n$ be 'n' observations occurs with frequencies $f_1, f_2, f_3, \ldots, f_n$ respectively then HM is defined as:

$$HM = \dfrac{\sum\limits_{i=1}^{n} f_i}{\dfrac{f_1}{x_1} + \dfrac{f_2}{x_2} + \ldots + \dfrac{f_n}{x_n}}$$

(ii)

$$\Rightarrow HM = \dfrac{\sum\limits_{i=1}^{n} f_i}{\sum\limits_{i=1}^{n} \dfrac{f_i}{m_i}}$$

Calculation of HM in Continuous Series

In continuous series HM can be calculated by replacing mid values (m_i) in place of x_i's in the equation (ii). Hence, HM is given by

$$\Rightarrow HM = \dfrac{\sum\limits_{i=1}^{n} f_i}{\sum\limits_{i=1}^{n} \dfrac{f_i}{m_i}}, \text{ where } m_i \text{ is the mid value of the } i\text{th class interval}$$

Uses

- The HM is used for computing the average rate of increase in profits of a concern.
- The HM is used to calculate the average speed at which a journey has been performed.

Merits

- Its value is based on all the observations of the data.
- It is less affected by the extreme values.
- It is suitable for further mathematical treatment.
- It is strictly defined.

Demerits

- It is not simple to calculate and easy to understand.
- It cannot be calculated if one of the observations is zero.
- The HM is always less than AM and GM.

Relation between AM, GM, and HM

The relation between AM, GM, and HM is given by

$$AM \geq GM \geq HM$$

Measures of Dispersion

The measures of central tendencies (i.e., means) indicate the general magnitude of the data and locate only the center of a distribution of measures. They do not establish the degree of variability or the spread out or scatter of the individual items and their deviation from (or the difference with) the means. Two distributions of statistical data may be symmetrical and have common means, medians and modes and identical frequencies in the modal class. Yet with these points in common they may differ widely in the scatter or in their values about the measures of central tendencies.' An average alone does not tell all the aspects of the series. It is hardly fully representative of a mass, unless we know the manner in which the individual item scatter around it. A further description of a series is necessary, if we are to gauge how representative the average is. From this discussion it concludes that emphasis should be given on the scatter or variability which is known as dispersion. In statistics, dispersion (also called variability, scatter, or spread) denotes how stretched or squeezed a distribution. There are different types of dispersion. They are as follows:

- The range
- Mean deviation
- Quartile deviation
- Variance
- Standard deviation

Range

The simplest methods of measuring dispersion is range. In any statistical series, the difference between the largest and the smallest values is called as the range. Range is quite a useful indication of how spread out the data is, but it has some serious limitations. This is because sometimes data can have outliers that are widely off the other data points. In these cases, the range might not give a true indication of the spread of data. It is extremely sensitive to outliers. A single data value can greatly affect the value of the range. In a lot of cases, however, data is closely clustered and if the number of observations is very large, then it can give a good sense of data distribution. Sometimes, we define range in such a way so as to eliminate the outliers and extreme points in the data set.

Thus, range (R) = L − S $\begin{cases} L = \text{Largest value of the series} \\ S = \text{Smallest value of the series} \end{cases}$

Coefficient of range: The relative measure of the range. It is used in the comparative study of the dispersion coefficient of range = $\frac{L - S}{L + S}$.

Example: (Individual series) find the range and the coefficient of the range of the following items: 110, 117, 140, 197, 200, 100, 100, 178, 255, 790.
Solution: R = L − S = 790 − 100 = 690
Coefficient of Range = L − S/L + S
= 690/890
= 0.775

Example: (Continuous series) find the range and its coefficient from the following data.

Table 10.19: Data table for range.

The weight in (kg) are	55–60	60–65	65–70	70–75	75–80
Frequency	20	11	9	12	8

Solution: R = L − S = 80 − 55 = 25

$$\text{Coefficient of range} = \frac{L-S}{L+S} = \frac{80-55}{80+55} = 0.185$$

Merits

- The simplest method among all methods of dispersion.
- Easy to calculate.
- Give quick and accurate result.
- Useful in evaluating quality control in health care service or some other situation where we have to project the total difference.

Limitations

- Not based on each and every observation.
- It is subject to fluctuation of considerable magnitude from sample-to-sample.
- Does not tells us the character of distribution.
- The range takes no accounts of the form of distribution only it shows the difference between lower and higher limits. So two totally different series range may be same if only the lower and upper limits are same. Hence, it is most unreliable measure of dispersion.

Percentile

A **percentile** (or a **centile**) is a measure used in statistics indicating the value below which a given percentage of observations in a group of observations fall. For example, the 20th percentile is the value (or score) below which 20% of the observations may be found. The nth percentile is that value (or size) such that n% of values of the whole data lies below it. For example, a score of 7% from the topmost score would be 93 the percentile as it is above 93% of the other scores.

Percentile range: It is used as one of the measure of dispersion. It is a set of data and is defined as = $P_{90} - P_{10}$ where P_{90} and P_{10} are the 90th and 10th percentile respectively. The semi-percentile range, i.e., $P_{90} - P_{10}/2$ can also be used but it is not common in use.

Quartiles

If we concentrate on two extreme values (as in the case of range), we do not get any idea about the scatter of the data within the range (i.e., the two extreme values). If we discard these two values the limited range thus available might be more informative. For this reason the concept of interquartile range is developed. It is the range which includes middle 50% of the distribution. Here, 1/4th (one quarter of the lower end) and 1/4th (one quarter of the upper end) of the observations are excluded.

Quartile is that value which divides the total distribution into four equal parts. So, there are three quartiles, i.e., Q_1, Q_2 and Q_3. Q_1, Q_2 and Q_3 are termed as first quartile, second quartile and third quartile or lower quartile, middle quartile and upper quartile respectively. Q_1 (quartile one)

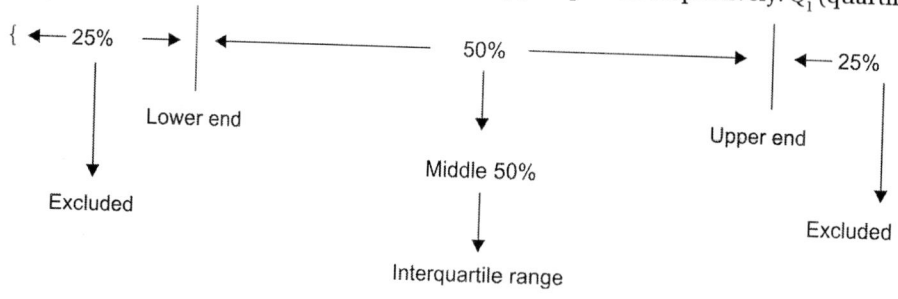

covers the first 25% items of the series and it divides the first half of the series into two equal parts. Q_2 (quartile two) is the median or middle value of the series and Q_3 (quartile three) covers 75% items of the series.

Quartile Deviation

It is based on the lower quartile Q_1 and the upper quartile Q_3. Quartile deviation (QD) means the semivariation between the upper quartiles (Q_3) and lower quartiles (Q_1) in a distribution. The difference Q_3-Q_1 is referred as the interquartile range. The difference divided by 2 is called semiinterquartile or the quartile deviation. Thus,

$$QD = \frac{Q_3 - Q_1}{2}$$

The quartile deviation is a slightly better measure of absolute dispersion than the range. But it ignores the observation on the tails. If we take difference samples from a population and calculate their quartile deviations, their values are quite likely to be sufficiently different. This is called sampling fluctuation. It is not a popular measure of dispersion. The quartile deviation calculated from the sample data does not help us to draw any conclusion (inference) about the quartile deviation in the population.

Coefficient of Quartile Deviation

A relative measure of dispersion based on the quartile deviation is called the coefficient of quartile deviation. It is defined as coefficient of quartile.
Coefficient of quartile deviation =

$$\frac{Q_3 - Q_1}{Q_3 - Q_1}$$

Calculation of Quartiles

The calculation of quartiles is done exactly in the same manner as it is in case of the calculation of median.

In case of individual and discrete series

Q_1 = Size of $\frac{i(N+1)}{4}$ th item of the series

$i = 1, 2, 3$

In Case of Continuous Series

Q_1 = Size of $\frac{iN}{4}$ th item of the series, $i = 1, 2, 3$

Interpolation formula for continuous series

$$Q_i = l_1 + \frac{l_2 - l_1}{f}\left(\frac{iN}{4} - c\right) \quad i = 1, 2, 3$$

Where,
l_1 = Lower limit of ith quartile class
l_2 = Upper limit of ith quartile class
c = Cumulative frequency preceding the ith quartile class
f = Frequency of ith quartile class.

Example:
Find the Q_1 and Q_3 of the following:
(a) 4, 5, 6, 7, 8, 9, 12, 13, 15, 10, 20

Answer:
(a) Values of the variable are in ascending order:
i.e. 4, 5, 6, 7, 8, 9, 10, 12, 13, 15, 20, So N = 11 (no. of values)

Q_1 = Size of $\frac{(N+1)}{4}$ th item of the series
= size of 3rd item = 6

Q_3 = Size of $\frac{3(N+1)}{4}$ th item of the series
= size of 9th item = 13

∴ Required Q_1 and Q_3 are 6 and 13 respectively.

Advantages

- Can be directly determined in case of open end class intervals without knowing the lower limit of lowest class and upper limit of the largest class.
- Can be calculated easily in absence of some data in a series.
- Not affected very much by the extreme items.
- Can be located graphically.

Disadvantages

- This are not easily understood by a common man. These are not well-defined and easy to calculate.
- This are not based on all the observations of a series.
- This cannot be computed if items are not given in ascending or descending order.
- This is affected very much by the fluctuation of sampling.
- The computation is not so easy in case of continuous series as the formula of interpolation is to be used.

Mean Deviation

Average deviations (mean deviation) is the average amount of variations (scatter) of the items in a distribution from either the mean or the median or the mode, average of absolute differences (differences expressed without plus or minus sign) between each value in a set of values, and the average of all values of that set. For example, the average (arithmetic mean or mean) of the set of values 1, 2, 3, 4, and 5 is (15 ÷ 5) or 3. The difference between this average (3) and the values in the set is 2, 1, 0, -1, and -2; the absolute difference being 2, 1, 0, 1, and 2. The average of these numbers (6 ÷ 5) is 1.2 which is the mean deviation. Also called mean absolute deviation, it is used as a measure of dispersion where the number of values or quantities is small, otherwise standard deviation is used.

Individual series: The mean deviation is calculated either from mean or median, but only median is preferred because when the signs are ignored, the sum of deviation of the sets taken from median is minimum. For calculating mean deviation the following steps can be followed **(Table 10. 20).**

Step 1: Find the mean or median of the given series.
Step 2: Find the **distance** of each value from that mean, median or mode. So using any one of three, find the deviations (differences) of the items of the series from them. The ith variable is x_i.
i.e. $x_i - \bar{x}$, x–Me
    Me = Median
Step 3: Find the absolute values of these deviations, i.e. ignore their positive (+) and negative (–) signs.
i.e. $|x_i - \bar{x}|, |x_i - Me|$
Step 4: Find the sum of these absolute deviations.
i.e. $\Sigma|x_i - \bar{x}|, \Sigma|x_i - Me|$
Step 5: Find the mean of those distances. The mean deviation can be calculated from the mean and median. The formula for mean deviation from mean and mean deviation from median are, respectively.

$$MD = \frac{\Sigma|x_1 - \bar{x}|}{N} \text{ and } \frac{\Sigma|x_1 - Me|}{N}$$

Note that:
* Generally MD obtained from the median is the best for the practical purpose.
* Coefficient of MD = MD/$\bar{x}$ or MD/Me

Example: Calculate mean deviation and its coefficient from median for a group of people having height in centimeter is: 140, 145, 143, 147, 149, 150, 152, 144, 156, 154, 158
Arranging in ascending order 140, 143, 144, 145, 147, 149, 150, 152, 154, 156, 158
Me = $\frac{n+1}{2}$ th term $n = 11$. So median is the sixth term which is 149.

Table 10.20: Calculation of mean deviation from median in individual series.

Sl. No.	Variables (x_i)	$|x_i - Me|$
1	140	9
2	145	4
3	143	6
4	147	2
5	149	0
6	150	1
7	152	3
8	144	5
9	156	7
10	154	5
11	158	9
		$\Sigma|x_i - Me| = 51$

$$MD = \frac{\Sigma |x_i - Me|}{N} = \frac{51}{11}$$

$$= 4.63$$

Coefficient of $MD = \frac{MD}{Me} = \frac{4.63}{49} = .09$

Another example of calculation of mean deviation from discrete series (Table 10.21).

Solution:

Table 10.21: Calculation of mean deviation from discrete series.

Size (x_i)	Frequency (f)	Cf	$|x_i - Me|$	$|x_i - Me|$
4	2	2	$|8-4| = 4$	$2 \times 4 = 8$
6	4	2+4 = 6	$|8-6| = 2$	$4 \times 2 = 8$
8	5	6+5 = 11	$|8-8| = 0$	$5 \times 0 = 0$
10	3	11+3 = 14	$|8-10| = 2$	$3 \times 2 = 6$
12	2	14+2 = 16	$|8-12| = 4$	$2 \times 4 = 8$
14	1	16+1 = 17	$|8-14| = 6$	$1 \times 6 = 6$
16	4	17+4 = 21	$|8-16| = 8$	$4 \times 8 = 32$
	n = 21			$|x_i - Me| = 68$

Calculations:

i. Median (Me) = Size of $\left(\frac{n+1}{2}\right)^{th}$ item $21\ 1^{th}$

= size $\left(\frac{21+1}{2}\right)^{th}$ item

= Size of 11th item.
Therefore, Median (Me) = 8

ii. $MD = \frac{\Sigma |x_i - Me|}{N} = \frac{68}{21} = 3.24$

Example: (Continuous series) calculate the mean deviation and the coefficient of mean deviation from the following data by using the mean **(Table 10.22).**
The number of patients admitted in a hospital.

Table 10.22: Calculation of the mean deviation in a continuous series.

Diff. age (in years)	No. of patients
0–5	449
5–10	705
10–15	507
15–20	281
20–25	109
25–30	52
30–35	16
35–40	4

Solution

Diff. age (in years)	Mid-values (x̄)	Frequency (f)	fx_i	|x_i - x̄|	f_i|x_i - x̄|
0–5	2.5	449	1122.5	8	3592
5–10	7.5	705	5287.5	3	2115
10–15	12.5	507	6337.5	2	1014
15–20	17.5	281	4917.5	7	1967
20–25	22.5	109	2452.5	12	1308
25–30	27.5	52	1430.0	17	884
30–35	32.5	16	520.0	22	352
35–40	37.5	4	150.0	27	108
		n = 2123	Σfx_i = 22217.5		Σf|x_i - x̄| = 11,340

Calculation

❖ $\bar{x} = \dfrac{\sum f_i x_i}{n} = \dfrac{22217.5}{2123} = 10.5 \text{ (approx.)}$

❖ $MD = \dfrac{\sum f_i |x_i - \bar{x}|}{n} = \dfrac{11440}{2123} = 5.4$

❖ Coefficient of MD $= \dfrac{M.D.}{\bar{x}} = \dfrac{5.4}{10.5} = 0.514$

Variance

The term variance was used to describe the square of the standard deviation. The concept of variance is of great importance in advanced work where it is possible to split the total into several parts, each attributable to one of the factors causing variations in their original series. The variance of a set of values, which we denote by σ^2. Variance is defined as follows: For individual series

$$\text{Variance} = \dfrac{\sum (x_i - \bar{x})^2}{n}$$

For grouped data is defined as $\sigma^2 = \sum f(x - \bar{x})^2 / n$ where $\bar{x}$ is the mean, x stands for each data value in turn, and f is the frequency with which data value, x, occurs. Note that $\sum f = n$.

The most important measure of variability is based on deviations of individual observations about the central value. For this purpose the mean usually serves as the center. Variance is the average squared deviation from the mean of a set of data. Variance measures how far a set of numbers is spread out. A variance of zero indicates that all the values are identical. Variance is always non-negative: The smaller the value of the variance indicates the more the cases are concentrated around the value of the mean the data points tend to be very close to the mean and hence to each other, while a high variance indicates that the data points are very spread out around the mean and from each other.

There are two distinct concepts that are both called 'variance'. One variance is a characteristic of a set of observations. The other is part of a theoretical probability distribution and is defined by an equation. When variance is calculated from observations, those observations are either measured from a real world system or generated by a theoretical probability distribution or other generating model. If all possible observations of the system are present then the calculated variance is called the population variance. Normally, however, only a subset is available, and the variance calculated from this is called the sample variance. The variance calculated from a sample is considered an estimate of the full population variance.

The population variance is the mean squared deviation from the population mean:

$$\sigma^2 = \frac{\sum_{i=1}^{N}(x_i - \mu)}{N}$$

Where,

σ^2 = the population variance
μ = the population mean
N = the total number of values in the population
x_i = the value of the ith observation
$\sum$ = a summation

Sample variance is defined as the sum of the squared deviations divided by $n-1$ which is computed to estimate the population variance.

The sample variance is calculated as follows:

$$s^2 = \frac{\sum_{i=1}^{N}(x_i - \bar{x})}{n-1}$$

Where,

s^2 = the sample variance
$\bar{x}$ = the sample mean
n = the total number of values in the sample
x_i = the value of the ith observation
$\sum$ = a summation

Sometime there is a doubt coming to mind why in sample variance we are dividing $n-1$ instead of n. This is because a sample is only part of the population and is not actually the whole picture. Because of that, statisticians found a way to compensate, by subtracting one from the total number of numbers in the data set. Also, variance will never be a negative number. Variance can only be zero if all of the numbers in the data set are the same. This is because there is zero difference in the numbers.

Standard Deviation

The standard deviation (SD) also represented by the Greek letter sigma σ or the Latin letter s) is a measure that is used to quantify the amount of variation or dispersion of a set of data values. Standard deviation is a measure of the dispersion of a set of data from its mean; more spread-apart data has a higher deviation. Standard deviation is calculated as the square root of variance.

The standard deviation gives researchers and statisticians an idea of how closely the data has fallen around the expected result. A low standard deviation indicates that the data points tend to be close to the mean (also called the expected value) of the set, while a high standard deviation indicates that the data points are spread out over a wider range of values. The standard deviation of a random variable, statistical population, data set, or probability distribution is the square root of its variance.

Thus, $SD = \sqrt{\dfrac{\sum (x_i - \bar{x})^2}{n}}$ for the ungrouped data.

Where, $\sum$ means 'sum of', x is a value in the data set, $\bar{x}$ is the mean of the data set, and n is the number of data points.

The standard deviation can be also calculated in grouped data. For the grouped data the formula for $SD = \sqrt{\dfrac{\sum f_i (x_i - \bar{x})^2}{n}}$ for the grouped data

where, $n = \sum f_i$

The steps for calculating standard deviation is as follows:

Step 1: Find the mean.
Step 2: For each data point, find the square of its distance to the mean.
Step 3: Sum the values from Step 2.
Step 4: Divide by the number of data points.
Step 5: Take the square root.

In case of grouped data we have to add the frequency column and the frequency will multiply with the square of its distance to the mean then we have to find the submission of all multiplication values. Then we have to divide by the number of data points and take the square root of whole.

Types

There are two different calculations for the SD: (i) Population standard deviation and (ii) Sample standard deviation. Which formula you use depends upon whether the values in your if some staff nurses are selected by using random sampling technique then sample standard will be used.

Population Standard Deviation

The standard deviation of a population gives researchers the amount of dispersion of data for an entire population of survey respondents. A population standard deviation represents a parameter, not a statistic. Parameters refer to a numerical property of a population. A statistic, conversely, means that a number can be computed from data. Researchers use statistics to estimate parameters. Population standard deviation dataset represent the standard deviation for the entire population. For example, if all staff nurses of a medical college hospital has been studied in such cases population standard deviation can be used.

The population standard deviation formula is:

$$\sigma = \sqrt{\dfrac{\sum (x - \mu)^2}{n}}$$

where,

σ = population standard deviation
Σ = represents the sum of
μ = population mean
n = number of scores in sample

Sample Standard Deviation

A standard deviation of a sample estimates the standard deviation of a population based on a random sample. The sample standard deviation, unlike the population standard deviation, is a statistic that measures the dispersion of the data around the sample mean. In statistics, 'mean' equals the average of a set of numbers; to obtain the mean, researchers add together a list of numbers and divide the total by the amount of numbers on the list. When a sample has been selected from a larger population then sample standard deviation has been used. For example, a study conducted on the attitude of nursing students towards patient care in Government Nursing School, Odisha. Here the students will be selected by following random sampling techniques from different Nursing Schools, Odisha. The sample standard deviation will represent the sample standard of whole population. To calculate the sample standard deviation, researchers divide the squared deviations by the number of data sets minus 1, then take the square root.

The **sample standard deviation formula** is:

$$s = \sqrt{\frac{\sum(x-\bar{x})^2}{n-1}}$$

where,

s = sample standard deviation
Σ = represents the sum of
$\bar{x}$ = sample mean
n = number of scores in sample

Merits

- It is rigidly defined and based on all observations.
- It is amenable for most prominently used in further statistical work. For example, in computing skewness, correlation, etc., use is made of standard deviation.
- It is not affected by sampling fluctuations of sampling than most other measures of dispersion.
- It is keynote in sampling and provides a unit of measurement for the normal distribution.
- It is less erratic.
- It is possible to calculate the combined standard deviation of two or more groups. This is not possible with any other measure.
- For comparing the variability of two or more distribution coefficient of variation is considered to be most appropriate and this is based on mean standard deviation.

Demerits

- It is difficult to understand and calculate.
- It gives greater weight to extreme values.

Measures of Relationship

Coefficient of Variation (CV)

To compare the variations (dispersion) of two different series, relative measures of standard deviation must be calculated. This is known as coefficient of variation or the coefficient of SD.
Its formula is:

$$CV = \frac{\sigma x}{\bar{x}} \times 100$$

Thus, it is defined as the ratio SD to its mean.

Remark: It is given as a percentage and is used to compare the consistency or variability of two more series. The higher the CV, the higher the variability and lower the CV, the higher is the consistency of the data.

Example: Calculate the standard deviation and its coefficient from the following data.

Table 10.23: Calculation of the standard deviation in individual series example.

A	10
B	12
C	16
D	8
E	25
F	30
G	14
H	11
I	13
J	11

Solution:

Table 10.24: Calculation of the standard deviation solution.

No.	x_i	$(x_i - \bar{x})$	$(x_i - \bar{x})^2$
A	10	−5	25
B	12	−3	9
C	16	+1	1
D	8	−7	49
E	25	+10	100
F	30	+15	225
G	14	−1	1
H	11	−5	16
I	13	−2	4
J	11	−4	16
n = 10	$\sum x_i = 150$		$\sum = |x_i - \bar{x}|^2 = 446$

Calculations

$$\bar{x} = \frac{\sum x_i}{n} = \frac{150}{10} = 15$$

$$SD(\sigma x) = \sqrt{\frac{\sum(x_i - \bar{x})^2}{n}} = \sqrt{\frac{446}{10}} = 6.7$$

$$\text{coefficient of SD} = \frac{\sigma x}{\bar{x}} = \frac{6.7}{15} = 0.45$$

Example: Calculate SD of the marks of 100 students **(Table 10.25)**.

Table 10.25: Calculation of the standard deviation in continuous series.

Marks	No. of students (f_i)	Mid-values (x_i)	$f_i x_i$	$f_i x_i^2$
0–2	10	1	10	10
2–4	20	3	60	180
4–6	35	5	175	875
6–8	30	7	210	1,470
8–10	5	9	45	405
	n = 100		$\sum f_i x_i = 500$	$\sum f_i x_i^2 = 2,940$

Solution:

$$\bar{x} = \frac{\sum f_i x_i^2}{n} = \frac{5,990}{1,000} = 5.99$$

$$SD(\sigma x) = \sqrt{\frac{\sum f_i x_i^2 - (x)^2}{n}} = \sqrt{\frac{38,770}{1000} - (5.99)^2}$$

$$= \sqrt{38.77 - 35.88} = \sqrt{2.89} = 1.7$$

Example: Calculate SD of the marks of 100 students.

Marks	No. of students (f_i)	Mid-values (x_i)	$f_i x_i$	$f_i x_i^2$
0–2	10	1	10	10
2–4	20	3	60	180
4–6	35	5	175	875
6–8	30	7	210	1,470
8–10	5	9	45	405
	n = 100		$\sum f_i x_i = 500$	$\sum f_i x_i^2 = 2,940$

Solution

- $\bar{x} = \dfrac{\sum f_i x_i}{n} = \dfrac{500}{1{,}000} = 0.5$

- $SD\ (\sigma x) = \sqrt{\dfrac{\sum f_i x_i^2 - (xy)^2}{n}}$

$= \sqrt{\dfrac{2{,}940}{100} - (5)^2} = \sqrt{29.40 - 25} = \sqrt{4.40}$

$x = 2.21$

Combined standard deviation: If two sets containing n_1 and n_2 items having means x_1 and x_2 and standard deviations σ_1 and σ_2 respectively are taken together then,

- Mean of the combined data is $\bar{x} = \dfrac{n_1 \bar{x}_1 + n_2 \bar{x}_2}{n_1 + n_2}$

- SD of the combined set is $\sigma = \sqrt{\dfrac{n_1(\sigma_1^2 + d_1^2) + n_2(\sigma_2^2 + d_2^2)}{n_1 + n_2}}$

Where, $d_1 = \bar{x}$ and $d_2 = \bar{x}_2 - \bar{x}$

Correlation

In conducting research the researcher has to find out the relationship between different variables. For example, when a researcher conducting a study on assessing the knowledge and practice of mothers of infants regarding supplementary feeding, here the researcher will analyzes whether the relationship between knowledge and practice of mothers of infants regarding supplementary feeding by using correlation analysis. Correlation is a statistical tool that helps to measure and analyze the degree of relationship between two variables. Correlation analysis deals with finding out the association between two or more variables. Correlation often used as means for prediction, which tells us how related two variables are. Generally, causation always implies correlation but correlation does not necessarily implies causation because there is the third variable possibility, i.e., there may be additional variable(s) that are causing the two things you are investigating to be related to each other. A correlation coefficient is a coefficient that illustrates a quantitative measure of some type of correlation and dependence, meaning statistical relationships between two or more random variables or observed data values.

Types of Correlation

The researcher classified the correlation as follows:
- **Positive correlation:** The correlation is said to be positive correlation if the values of two variables changing with same direction. If x and y have a positive linear correlation, it indicates a relationship between x and y variables such that as values for x increases, values for y also increase, e.g., height and weight.
- **Negative correlation:** The correlation is said to be negative correlation when the values of variables change with opposite direction. Negative values indicate a relationship between x and y such that as when the values of x increase, the values of y decrease, e.g., anxiety and result score in examination.

- ❖ **No correlation:** If there is no linear correlation or a weak linear correlation, r is close to 0. A value near zero means that there is a random, nonlinear relationship between the two variables.
- ❖ **Linear correlation:** Correlation is said to be linear when the direction of a linear relationship between two variables exists means the amount of change in one variable tends to bear a constant ratio to the amount of change in the other. The graph of the variables having a linear relationship will form a straight line.
- ❖ **Nonlinear correlation:** The correlation would be nonlinear if the direction of a linear relationship between two variables does not exist means the amount of change in one variable does not bear a constant ratio to the amount of change in the other variable.
- ❖ **Simple correlation:** Under simple correlation problem there are only two variables are studied.
- ❖ **Multiple correlation:** Under multiple correlation three or more than three variables are studied.
- ❖ **Partial correlation:** Analysis recognizes more than two variables but considers only two variables keeping the other constant.
- ❖ **Total correlation:** This is based on all the relevant variables, which is normally not feasible.

Correlation can directly display in scatter diagram or it can be find out by computing correlation coefficient.

Scatter Diagram

Scatter diagram is a graph of observed plotted points where each points represents the values of x and y as a coordinate. It portrays the relationship between these two variables graphically. Scatter points are not joined and there is no frequency table. If the data points make a straight line going from the origin out to high x- and y-values, then the variables are said to have a positive correlation. If the line goes from a high-value on the y-axis down to a high-value on the x-axis, the variables have a negative correlation. A perfect positive correlation is given the value of 1. A perfect negative correlation is given the value of -1. If there is absolutely no correlation present the value given is 0. The closer the number is to 1 or -1, the stronger the correlation, or the stronger the relationship between the variables. The closer the number is to 0, the weaker the correlation. So something that seems to kind of correlate in a positive direction might have a value of 0.67, whereas something with an extremely weak negative correlation might have the value (**Figs. 10.16 A to G**).

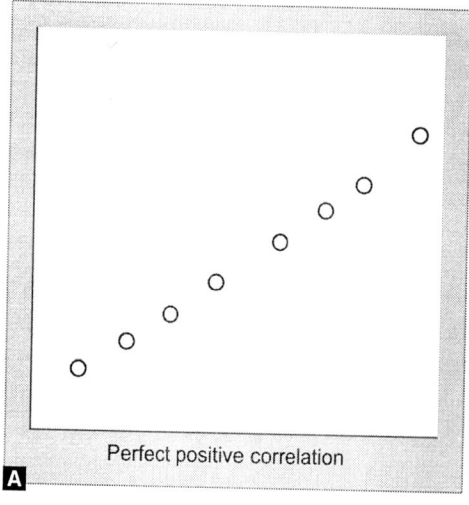
Perfect positive correlation
A

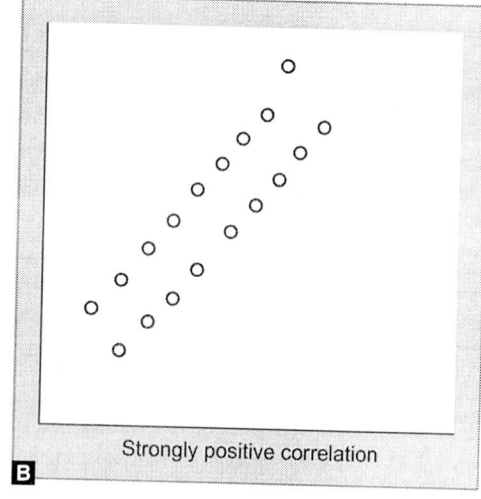
Strongly positive correlation
B

Figs. 10.16A and B

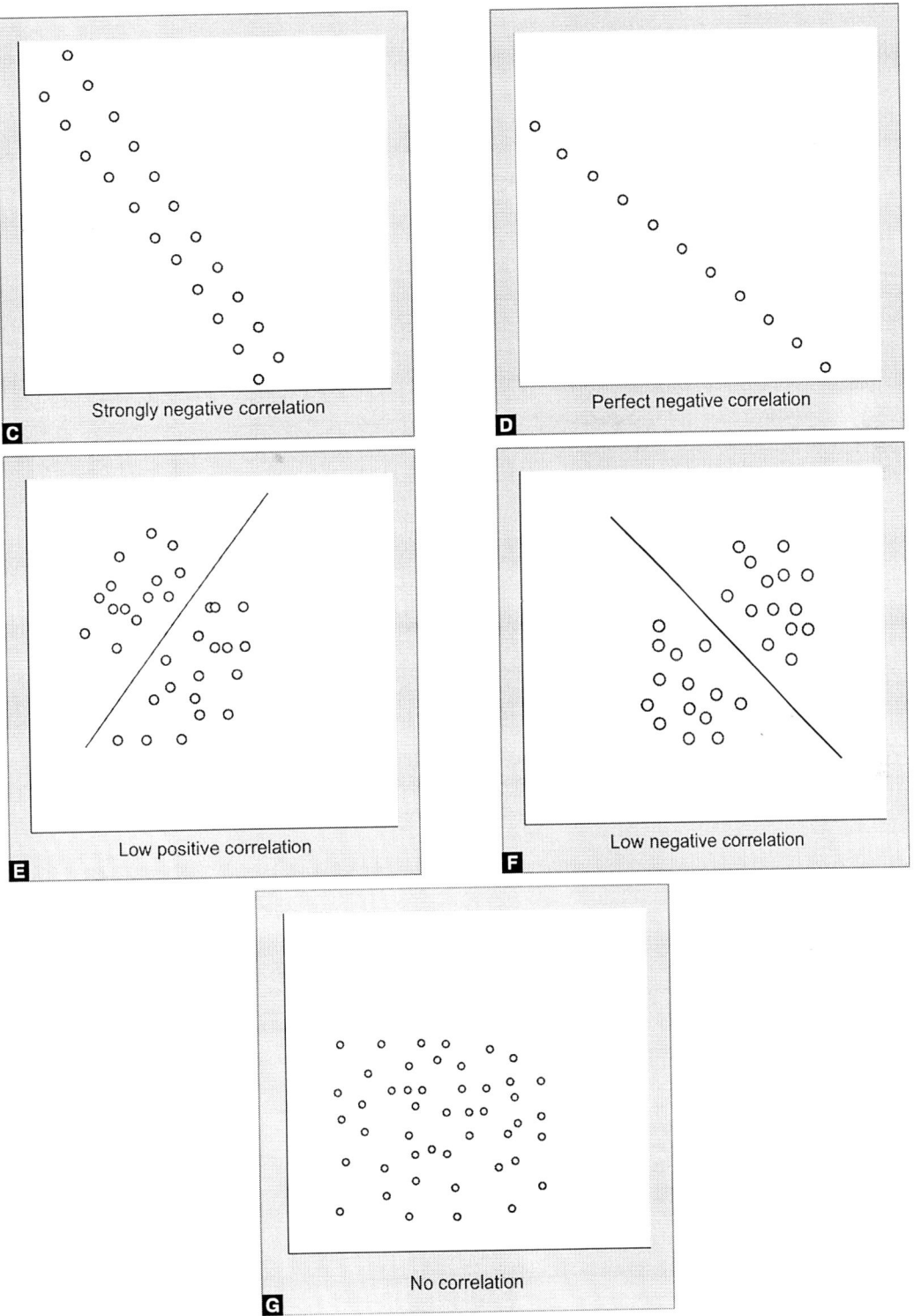

Figs. 10.16C to G
Figs. 10.16A to G: Scatter diagrams.

Advantages

- Simple and nonmathematical method.
- Not influenced by the size of extreme item.
- First step in investing the relationship between two variables.
- It can help identify trends in the data by a positive correlation, negative correlation, or no correlation.
- Retains exact data values and sample size.

The Graph is Straightforward Towards Observation

Scatter plots show the minimum, maximum, and outlier(s) of the data set.

Disadvantages

- Although a scatter plot can help you to see relationships in the data, it is sometimes difficult to tell if the correlation is positive, negative, or if there is not one. It cannot adopt an exact degree of correlation. Flat trend line gives inconclusive results.
- The scatter plot makes it hard to see the data because there are no graph lines to see exactly where the point is.
- Data on both axes should be continuous.
- The method is not applicable to show the relation of more than two variables.
- Number of observations is limited.
- They are used to plot only for the quantitative variable which are numerically comparable.
- External values are not influenced to change the correlation of data.

Correlation Coefficient (Table 10.26)

Pearson's correlation coefficient is the covariance of the two variables divided by the product of their standard deviations. The form of the definition involves a 'product moment', i.e., the mean (the first moment about the origin) of the product of the mean adjusted random variables. Pearson product-moment correlation coefficient also known as r, R, or Pearson's r, a measure of the strength and direction of the linear relationship between two variables, i.e., defined as the (sample) covariance of the variables divided by the product of their (sample) standard deviations. The correlation coefficient r is known as Pearson's correlation coefficient as it was discovered by Karl Pearson. Pearson's correlation coefficient returns a value of between -1 and $+1$. A -1 means there is a strong negative correlation and $+1$ means that there is a strong positive correlation.

Table 10.26: Correlation value table.

r value =	
+.70 or higher	Very strong positive relationship
+.40 to +.69	Strong positive relationship
+.30 to +.39	Moderate positive relationship
+.20 to +.29	Weak positive relationship
+.01 to +.19	No or negligible relationship
0	No relationship
−.01 to −.19	No or negligible relationship
−.20 to −.29	Weak negative relationship
−.30 to −.39	Moderate negative relationship
−.40 to −.69	Strong negative relationship
−.70 or higher	Very strong negative relationship

The formula for finding correlation coefficient is

$$r = \frac{n(\Sigma xy)-(\Sigma x)(\Sigma y)}{\sqrt{[n(\Sigma x^2)-(x)^2[n(y^2)-(\Sigma y)^2]}}$$

The convenient way of interpreting the value of correlation coefficient is to use of square of coefficient of correlation which is called coefficient of determination.

The coefficient of determination = r^2. Suppose: $r = 0.9$, $r^2 = 0.81$ this would mean that 81% of the variation in the dependent variable has been explained by the independent variable r = 0.30. It does not mean that the first correlation is twice as strong as the second the 'r' can be understood by computing the value of r^2.

When, $r = 0.60$ $r^2 = 0.36$ -----(1)
        $r = 0.30$ $r^2 = 0.09$ -----(2)

This implies that in the first case 36% of the total variation is explained whereas in second case 9% of the total variation is explained.

Spearman's Rank Correlation Coefficient

- When statistical series in which the variables under study are not capable of quantitative measurement but can be arranged in serial order, in such situation Pearson's correlation coefficient cannot be used in such case Spearman's rank correlation can be used. Rank correlation, the study of relationships between rankings of different variables or different rankings of the same variable. Spearman's rank correlation coefficient, a measure of how well the relationship between two variables can be described by a monotonic function. It is a nonparametric measure of correlation.

Which makes use of the two sets of ranks that may be assigned to the sample values of x and y.

Where,
$R = 1 - (6 \Sigma D^2)/N(N^2 - 1)$
R = Rank correlation coefficient.
D = Difference of rank between paired item in two series.
N = Total number of observation.

- Rank the values of X from 1 to n where n is the numbers of pairs of values of X and Y in the sample.
- Rank the values of Y from 1 to n.
- Compute the value of d for each pair of observation by subtracting the rank of Y from the rank of X.

Square each d and compute Σd^2 which is the sum of the squared values.

In a study of the relationship between level education and income **(Table 10.27)** the following data was obtained. Find the relationship between them and comment.

Table 10.27: Correlation between level of education and income.

Sample numbers	Level education (X)	Income (Y)
A	Preparatory	25
B	Primary	10
C	University	8
D	Secondary	10
E	Secondary	15
F	Illiterate	50
G	University	60

	(X)	(Y)	Rank X	Rank Y	d	d²
A	Preparatory	25	5	3	2	4
B	Primary	10	6	5.5	0.5	0.25
C	University	8	1.5	7	-5.5	30.25
D	Secondary	10	3.5	5.5	-2	4
E	Secondary	15	3.5	4	-0.5	0.25
F	Illiterate	50	7	2	5	25
G	University	60	1.5	1	0.5	0.25

Computing rank correlation coefficient by using formula

$R = 1 - (6 \sum D^2)/N(N^2 - 1)$
$= 1 - 6 \times 64/7(48)$
$= -0.1$ (which denote very weak negative correlation).

There is an indirect weak correlation between level of education and income.

Like Pearson's correlation coefficient, the value of rank correlation coefficient 'R' ranges from -1 to +1. If R = +1, then there is complete agreement in the order of the ranks and the ranks are in the same direction. If R = -1, then there is complete agreement in the order of the ranks and the ranks are in the opposite direction. If R = 0, then there is no correlation.

Regression Analysis

Regression analysis is a statistical process for estimating the relationships among variables. It includes many techniques for modeling and analyzing several variables, when the focus is on the relationship between a dependent variable and one or more independent variables or predictors. More specifically, regression analysis helps one to understand how the typical value of the dependent variable or criterion variable changes when anyone of the independent variables is varied, while the other independent variables are held fixed. Regression analysis is widely used for prediction and forecasting. Regression analysis is also used to understand which among the independent variables are related to the dependent variable, and to explore the forms of these relationships. In restricted circumstances, regression analysis can be used to infer causal relationships between the independent and dependent variables. Generally, speaking; regression refers to the prediction of one variable from our knowledge of another variable. We label the variable that is being predicted as the Y variable and refer to it as the **criterion variable** and the variable that we are predicting from as the X variable and refer to it as the **predictor variable.** Correlation is a specialized procedures from a larger family of regression procedures. Regression procedures examine the relationship between two or more sets of paired variables. The basic linear regression formula **y = a + bx**. Where, *y* is the set of dependent variable values, **b** is the intercept, the value of y when *x* is 0, **a** is the change in *y* for each unit of *x*. The regression line is a graphical display of the relation between the values on the predictor variable and predicted values on the criterion variable. It is similar to the scatter plot used to display correlations. Regression uses a variable (*x*) to predict some outcome variable (*y*) and it tells you how values in y change as a function of changes in values of x.

Linear regression establishes a relationship between dependent variable (Y) and one or more independent variables (X) using a best fit straight line (also known as regression line) **(Fig. 10.17)**.

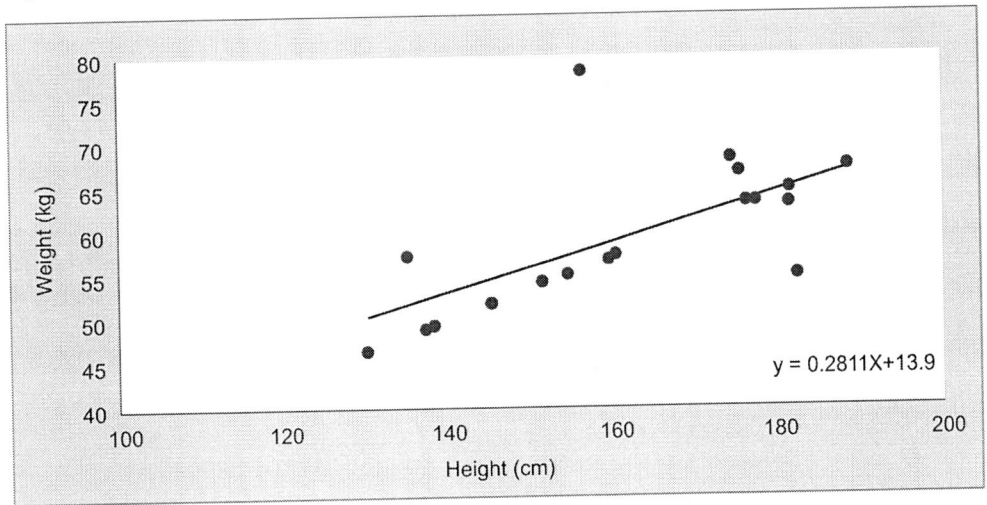

Fig. 10.17: Regression line.

The difference between simple linear regression and multiple linear regression is that, multiple linear regression has more than one independent variables, whereas simple linear regression has only one independent variable.

Regression Definition

A regression is a statistical analysis assessing the association between two variables. It is used to find the relationship between two variables.

Regression Formula

Regression Equation (y) = a + bx Slope (b) = $(N\Sigma XY - (\Sigma X)(\Sigma Y))/(N\Sigma X^2 - (\Sigma X)^2)$ **Intercept (a)** = $(\Sigma Y - b(\Sigma X))/N$. where, x and y are the variables. b = The slope of the regression line, a = The intercept point of the regression line and the y axis. N = Number of values or elements, X = First score, Y = Second score, ΣXY = Sum of the product of first and second scores, ΣX = Sum of first scores, ΣY = Sum of second scores, ΣX^2 = Sum of square first scores.

$$b = \frac{n(\Sigma xy)(x^2) - (\Sigma x)(xy)}{n(\Sigma x^2) - (\Sigma x)^2}$$

Assuming that you have decided that you can have a regression equation because there is significant linear correlation between the two variables, the equation becomes: $y' = ax + b$ or $y' = a + bx$ (some books use y-hat instead of y-prime).

a is the slope of the regression line: $a = \dfrac{n(\Sigma xy)(x^2) - (\Sigma x)}{n(\Sigma x^2) - (\Sigma x)^2}$

b is the y-intercept of the regression line: $b = \dfrac{(\Sigma y)(\Sigma x^2) - (\Sigma x)(\Sigma xy)}{n(\Sigma x^2) - (\Sigma x)^2}$

Regression Example (Table 10.28)

To find the simple or linear regression of

Table 10.28: Calculation of linear regression.

X value	Y value
60	3.1
61	3.6
62	3.8
63	4
65	4.1

To find regression equation, we will first find slope, intercept and use it to form regression equation.

Step 1

Count the number of values. N = 5

Step 2

Find XY, X^2 (see the **Table 10.29**).

Table 10.29: Calculation of linear regression.

X value	Y value	X × Y	X^2
60	3.1	60 × 3.1 = 186	60 × 60 = 3600
61	3.6	61 × 3.6 = 219.6	61 × 61 = 3721
62	3.8	62 × 3.8 = 235.6	62 × 62 = 3844
63	4	63 × 4 = 252	63 × 63 = 3969
65	4.1	65 × 4.1 = 266.5	65 × 65 = 4225

Step 3

Find ΣX, ΣY, ΣXY, ΣX^2. $\Sigma X = 311$ $\Sigma Y = 18.6$ $\Sigma XY = 1159.7$ $\Sigma X^2 = 19359$.

Step 4

Substitute in the above slope formula given. Slope (b) = $(N\Sigma XY - (\Sigma X)(\Sigma Y))/(N\Sigma X^2 - (\Sigma X)^2)$ = $((5) \times (1159.7) - (311) \times (18.6))/((5) \times (19359) - (311)^2)$ = $(5798.5 - 5784.6)/(96795 - 96721)$ = $13.9/74 = 0.19$

Step 5

Now, again substitute in the above intercept formula given. Intercept (a) = $(\Sigma Y - b(\Sigma X))/N$ = $(18.6 - 0.19(311))/5 = (18.6 - 59.09)/5 = -40.49/5 = -8.098$.

Step 6

Then substitute these values in regression equation formula. Regression equation (y) = a + bx = −8.098 + 0.19x. Suppose if we want to know the approximate y value for the variable x = 64. Then we can substitute the value in the above equation. Regression equation(y) = a + bx = −8.098 + 0.19 (64). = −8.098 + 12.16 = 4.06. This example will guide you to find the relationship between two variables by calculating the regression from the above steps. Difference between correlation and linear regression is summarized in **Table 10.30**.

Table 10.30: Differences between correlation and linear regression.

Correlation	Linear regression
Correlation examines the relationship between two variables using a standardized unit. However, most applications use raw units as an input.	Regression examines the relationship between one dependent variables and one or more independent variables. Calculations may use either raw unit values, or standardized as input.
The calculation is symmetrical, meaning that the order of comparison does not change the result.	The calculation is not symmetrical. So one variable is assigned the dependent role (the values being predicted) and one or more the independent role (the values hypothesize to impact the dependent variable).
Correlation coefficients indicate the strength of a relationship.	Regression shows the effect of one unit change in an independent variable on the dependent variable.
Correlation removes the effect of different measurement scales. Therefore, comparison between different models is possible since the rho coefficient is in standardized units.	Linear regression using raw unit measurement scales can be used to predict outcomes.

INFERENTIAL STATISTICS

Inferential statistics, which are based on the laws of probability, provide a means for drawing conclusions about a population, given data from a sample. With inferential statistics, researchers estimate population parameters from sample statistics. These probabilistic estimates involve some error, but inferential statistics provide a framework for making judgments about their reliability in a systematic, objective fashion.

It helps in drawing inference from the data, for example, finding the association and difference between two or more variables with the help of parametric and nonparametric test.

To estimate population parameters, inferential statics uses representative samples. As we knew in probability samples are the best way to get representative samples. Inferential statistics are based on the assumption of random sampling from populations. Even when random sampling is used, however, sample characteristics are seldom identical to population characteristics. This statistics used to test hypothesis which have been developed at the beginning of the study. When a researcher will determine randomly two sample from the same population, the mean value of two sample can also differ from one another. The tendency for statistics to fluctuate from one sample to another is known as sampling error. The challenge for researchers is to determine whether sample values are good estimates of population parameters. This statistics helps the researcher to determine whether the difference found between experimental and control group is true difference or only by a chance. Before learning different types of tests for significance lets explain some important concepts related to inferential statistics.

Concepts Related to Inferential Statistics

Parametric Tests

A statistical test, in which specific assumptions are made about the population parameter, is known as parametric test. Parametric tests assume a normal distribution of values, or a "bell-shaped curve." For example, height is roughly a normal distribution in that if you were to graph height from a group of people, one would see a typical bell-shaped curve. Parametric tests are used only where a normal distribution is assumed. The most widely used tests are the t-test (paired or unpaired), ANOVA (one-way non-repeated, repeated; two-way, three-way), linear regression and Pearson rank correlation. In the parametric test, the test statistic is based on distribution. In the parametric test, it is assumed that the measurement of variables of interest is done on interval or ratio level.

Nonparametric Test

The nonparametric test is defined as the hypothesis test which is not based on underlying assumptions, i.e., it does not require population's distribution to be denoted by specific parameters. The test is mainly based on differences in medians. Hence, it is alternately known as the distribution-free test. The test assumes that the variables are measured on a nominal or ordinal level. Nonparametric tests are used when continuous data are not normally distributed or when dealing with discrete variables. Most widely used examples are chi-squared, Fisher's exact tests, Wilcoxon's matched pairs, Mann–Whitney U-tests, Kruskal–Wallis tests and Spearman rank correlation. It is used when the independent variables are nonmetric. The test statistic is arbitrary.

P-value Approach

The *P*-value approach involves determining "likely" or "unlikely" by determining the probability — assuming the null hypothesis were true — of observing a more extreme test statistic in the direction of the alternative hypothesis than the one observed. If the *P*-value is small, say less than (or equal to) α, then it is "unlikely." And, if the *P*-value is large, say more than α, then it is "likely."

If the *P*-value is less than (or equal to) α, then the null hypothesis is rejected in favor of the alternative hypothesis. And, if the *P*-value is greater than α, then the null hypothesis is not rejected.

Specifically, the four steps involved in using the *P*-value approach to conducting any hypothesis test are:

1. Specify the null and alternative hypotheses.
2. Using the sample data and assuming the null hypothesis is true, calculate the value of the test statistic. Again, to conduct the hypothesis test for the population mean μ, we use the *t*-statistic $t^* = \bar{x} - \mu s/n\sqrt{}$ which follows a *t*-distribution with $n - 1$ degrees of freedom.
3. Using the known distribution of the test statistic, calculate the **P-value**: "If the null hypothesis is true, what is the probability that we'd observe a more extreme test statistic in the direction of the alternative hypothesis than we did?" (Note how this question is equivalent to the question answered in criminal trials: "If the defendant is innocent, what is the chance that we'd observe such extreme criminal evidence?")
4. Set the significance level, α, the probability of making a Type I error to be small — 0.01, 0.05, or 0.10. Compare the *P*-value to α. If the *P*-value is less than (or equal to) α, reject the null hypothesis in favor of the alternative hypothesis. If the P-value is greater than α, do not reject the null hypothesis.

Hypothesis-Testing Procedures

Each statistical test described in this chapter has a particular application, but the overall process of testing hypotheses is basically the same. The steps are as follows:

1. *Making a formal statement:* The step consists in making a formal statement of the null hypothesis ($H0$) and also of the alternative hypothesis (Ha). This means that hypotheses should be clearly stated, considering the nature of the research problem. If the hypothesis is already developed then the researcher has to decide whether a parametric test is justified, which levels of measurement were used, whether a between-groups test is needed, and how many groups are being compared based on that the test will be decided.
2. *Establish the level of significance:* Researchers establish the criterion for accepting or rejecting the null hypothesis before analyzes are undertaken. A level of .05 is usually acceptable. The hypotheses are tested on a predetermined level of significance and as such the same should be specified. Generally, in practice, either 5% level or 1% level is adopted for the purpose. The factors that affect the level of significance are: (a) the magnitude of the difference between sample means; (b) the size of the samples; (c) the variability of measurements within samples; and (d) whether the hypothesis is directional or nondirectional.
3. After deciding the level of significance, the next step in hypothesis testing is to select a one-tailed or two-tailed test. In most cases, a two-tailed test should be used, but in some cases a one-tailed test may be warranted. A one-tailed test is a statistical test in which the critical area of a distribution is one-sided so that it is either greater than or less than a certain value, but not both. If the sample being tested falls into the one-sided critical area, the alternative hypothesis will be accepted instead of the null hypothesis.
4. *Compute a test statistic*: Using collected data, researchers calculate a test statistic using appropriate computational formulas given, or the researcher can instruct a computer to calculate the statistic. The test statistics is computed as per selected formula.
5. *Calculate the degrees of freedom* (symbolized as *df*): Degrees of freedom is a concept that refers to the number of observations free to vary about a parameter. The concept is too complex for full elaboration here, but fortunately *df* is easy to compute. The degree of freedom calculation varies based on the type of test.
6. *Obtain a tabled value for the statistical test*: There are theoretical distributions for all test statistics. These distributions enable researchers to determine whether obtained values of the test statistic are beyond the range of what is probable if the null hypothesis were true. Researchers examine a table for the appropriate test statistic and obtain the critical value corresponding to the degrees of freedom and significance level.
7. *Compare the test statistic with the tabled value*: In the final step, researchers compare the value in the table with the value of the computed test statistic. If the absolute value of the test statistic is *larger* than the tabled value, the results are statistically significant. If the computed value is *smaller*, the results are nonsignificant.

USE OF COMPUTER IN QUANTITATIVE DATA ANALYSIS

Microsoft Excel

As a coding sheet, excel can be used not only for data entry, manipulation and presentation but it also offers a suite of statistical analysis functions and other tools that can be used to run descriptive statistics like calculating frequency, percentage, mean, standard deviation and to perform several different and useful inferential statistical tests, such as chi-square test, ANOVA, regression analysis which are widely used in nursing research. In addition, it provides all of the standard spread sheet functionality, which makes it useful for other analysis and data manipulation tasks, including generating graphical and other presentation formats. Finally, even if using modified statistical software, excel can be helpful when preparing data for analysis in those packages. The limitations of Microsoft excel is it does not cover many of the more advanced statistical techniques that are used in research. More surprisingly, it lacks some common tools (such as boxplots) that are widely taught in basic statistics. The extensive range of graph (chart) templates is also criticized for encouraging bad practice in data presentation through inappropriate use of color, 3-D display, etc. Though many basic analysis projects involved and successfully completed of exploration of primarily data, calculation of descriptive and simple inferential statistics by using standard Excel still more advanced projects, especially those involving multivariate analysis are more challenging research in such cases it is worth considering using specialist analysis software such as IBM, SPSS.

Data Analysis Menu Dialogue Box in Excel

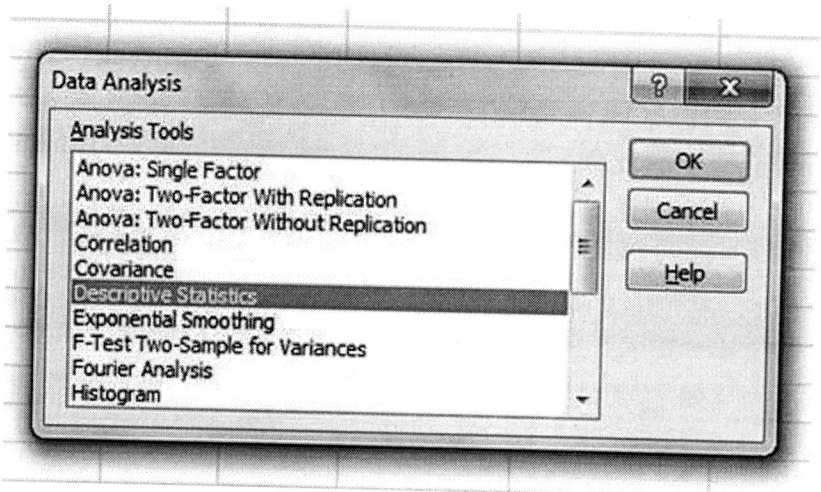

Descriptive Statistics Output for Variable Age

	A	B	C
1	Age		
2			
3	Mean	30.5	
4	Standard Error	2.200207	
5	Median	31	
6	Mode	28	
7	Standard Deviation	7.621739	
8	Sample Variance	58.09091	
9	Kurtosis	-0.81553	
10	Skewness	-0.12122	
11	Range	24	
12	Minimum	18	
13	Maximum	42	
14	Sum	366	
15	Count	12	
16			

SPSS

Originally this is known as statistical package for social science. The SPSS software package was created for the management and statistical analysis of social science data. It was originally launched in 1968 by SPSS Inc., and was later acquired by IBM in 2009. SPSS is used by market researchers, health researchers, survey companies, government entities, education researchers, marketing organizations, data miners, and many more for the processing and analyzing of survey data. These techniques are used to analyze, transform, and produce a characteristic pattern between different data variables. In addition to it, the output can be obtained through graphical representation so that a user can easily understand the result. The statistics you can calculate by this software programs are descriptive statistics, including methodologies, such as frequencies, cross tabulation, and descriptive ratio statistics. Bivariate statistics, including methodologies such as analysis of variance (ANOVA), means, correlation, and nonparametric tests. Numeral outcome prediction such as linear regression.

Prediction for identifying groups, including methodologies, such as cluster analysis and factor analysis can be possible through these software programs. There are mainly three types of windows in SPSS:
1. Data editor window
2. Output window
3. Syntax window

Whenever SPSS is opened, it opens a Data editor window and an Output window. Syntax window opens only if we paste a command. In SPSS software there are two views used for data analysis: (1) data view and (2) variable views. Data view is just like spread sheet. In data view each rows represent one subject/participants/things and each column one variable.

	VAR000 01	VAR000 02	var	var	var	var	var
1	1.00	4.00					
2	2.00	5.00					
3	3.00	6.00					
4							
5							
6							
7							
8							
9							
10							

In above picture the variables can just entered as variable 1,2 like that but in variable view the variables can be actually renamed. When naming a variable, name should start with alphabets only, name can be mixture of alphabets, numerals and special characters, name cannot have blanks in between and name cannot be repeated. The name cannot begin with a number, cannot begin with a special character like @,#, etc.

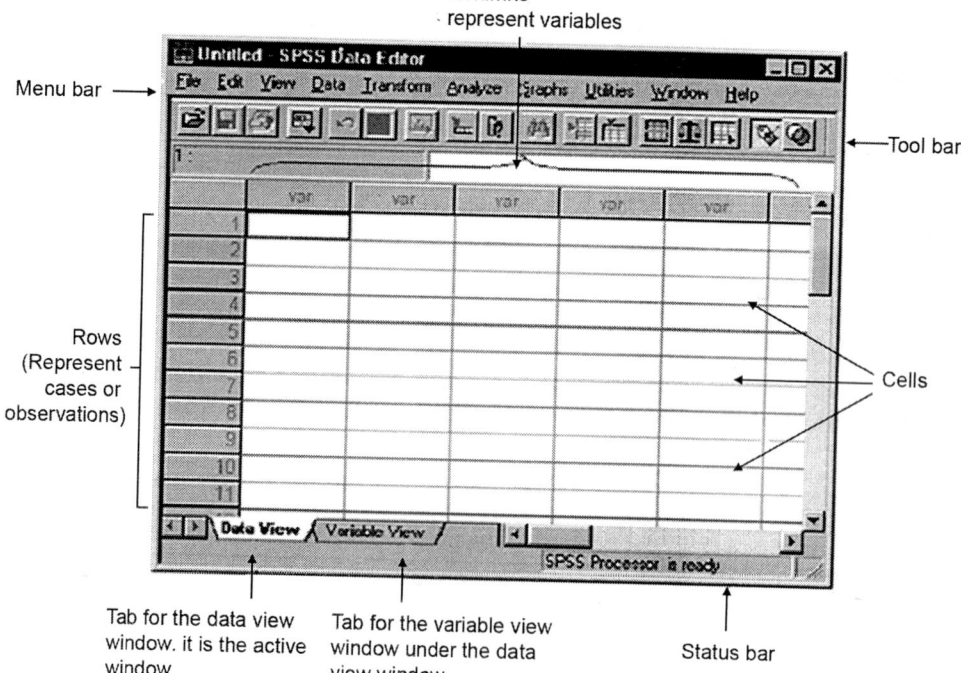

Chapter 10: Analysis of Data and Application of Biostatistics in Nursing Research

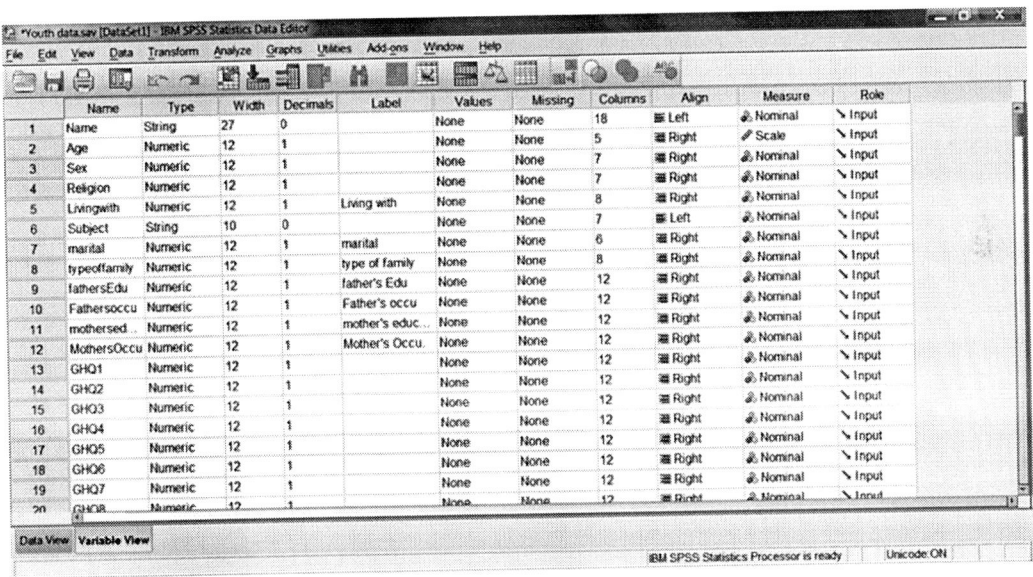

Difference between SPSS and Microsoft Excel

Excel is spread sheet software, SPSS is statistical analysis software. In Excel, you can perform some statistical analysis but SPSS is more powerful. When it comes to organizing and managing your data, the SPSS software offers the user a lot of control. Since the software remembers the location of the variables and cases, it provides quicker and accurate data analysis. In SPSS every column is one variable, Excel does not treat columns and rows in that way (**Table 10.31**).

Table 10.31: Comparison of SPSS and Excel.

Basis for comparison	SPSS	Excel
Definition	The full form of SPSS is statistical package for social science, a tool formulated for statistical analysis of data	Microsoft's product used for data entry and data manipulation to store some information
Usage	Statistical calculations and manipulation of data as per IBM SPSS allows to perform complex analytics, such as factor analysis, logistic regression, cluster analysis, etc. guidelines	Managing and storing data with formulated operations defined by microsoft. In excel, only some statistical analysis is possible
Benefits	Speed and performance	Reduction in data redundancy
Real time usage	Usage of advanced and ultra-fast devices like supercomputers	Maintenance and handling of large volumes of customer data
Academics	Exists since from many years under the SPSS umbrella now under IBM	Exists and evolved with developing branch of science and technology
Industry	Data scientist/analyst are the professions to become after studying in this field	Data scientist/analyst are the professions to become after studying in this field
Applications	Applies to all technical industries and large-scale companies	Applies to companies where large-scale sensitive data is to be managed
Field	Covers entire technological field which is a superset of data science	A subset of computer science where the study of data is done by using different methods and technologies

Chi-square Test

A chi-squared test, also referred to as χ^2 test (or chi-square test), is any statistical hypothesis test in which the sampling distribution of the test statistic is a chi-square distribution when the null hypothesis is true. Chi-squared tests are often constructed from a sum of squared errors, or through the sample variance. Chi-square is a statistical test commonly used to compare observed data with data we would expect to obtain according to a specific hypothesis. It is used to determine whether there is a significant difference between the expected frequencies and the observed frequencies in one or more categories, do the number of individuals or objects that fall in each category differ significantly from the number you would expect? Is this difference between the expected and observed due to sampling error, or is it a *real* difference? The chi-square statistic is most commonly used to evaluate tests of independence when using a cross tabulation (also known as a bivariate table). Cross tabulation presents the distributions of two categorical variables simultaneously, with the intersections of the categories of the variables appearing in the cells of the table. The test of independence assesses whether an association exists between the two variables by carefully examining the pattern of responses in the cells; calculating the chi-square statistic and comparing it against a critical value from the chi-square distribution allows the researcher to assess whether the association seen between the variables in a particular sample is likely to represent an actual relationship between those variables in the population. In statistics, there are two types of variables: numerical (countable) variables and non-numerical (categorical) variables. The chi-squared statistic is a single number that tells you how much disparity exists between the real, or observed counts of a categorical variable and the counts you would expect if there were no relationship at all in the population. Chi-square statistics can only be used on numbers. They cannot be used for percentages, proportions, means or similar statistical value. For example, if you have 10% of 200 people, you would need to convert that to a number (20) before you can run a test statistic. Chi-square test enables us to explain whether or not two attributes are associated. For instance, we may be interested in knowing whether a new medicine is effective in controlling fever or not, chi-square test will helps us in deciding this issue. In such a situation, we proceed with the null hypothesis that the two attributes (viz., new medicine and control of fever) are independent which means that new medicine is not effective in controlling fever. On this basis we first calculate the expected frequencies and then work out the value of c2. If the calculated value of c2 is less than the table value at a certain level of significance for given degrees of freedom, we conclude that null hypothesis stands which means that the two attributes are independent or not associated (i.e., the new medicine is not effective in controlling the fever). But if the calculated value of c2 is greater than its table value, our inference then would be that null hypothesis does not hold good which means the two attributes are associated and the association is not because of some chance factor but it exists in reality (i.e., the new medicine is effective in controlling the fever and as such may be prescribed). It may, however, be stated here that c2 is not a measure of the degree of relationship or the form of relationship between two attributes, but is simply a technique of judging the significance of such association or relationship between two attributes.

Chi-square Test Requirements

- Quantitative data
- One or more categories
- Independent observations
- Adequate sample size (at least 10)
- Simple random sample
- Data in frequency form
- All observations must be used

The Steps of Chi-square Analysis

1. Draw a contingency table.

Table 10.32: Association of malnutrition with economic status.

Smoking	Lung cancer		Total
	Yes	No	
Yes	70	6930	7000
No	3	2997	3000
	73	9927	10000

2. Enter the observed frequencies or counts (O).
3. Write the expected frequency into the appropriate box in the table.
   The formula for expected frequencies is:
   E = row total × column total/grand total
4. Calculate totals (in the margins).

Check: Expected frequencies (E) marginal totals are the same as for observed frequencies (O). Eyeball the contingency table, noting where the differences between O (observed) and E (expected) values occur. *If they are close to each other, the levels of the independent (predictor) variable are not having an effect.*

5. Find out chi-square value $\chi^2 = \sum \dfrac{(O - E)^2}{E}$

$$\chi^2 = \sum \dfrac{(O_i - E_i)^2}{E_i}$$

6. Determine the null hypothesis or alternate hypothesis
*Null (H0): Two variables are independent alternate (H1): Two variables are not independent. Calculate the expected value matrix.

Expected Frequencies

Let us take an example of 3 × 3 contingency table. The method will be directly applicable to any similar problem. The following **Table 10.33** refers to find out association of malnutrition with socioeconomic status.

Table 10.33: Association of malnutrition with socioeconomic status.

Degree of malnutrition present socioeconomic status	Mild	Moderate	Severe	Total
High income group	11	6	4	21
Moderately income group	12	7	7	26
Poor group	7	7	14	28
Total	30	20	25	75

To find the expected frequencies, we assume independence of the rows and columns. To get the expected frequency corresponding to the 11 we look at row total (21) and column total (30), multiply them, and then divide by the overall total (75). So the expected frequency is:

$$\dfrac{21 \times 30}{75} = 8.4$$

So, to complete the expected table, draw up another table similar to that above and having the same row and column totals. For each entry in this table, we simply calculate (row total × column total)/75. The completed table on expected frequency is:

Table 10.34: Association of malnutrition with economic status by expected frequency.

Degree of malnutrition present socioeconomic status	Mild	Moderate	Severe	Total
High income group	8.4	5.6	7.0	21
Moderately income group	10.4	6.9	8.7	26
Poor group	11.2	7.5	9.3	28
Total	30	20	25	75

The number of degrees of freedom is calculated for an m-by-n table as:
(m – 1) (n – 1), so in this case (3 – 1) (3 – 1) = 2 × 2 = 4.
To calculate χ^2 we then have a further table:

Table 10.35: Chi-square table with expected and observed value.

O	E	|O – E|	|O – E|²/E
11	8.4	2.6	0.805
6	5.6	0.4	0.0286
4	7	3	1.2857
12	10.4	1.6	0.246
7	6.9	0.1	0.0014
7	8.7	1.7	0.332
7	11.2	4.2	1.575
7	7.5	0.5	0.033
14	9.3	4.7	2.375
			Total = 5.96 = χ^2

The tabular 95% value of χ^2 (degrees of freedom = 4) is 9.49, so the value of χ^2 that we obtained (5.96) is not significant at the 5% level. We conclude that the state of the pitch does not affect the performance of the team.

The Simplest Method of Chi-Square Analysis in 2 × 2 Table

For a 2 × 2 contingency table the Chi-square statistic is calculated by the formula:
$x^2 = N(ad - bc)^2 / (a + c)(b + d)(a + b)(c + d)$ which is clear by the table given below.

Variable 2	Data type 1	Data type 2	Totals
Category 1	a	b	a + b
Category 2	c	d	c + d
Total	a + c	b + d	a + b + c + d = N

For the above table let's take an example of a drug trial in increasing heart rate.

Suppose a researcher conducted a drug trial on a group of animals and hypothesized that the animals receiving the drug would show increased heart rates compared to those that did not receive the drug, then he/she conduct the study and collect the following data:

Ho: The proportion of animals whose heart rate increased is independent of drug treatment.
Ha: The proportion of animals whose heart rate increased is associated with drug treatment.

	Heart rate increased	No heart rate increase	Total
Treated	36	14	50
Not treated	30	25	55
Total	66	39	105

Chi-square = $105[(36)(25)-(14)(30)]^2/(50)(55)(39)(66) = 3.418$

For calculating x^2 we need degree of freedom. A simple rule for calculating degrees of freedom in a 2 × 2 table is (number of columns minus one) × (number of rows minus one).

df = (rows − 1)(columns−1)
df = (2 − 1)(2 − 1) = 1

We now have our Chi square statistic (x^2 = 3.418), our predetermined level of significance is 0.05, and our degrees of freedom (df) = 1. Entering the chi-square distribution table with 1 degree of freedom. The obtained value of 3.418 is less than the cut off of value 3.84, shown on the table at the .05 level. Therefore, $p < .05$. So null hypothesis is accepted. In other words, there is no statistically significant difference in the proportion of animals whose heart rate increased.

t-test

Theoretical test done on T-distribution was done by WS Gosset in the early 1900. Gosset was employed by Guinness and Sons at Doublin bravery, Ireland which did not permit employees to publish research findings under their own names so Gosset adopted the pen name 'STUDENT' and published his findings under this name. Thereafter the T-distribution is commonly called as student's T-distribution or student's distribution. A t-test's statistical significance indicates whether or not the difference between two groups' averages most likely reflects a 'real' difference in the population from which the groups were sampled. A t-test is an analysis of two populations means through the use of statistical examination; a t-test with two samples is commonly used with small sample sizes, testing the difference between the samples when the variances of two normal distributions are not known. A t-test looks at the t-statistic, the t-distribution and degrees of freedom to determine the probability of difference between populations; the test statistic in the test is known as the t-statistic.

One Sample t-test

One sample t-test is a statistical procedure used to examine the mean difference between the sample and the known value of the population mean. In one sample t-test, we know the population mean. We draw a random sample from the population and then compare the sample mean with the population mean and make a statistical decision as to whether or not the sample mean is different from the population mean. We can use this analysis, e.g., when we take a sample from the city and we know the mean of the country (population mean). If we want to know whether the city mean differs from the country mean, we will use the one sample t-test.

In one sample t-test, to test the significance of the mean of a random sample, the t-statistics is given by:

$$t = \frac{\bar{x} - \mu}{S} \times \sqrt{n}$$

Where, $S = \sqrt{\frac{(x - \bar{x})^2}{n - 1}}$

and $\bar{x}$ = Mean of the sample
μ = The actual or hypothetical mean of the population.
s = Standard deviation of the sample.

If the calculated value of 't' always positive exceeds to 0.05 we say that the difference between $\bar{x}$ and μ is significant at 5% level. If it exceeds 0.01 then it is significant at 1% level. If 't'<0.05 then it is less significant at 5% level and if 't' > 0.05% then it is more significant at 5% level.

Example:
A pharmacy company for determining expiry dates of certain drugs claims that his drugs have mean potency for 25 months with a SD of 5 months. A random sample of 6 such drugs gave the following potency values. Can you regard the company's claim to be valid at 1% significant level?

1-24
2-26
3-30
4-20
5-20
6-18

Solution:
Let us take hypothesis that there is no significant difference between mean potency of drugs in sample and that of the population.

x	$x - \bar{x}$	$(x - \bar{x})^2$
24	1	1
26	3	9
30	7	49
20	-3	9
20	-3	9
18	-5	25

$$\bar{x} = \frac{24 + 26 + 30 + 20 + 20 + 18}{6}$$

$\bar{x}$ = 23 = sample mean
μ = 25 (population mean)

$$S = \sqrt{\frac{\sum(x - \bar{x})^2}{n - 1}} = \sqrt{\frac{102}{5}} = 4.51$$

$$t = \frac{\bar{x} - \mu}{S} \times \sqrt{n} = \frac{23 - 25}{4.51} \times \sqrt{x} = 0.44 \times 2.44 = 1.08$$

Degree of freedom = $(n - 1) = 6 - 1 = 5$

't' at 0.01 = 4.03

Hence, the hypothesis is accepted as the company's claim is not valid at 1% level significance. Unpaired and paired two-sample t-tests.

Paired Sample t-test

In **paired sample** hypothesis testing, a sample from the population is chosen and two measurements for each element in the sample are taken. Each set of measurements is considered a sample. Unlike the hypothesis testing studied so far, the two samples are not independent of one another. Paired samples are also called matched samples or repeated measure. The paired t-test calculates a sample of matched pairs of similar units the difference within each before-and-after pair of measurements, determines the mean of these changes, and reports whether this mean of the differences is statistically.

Steps

Set up hypothesis: We set up two hypotheses. Generally in experimental studies we consider null hypothesis. For example, in a study 'evaluate the effectiveness of SIM on knowledge of staff nurses regarding infection prevention in labor room' the null hypothesis is there is no significant association between per and postknowledge score of staff nurses regarding infection prevention in labor room.

Select the level of significance: The level of significance determines the percentage of error a researcher can allow after making the hypothesis, we choose the level of significance. In most of the cases, significance level is 5%, in medicine to evaluate the effectiveness of a treatment, the significance level is set at 1%.

Calculate the parameter: To calculate the parameter we will use the following formula:

$$t = \frac{\bar{d}}{\sqrt{s^2/n}}$$

where, d bar is the mean difference between two samples, s^2 is the sample variance, n is the sample size and t is a paired sample t-test with n–1 degrees of freedom. An alternate formula for paired sample t-test is:

$$t = \frac{\sum d}{\sqrt{\frac{n(\sum d^2) - (\sum d)^2}{n-1}}}$$

Testing of hypothesis or decision making: After calculating the parameter, we will compare the calculated value with the table value. If the calculated value is greater than the table value, then we will reject the null hypothesis for the paired sample t-test. If the calculated value is less than the table value, then we will accept the null hypothesis and say that there is no significant mean difference between the two paired samples.

Assumptions

- Only the matched pairs can be used to perform the test.
- Normal distributions are assumed.
- The variance of two samples is equal.
- Cases must be independent of each other.

Unpaired t-test

An unpaired t-test is used to compare two population means. The following notation will be used throughout this leaflet:

The independent samples t-test is used when two separate sets of independent and identically distributed samples are obtained, one from each of the two populations being compared. For example, suppose we are evaluating the effect of a medical treatment, and we enroll 100 subjects into our study, then randomly assign 50 subjects to the treatment group and 50 subjects to the control group. In this case, we have two independent samples and would use the unpaired form of the t-test.

Testing difference between 2 means of independent random samples of size n_1 and n_2 with means $\bar{x}_1$ and $\bar{x}_2$ and SD s_1 and s_2. This may be integrated in testing the hypothesis that the sample came from the same normal population with early

Symbolically $= \dfrac{\bar{x}_1 - \bar{x}_2}{S} \times \sqrt{\dfrac{n_1 n_2}{n_1 + n_2}}$

S = Combined SD

The value is calculated as $S = \sqrt{\dfrac{\sum(x_1 - \bar{x}_1)^2 + \sum(x_2 - \bar{x}_2)^2}{n_1 + n_2 - 2}}$

Where, DF = $n_1 + n_2 - 2$ (degree of freedom).

Example:
Two drugs are used on 5 and 7 patients for reducing their weight. Drug A was imported and drug B is indigenous. The decrease in weight after using the drugs for 6 months was as follows. Find out if there is any significant difference in efficiency of two drugs?

Drug A	Drug B
10	8
12	9
13	12
11	14
14	15
	10
	9

Solution:
Let us assume that there is no significant difference in the efficacy of two drugs.

Table 10.36: 't' test to find out efficacy between two drugs.

x	y	x−$\bar{x}$	y−$\bar{y}$	(x−$\bar{x}$)²	(y−$\bar{y}$)²
10	8	−2	−3	4	9
12	9	0	−2	0	4
13	12	1	1	1	1
11	14	−1	3	1	9
14	15	2	4	4	16
	10		−1		1
	9		−2		4

$\bar{x} = 60/5 = 12$
$\bar{y} = 77/7 = 11$

$$S = \sqrt{\frac{\sum(x-\bar{x})^2 + \sum(y-\bar{y})^2}{n_1 + n_2 - 2}} = \sqrt{\frac{10 + 44}{5 + 7 - 2}} = \sqrt{\frac{54}{10}} = \sqrt{5.4} = 2.32$$

$$t = \frac{(\bar{x}-\bar{y})}{S} \times \sqrt{\frac{n_1 + n_2}{n_1 n_2}} = \frac{12 - 11}{2.32} \times \sqrt{\frac{5 \times 7}{5 + 7}} = 0.43 \times 1.70 = 0.73$$

Degree of freedom = $(n_1 + n_2 - 2) = (5 + 7 - 2) = 10$

❖ Tabulated value is 2.23 for 0.05 or 5% significance for DF 10.
The tabulated value is more than the calculated value. So there is no significance. Thus, hypothesis is accepted that there is no significant difference on the efficacy of 2 drugs.

Analysis of Variance

Analysis of variance (ANOVA) is a collection of statistical models used to analyze the differences among group means and their associated procedures (such as 'variation' among and between groups), developed by statistician and evolutionary biologist Ronald Fisher in 1918 and is the extension of the *t* and the *z*-test. This test is also called the Fisher analysis of variance, which is used to do the analysis of variance between and within the groups whenever the groups are more than two. In the ANOVA setting, the observed variance in a particular variable is partitioned into components attributable to different sources of variation. In its simplest form, ANOVA provides a statistical test of whether or not the means of several groups are equal, and therefore generalizes the *t*-test to more than two groups. ANOVAs are useful for comparing (testing) three or more means (groups or variables) for statistical significance. It is conceptually similar to multiple two-sample *t*-tests, but is less conservative (results in less type I error) and is therefore suited to a wide range of practical problems. The analysis of variance frequently referred to by the contraction ANOVA is a statistical technique especially designed to test whether the means of more than 2 quantitative populations are equal. It consists of classifying and cross classifying statistical results and testing whether the means of a specified classification defers significantly. In this way it is determined whether the given classification is important in affecting the results. The logic behind this procedure has to do with how much variance there is in the population. ANOVA can be used in three ways: one-way ANOVA, two-way ANOVA, and *n*-way multivariate ANOVA.

Definition

A statistical measure that analyzes the variance of two or more comparable series or sample through the F-test technique to ascertain whether the difference in mean values is significant or not and whether the different samples under study are drawn from same universe or from different universe is the same or not.

One-way

When we compare more than two groups, based on one factor (independent variable), this is called one-way ANOVA. For example, it is used if a manufacturing company wants to compare the productivity of three or more employees based on working hours.

Two-way

When a researcher compare more than one group based on more than one factors then two way ANOVA can be adopted, e.g., when a researcher wants to compare the productivity of company based on two factors (two independent variables), i.e., the working hours and working conditions, then two-way (factorial) ANOVA analysis can be done to find out association.

N-way

When the factor comparison is taken, then it said to be n-way ANOVA. For example, in productivity measurement if a company takes all the factors for productivity measurement, then it is said to be n-way ANOVA.

Classical ANOVA for balanced data does three things at once:

- As exploratory data analysis, an ANOVA is an organization of an additive data decomposition, and its sums of squares indicate the variance of each component of the decomposition (or, equivalently, each set of terms of a linear model).
- Comparisons of mean squares, along with an F-test ... allow testing of a nested sequence of models.
- Closely related to the ANOVA is a linear model fit with coefficient estimates and standard errors.

Assumptions of ANOVA

To use the ANOVA test we made the following assumptions:

- Each group sample is drawn from a normally distributed population.
- All populations have a common variance.
- All samples are drawn independently of each other.
- Within each sample, the observations are sampled randomly and independently of each other.
- Factor effects are additive.
  - It may be noted that theoretical speaking whenever any of the assumptions is not met the analysis of variance technique cannot be employed to yield valid inferences.
  - It is indeed fortunate that many economic and business expressed to confirm at least approximately to this premises.
  - In some cases of experimental work departure from assumptions also exists. In such situations the analysis of variance can still applied after a transformation of data.

Techniques of ANOVA

These days, researchers are using ANOVA in many ways. The use of ANOVA depends on the research design. Commonly, researchers are using ANOVA in three ways: one-way ANOVA, two-way ANOVA, and N-way multivariate ANOVA.

For the sake of priority the technique of analysis of variance has been discussed separately

- One-way classification
- Two-way classification

One-way Classification

When we compare more than two groups, based on one factor (independent variable), this is called one-way ANOVA. For example, it is used if a manufacturing company wants to compare the productivity of three or more employees based on working hours. This is called one-way ANOVA.

In this the data are classified according to only one criterion. The null hypothesis is:
$H_0 = \mu_1 = \mu_2 = \mu_3 = \ldots = \mu_k$
$H_1 = \mu_1 \neq \mu_2 \neq \mu_3 \neq \ldots \neq \mu_k$

Calculate Variance Between the Samples

- The variance between samples measures the difference between the sample mean of each group and the overall mean weight by the number of observations in each group.
- The variance between samples taken to account the random variations from observation to observation.
- It also measures difference from one group to another.
- The sum of squares between the samples is denoted by 'SSC'.

Process of Calculation

- Calculate the mean of each sample, i.e., $\bar{x}_1$ and $\bar{x}_2$.
- Calculate the grand mean $\bar{\bar{x}}$. Its value is obtained as follows:

$$\bar{\bar{x}} = \frac{\bar{x}_1 + \bar{x}_2 + \bar{x}_3 + \ldots + \bar{x}_k}{n_1 + n_2 + n_3 + \ldots + n_k}$$

- Take the difference between the means of the variance samples and grand average.
- Square these deviations and obtain the total which will give sum of squares between the samples.
- Divide the total sum of squares obtained in above step by the degrees of freedom. Here the DF will be 1 less than the number of samples (n – 1).

Calculate the Variance Within the Samples

The variance (sum of squares) within samples measured those intersample differences due to chance only. It is denoted by 'SSE'.
'SSE' = sum of squares within the sample.

Steps

- Calculate the mean value of each samples $\bar{x}_1, \bar{x}_2$…etc.
- Take the deviations of the various items in a sample from the mean values of the respective samples.
- Square these deviations and obtain the total which gives the sum of the squares within the samples.
- Divide the total obtained sum of squares above step by 'DF' is obtained by deduction from total number of items by the number of samples, i.e., DF = N – K
  where, K = Number of samples
  N = Number of all observations

$$\text{Calculate the ratio 'F'} = \frac{\text{Between column variance}}{\text{Within column variance}} = \frac{s_1^2}{s_2^2}$$

Chapter 10: Analysis of Data and Application of Biostatistics in Nursing Research

Compare the Calculated Value with the Tabulated Value
* We take 5% of level of significance.
* If the calculated F > tabulated F = Significance difference in sample means, i.e., it is not arisen due to fluctuations of simple sampling or in other words the samples do not come from the sample population.
* In the other hand if the calculated value F < tabulated value then the difference is not significant and has arisen due to fluctuations of simple sampling.

Analysis of variance table, ANOVA with one-way calculation **(Table 10.37)**

Table 10.37: ANOVA with one-way calculation.

Square of variation	SS (sum of squares)	Degree of freedom	MS (mean square)	Variance ratio of 'F'
Between samples	SSC	C–1	MSC – SSC/C – 1	
Within samples	SSE	N–C	MSE – SSE/N – C	
Total	SST	N–1		MSC/MSE

[SST: total sum of squares of variations; SSC: sum of squares between samples (column); SSE: sum of squares within samples (rows); MSC: mean sum squares between samples; MSE: mean sum squares within samples; C: column; N: total sample size]

Example:
To assess the significance of possible variations in performance in certain test between the nursing colleges of a city. A common test was given to a number of students taken at random from the MSc class of each of the four colleges concern. The results are given below:

Table 10.38: ANOVA with one-way calculation.

A	B	C	D
8	12	18	13
10	11	12	9
12	9	16	12
8	14	6	16
7	4	8	15

Solutions:
* Sample means are as follows:
  $\bar{x}_1 = 45/5 = 9$
  $\bar{x}_2 = 50/5 = 10$
  $\bar{x}_3 = 60/5 = 12$
  $\bar{x}_4 = 65/5 = 13$

- **Grand mean** $= \bar{\bar{x}} = \dfrac{\bar{x}_1 + \bar{x}_2 + \bar{x}_3 + \bar{x}_4}{4} = \dfrac{44}{4} = 11$
- **Variations between samples:**

$(x_1 - \bar{\bar{x}})^2$	$(\bar{x}_2 - \bar{\bar{x}})^2$	$(\bar{x}_3 - \bar{\bar{x}})^2$	$(\bar{x}_4 - \bar{\bar{x}})^2$
4	1	1	4
4	1	1	4
4	1	1	4
4	1	1	4
4	1	1	4
Total 20	5	5	20

Sum of the squares between the samples = 20 + 5 + 5 + 20 = 50
Mean sum of squares between the sample is 50/4 – 1 = 16.7

- **Variance within samples:**

$(\bar{x}_1 - \bar{\bar{x}})^2$	$(\bar{x}_2 - \bar{\bar{x}})^2$	$(\bar{x}_3 - \bar{\bar{x}})^2$	$(\bar{x}_4 - \bar{\bar{x}})^2$
1	4	36	0
1	1	0	16
9	1	16	1
1	16	36	9
4	36	16	4
Total 16	58	104	30

Total sum of squares within samples = 16 + 58 + 104 + 30 = 208
Mean sum of squares within the samples = 208/20 – 4 = 13

Sources of variance	Sum of squares	DF	Mean square
Between samples	50	3	16.7
Within samples	208	16	13
Total	258	19	29.7

$$F = \dfrac{\text{Variance between samples}}{\text{Variance within samples}} = \dfrac{16.7}{13} = 1.28$$

- The table value of 'F' for $DF_1 = 3$
  $DF_2 = 16$
- At 5% level the significance is 3.24.
- The calculated 'F' < tabulated 'F' hence the difference mean values of the samples could have come from the same universe.

Two-way Classification

When a researcher compare more than one group based on more than one factors, then two way ANOVA can be adopted, e.g., a nurse researcher conducting a study on effects of back massage and warm compress on labor pain of prime and multigravida mothers. Here, she has to compare more than one factor (back massage and warm compress) with two groups (prime and multigravida mothers). This is a great way to control for extraneous variables as you are able to add them to the design of the study. In one factor analysis of variance expressed above the treatments constitute different levels of single factor which is controlled in the experiment. These are however at many situations in which two response variables of interest may be affected by more than one factor. For example, sale of cosmetics in condition to being affected by the paint of sale displayed. The number of competitive products sold by the store, e.g., hospital resource enlargement, establishment might have been affected by changes, the size and the location of the store. Similarly petrol mileage may be affected by the type of car driven. The way it is driven and its condition and the brand of petrol used.

In a two-way classification the data are classified according to two different criteria/factor. The procedure for analysis of variance in somewhat different than the following while dealing with the problem of one-way classification. The two-way classification analysis of variance is given in **Table 10.39**.

Table 10.39: ANOVA with two-way classification.

Sources of variance	Sum of squares	Degree of freedom	Mean sum of squares	Ratio of 'F'
Between columns	SSC	c–1	MSC = SSC/(c–1)	MSC/MSE
Between rows	SSR	r–1	MSR = SSR/(r–1)	MSR/MSE
Residence on error	SSE	(c–1)(r–1)	MSE = SSE/(c–1)(r–1)	
Total	SST	n–1		

(SSC: sum of squares between columns; SSR: sum of squares between rows; SSE: sum of squares due to error; SST: total sum of squares; MSC: mean sum squares between column; MSR: mean sum squares within the rows; MSE: mean sum of squares due to error)

The sum of squares for the source residual n's obtained by subtracting from the total sum of squares between columns and rows.
i.e., SSE = SST –(SSC + SSR)
The total number of degrees of freedom = (n–1) or (cr–1)
where, 'c' = Number of columns
'r' = Number of rows
Number of degrees of freedom between columns (c–1)
Number of degrees of freedom between rows (r–1)
Number of degrees of freedom for residual = (c–1)(r–1)

- The total sum of squares, sum of squares for below columns and sum of squares for between rows one obtained in the same way as before.
- Residues on error sum of square = Total sum of square – (sum of squares between columns + sum of squares between rows).

* The 'F' values are calculated as follows:

  - $F(df_1, df_2) = \dfrac{MSC}{MSE}$
    $df_1 = c-1$
    $df_2 = (r-1)(c-1)$

  - $f(df_1, df_2) = \dfrac{MSR}{MSE}$

  - $df_1 = (r-1), df_2 = (r-1)(c-1)$

  It should be carefully noted that DF_1 may not be same in both cases, in one case $DF_1 = (r-1)$ in another it is $DF_1 = (r-1)$.

Interpretation

The calculated values of 'F' are compared with table value if the calculated values at pre-assigned level of significance. The null hypothesis is rejected otherwise accepted.

Example:

A tea company has appointed four salesman named A, B, C, D and observed their sales in three different seasons like Summer, Winter and Monsoon. The sales of the four sales man in lakhs are given in the following table. Perform a two-way ANOVA on that.

Seasons	Treatment			
	A	B	C	D
Summer	38	40	41	39
Winter	45	42	49	36
Monsoon	40	38	42	42

The above data are classified according to criteria like salesman and seasons, etc., in order to simplify the classification we code the data by subtracting 40 from each figure.

* Let us take the hypothesis that there is no significance difference in the performance of the salesman. There is no significance variation in the sales between different seasons.

Seasons	A	B	C	D	Total
Summer	-2	0	1	-1	-2
Winter	5	2	9	-4	12
Monsoon	0	-2	2	2	2
Total	3	0	12	-3	Grand total T = 12

Correlation factor = $T^2/N = 12^2/12 = 12$ (where T = Grand total, N = Total number of items)

Sum of squares between treatments =

$= \dfrac{3^2}{3} + \dfrac{0^2}{3} + \dfrac{12^2}{3} + \dfrac{-3^2}{3} - \dfrac{T^2}{N} = \dfrac{9}{3} + 0 + \dfrac{144}{3} + \dfrac{9}{3} - 12 = 42$

The degree of freedom (c–1) = 4–1 = 3
* The sum of squares between the salesman =

$$\frac{-2^2}{4} + \frac{12^2}{4} - \frac{T^2}{N} = 1 + 36 + 1 - 12 = 26$$

* Degree of freedom (r-1) = 3-1 = 2
* Total sum of squares =
  $(-2)^2 + (5)^2 + (0)^2 + (0)^2 + (2)^2 + (-2)^2 + (1)^2 + (9)^2 + (2)^2 + (-1)^2 + (-4)^2 + (2)^2 - T^2/N =$
  $4 + 25 + 4 + 4 + 1 + 81 + 4 + 1 + 16 + 4 - 12 = 144 - 12 = 132$

Sources of variance	Sum of squares	Degree of freedom	Mean sum of squares	Ratio of 'F'
Between columns	SSC – 42	(c–1) = 3	SSC/(c–1) = 14	14/10.6 = 1.32
Between rows	SSR – 26	(r–1) = 2	SSR/(r–1) = 13	13/10.6 = 1.22
Residual errors	SSE – 64	(c–1)(r–1) = 6	MSE = SSE/(r–1) (c–1) = 10.6	
Total	SST= (SSC+SSR) = 132			

* For DF(3,6) at 'F'$_{0.05}$ = 4.76 (ANOVA table two-way classification) and for DF(2,6) at 'F'$_{0.05}$ = 5.14.
* Calculated value is less than the tabulated value so null hypothesis is accepted. Hence, there is no significance difference in the performance of the salesman and there is no significance variation in sales between different seasons.

Analysis of Covariance

Analysis of covariance (ANCOVA) is an extension of ANOVA that provides a way of statistically controlling the (linear) effect of variables one does not want to examine in a study. These extraneous variables are called covariates, or control variables. (Covariates should be measured on an interval or ratio scale). ANCOVA allows you to remove covariates from the list of possible explanations of variance in the dependent variable. ANCOVA does this by using statistical techniques (such as regression to partial out the effects of covariates) rather than direct experimental methods to control extraneous variables. ANCOVA is used in experimental studies when researchers want to remove the effects of some antecedent variable. For example, pretest scores are used as covariates in pretest post-test experimental designs. ANCOVA is also used in nonexperimental research, such as surveys or nonrandom samples, or in quasi-experiments when subjects cannot be assigned randomly to control and experimental groups. ANCOVA can be used to increase statistical power (the ability to find a significant difference between groups when one exists) by reducing the within-group error variance. In order to understand this, it is necessary to understand the test used to evaluate differences between groups, the F-test. The F-test is computed by dividing the explained variance between groups (e.g., gender difference) by the unexplained variance within the groups.

A One-way Analysis of Covariance

It evaluates whether population means on the dependent variable are the same across levels of a factor (independent variable), adjusting for differences on the covariate, or more simply stated, whether the adjusted group means differ significantly from each other. With a one-way analysis of covariance, each individual or case must have scores on three variables: a factor or independent variable, a covariate, and a dependent variable. The factor divides individuals into two or more groups or levels, while the covariate and the dependent variable differentiate individuals on quantitative dimensions. The one-way ANCOVA is used to analyze data from several types of studies; including studies with a pretest and random assignment of subjects to factor levels, studies with a pretest and assignment to factor levels based on the pretest, studies with a pretest, matching based on the pretest, and random assignment to factor levels, and studies with potential confounding.

Purpose

- In experimental designs, to control for factors which cannot be randomized but which can be measured on an interval scale.
- In observational designs, to remove the effects of variables which modify the relationship of the categorical independents to the interval dependent.
- In regression models, to fit regressions where there are both categorical and interval independents. This third purpose has become displaced by logistic regression and other methods.
- **Covariate** (also called a 'concomitant' or 'confound' variable) a variable that a researcher seeks to control.
- **Extraneous variable** (sometimes called 'nuisance variable') any condition not part of a study (that is, one in which researchers have no interest) but that could have an effect on the study's dependent variable.

$$F = \frac{\text{Mean sum between the group}}{\text{Mean sum within the group}}$$

- If this value is larger than a critical value, it is concluded that there is a significant difference between groups.

Assumptions

- The cases represent a random sample from the population, and the scores on the dependent variable are independent of each other, known as the assumption of independence.
- The dependent variable is normally distributed in the population for any specific value of the covariate and for any one level of a factor (independent variable), known as the assumption of normality.
- The variances of the dependent variable for the conditional distributions are equal, known as the assumption of homogeneity of variance.

Multivariate Analysis of Covariance

Multivariate analysis of covariance (MANCOVA) is a statistical technique that is the extension of analysis of covariance (ANCOVA). Basically, it is the multivariate analysis of variance (MANOVA) with a covariate(s). It is an extension of common analysis of variance (ANOVA). It is a statistical test procedure for comparing means of several groups unlike ANOVA. It uses the variance and covariance between variables in testing the statistical significance of mean differences. It is generalized form of univariant analysis of variance. It is used when there are more than two variables.

In MANCOVA, we assess for statistical differences on multiple continuous dependent variables by an independent grouping variable, while controlling for a third variable called the covariate; multiple covariates can be used, depending on the sample size. Covariates are added so that it can reduce error terms and so that the analysis eliminates the covariates' effect on the relationship between the independent grouping variable and the continuous dependent variables.

In multivariate analysis of covariance (MANCOVA), all assumptions are the same as in MANOVA, but one more additional assumption is related to covariate.

Characteristics

- It helps to answer among the independent variables and what are interaction among the dependent variables.
- Do changes in the independent variables have significant effect on dependent variables.

Assumptions

- **Independent random sampling:** MANCOVA assumes that the observations are independent of one another, there is not any pattern for the selection of the sample, and that the sample is completely random.
- **Level and measurement of the variables:** MANCOVA assumes that the independent variables are categorical and the dependent variables are continuous or scale variables. Covariates can be either continuous, ordinal, or dichotomous.
- **Absence of multicollinearity:** The dependent variables cannot be too correlated to each other. Tabachnick and Fidell (2012) suggest that no correlation should be above r= .90.
- **Normality:** Multivariate normality is present in the data.
- **Homogeneity of variance:** Variance between groups is equal.
- **Relationship between covariate(s) and dependent variables:** In choosing what covariate(s) to use, it is common practice to assess if a statistical relationship exists between the covariate(s) and the dependent variables which can be done through.
- The response variables are continuous.
- The residuals follow the multivariate-normal probability distribution with means equal to zero.
- The variance-covariance matrices of each group of residuals are equal.
- The individuals are independent.

PROBABILITY

Probability of a given event is an expression of the likelihood of chance of occurrence of that an event. Probability is quantified as a number between 0 and 1 (where 0 indicates impossibility and 1 indicates certainty). The higher the probability of an event, the more certain that the event will occur. The literally meaning of probability is a chance or possibility or likelihood of chance of occurrence. Mathematically, it is a number which is expressed either in the form of a fraction, percentage or a decimal.

Certain Terms in Probability

Experiment/Observation
It is an operation which produces some results or outcome. For example, a coin is tosses once, a dice is rolled twice.

Sample Space
- It is a set of all possible results/outcome of an experiment.
  S = Sample point.
- Each one of the possible results of an experiment represented as an element of a sample space is called sample point.
  For example, a coin is tossed twice
  S = {HH, TH, HT, TT}
  Here {HH, TH, HT, TT} are the events.

Theoretical Distribution

The probability distribution of a random variable may be:
- Theoretical listing of outcomes and probability which can be obtained from a mathematical model representing some phenomena of interest.
- A subjective listing of outcomes associated with subjective probabilities representing the degree of conviction of the decision maker as to the likelihood of the possible outcomes.
  For example, marks 0–10, 10–20, 20–30, 30–40, 40–50
  Frequency 10 18 15 16
- The above example clearly shows that the observed frequency distribution are obtained by grouping data.

Types of Theoretical Distribution

The types of theoretical distribution are:
- Binomial distribution
- Multinomial distribution
- Negative binomial distribution
- Poisson distribution
- Hypergeometric distribution
- Normal distribution
  Among these, the first and last one is continuous one.

Normal Distribution

- The binomial and the Poisson distributions as described above are the most useful theoretical distribution for discrete variables, i.e., they are related to the occurrence of distinct events.
- In order to have mathematical distribution, suitable for dealing with quantities whose magnitude is continuous variable, a continuum distribution is needed.
- The normal distribution is called normal probability distribution, happens to be most useful theoretical distribution for theoretical variables.
- The normal distribution was first described by Abraham De Moivre as the limiting form of binomial distribution in 1718.

$$(p+q)^n \; q^n + nc_r p^n q^{n-1} + n_{(r-1)} p^2 q^n$$

- Normal distribution was rediscovered by Gauss in 1809 and by Caplace in 1812.
- The normal distribution is an approximation to binomial distribution, whether or not p = q, the binomial distribution tends to the form of the continuous curve and when n becomes large, at least for the material part of the range as a matter of fact.
- The correspondence between the binomial and the curve is surprisingly close even for comparatively low values of 'n' proved that p and q are fairly nearly equal.
- The limiting frequency curve obtained as n becomes large.
- The normal distribution

$$p(x) = \frac{1}{\delta\sqrt{2\pi}} e^{-\frac{(x-\mu)^2}{2\delta^2}}$$

Where,
x = Values of the continuous random variable
μ = Mean of the normal random variable
e = Mathematical constant
    (Approximately 2.7183)
π = 22/7 (Mathematical constant)
δ = Standard deviation

- The normal distribution can have different shapes depending upon different values of means and standard deviation, but there is one and only one normal distribution for any given pair of values for mean (μ) and standard deviation (δ).
- Normal distribution is a limiting case binomial distribution.
  Where,
  - $n \longrightarrow \infty$
  - Neither p nor q is very small.
- Normal distribution is a limiting case of Poisson distribution where its mean is very large.
- The mean of a normally distributed population lies at the center of its curve.
- The 2 tails of the probability extends infinitely and never cross the horizontal axis. Which implies a positive probability for finding values of the random variable within any range of $-\infty$ to $+\infty$.

Computation of normal probability curve: If a coin is tossed unbiased it will fall either head (H) or tail (T). This the probability of appearing a head is one chance in two. So the probability ratio of H is ½ and T is ½.

Thus, $(H+T)^1 = H\frac{1}{2} + T\frac{1}{2} = 1.00$

Likewise of we shall toss two coins, coin x and coin y there are four possible ways of falling.

1		2		3		4	
x	y	x	y	x	y	x	y
H	H	T	H	H	T	T	T

Thus the four possible ways are–both x and y may fall H, x may fall T and y H, x may fall H and yT or both may fall T.

Expressed in ratios
Probability of two heads = ¼
Probability of two tails = ¼
Probability of one H and one T = ¼
Probability of one T and one H = ¼
Thus the submission ratios are ¼ + ½ + ¼ = 1.00

The expected appearance of heads and tails of two coins can be expressed as:
$(H + T)^2 = H^2 + 2HT + T^2$

If we shall increase the number of coins to three, i.e. x, y and z, there can be eight possible arrangements.

1	2	3	4	5	6	7	8
x y z	x y z	x y z	x y z	x y z	x y z	x y z	x y z
H H H	H H T	H T H	T H H	H T T	T H T	T T H	T T T

The expected appearance of heads and tails of coins can be expressed as:

$(H + T)^3 = H^3 + 3H^2T + 3HT^2 + T^3$

where,

1 H^3 = Three heads; one out of 8; probability ratio = $\dfrac{1}{8}$

3 H^2T = Two heads 1 tail; 3 out of 8; probability ratio = $\dfrac{3}{8}$

3 HT^2 = 1 heads 2 tails; 3 out of 8; probability ratio = $\dfrac{1}{8}$

Total = 1

In this way we can determine the probability of different combinations of heads and tails of any number of coins.

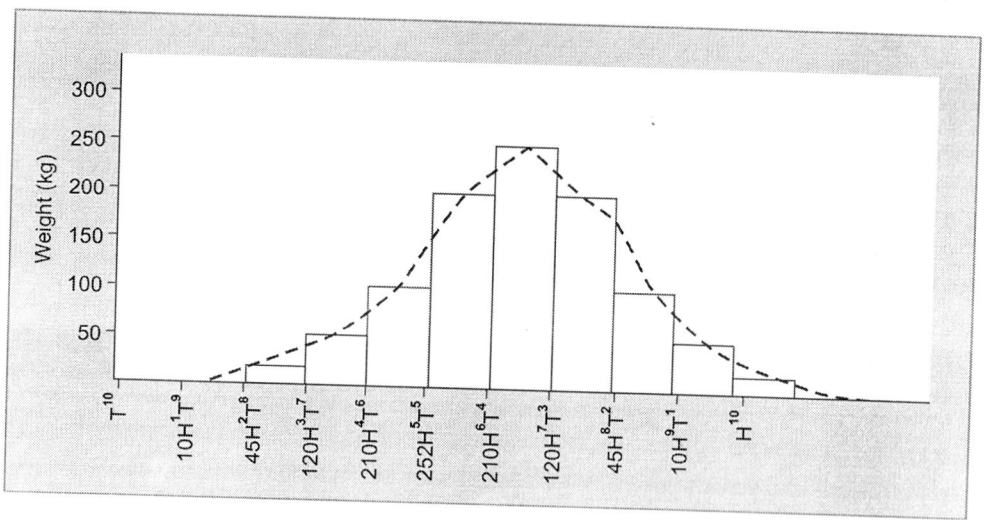

Fig. 10.18: Probability curve obtained from the expansion of $(H + T)^{10}$.

Thus the **Figure 10.18** we obtained from toss of 10 coins $(H + T)^{10}$ is a symmetrical many sided polygon.

And if we shall go on increasing the number of coins, with each increase the polygon would exhibit a perfectly smooth surface line which is called as normal probability curve. Normal probability curve, is bell-shaped curve and a graph representing a distribution of scores. Laplace and Gauss (1777–1855), derived the normal probability curve independently, so the curve is also known as Gaussian curve in the honor of Gauss.

Normal probability curve is the frequency polygon of any normal distribution. It is an ideal symmetrical frequency curve and is supposed to be based on the data of a population **(Fig. 10.19)**.
* The normal distribution can have different shapes depending upon different values of means and standard deviation, but there is one and only one normal distribution for any given pair of values for mean (μ) and standard deviation (δ). Normal distribution is a limiting case binomial distribution where
  - $n \longrightarrow \infty$
  - Neither p nor q is very small.
* Normal distribution is a limiting case of Poisson distribution where its mean is very large.
* The mean of a normally distributed population lies at the center of its curve.
* The 2 tails of the probability extends infinitely and never cross the horizontal axis. Which implies a positive probability for finding values of the random variable within any range of $-\infty$ to $+\infty$.

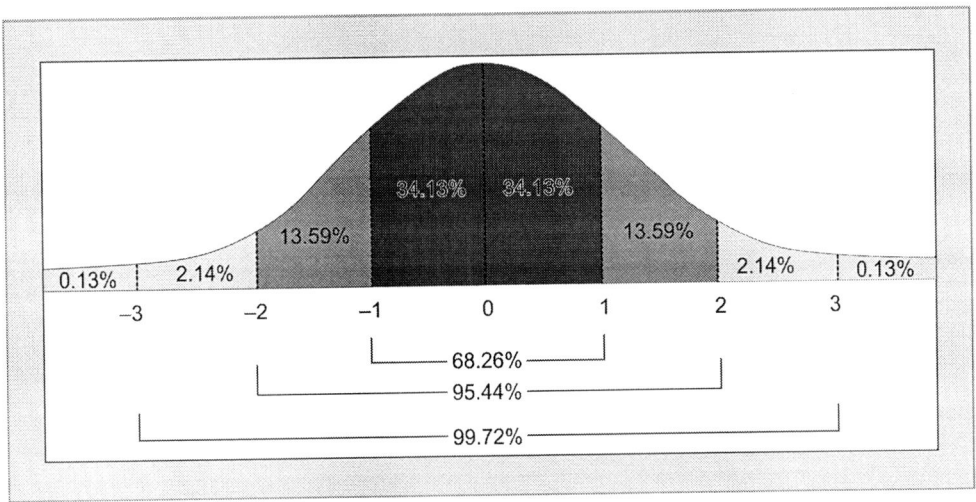

Fig. 10.19: Normal probability distribution.

Characteristics of Normal Probability Curve

Some of the major characteristics of normal probability curve are as follows:
* The normal distribution curve is bell-shaped and symmetrical in its appearance. The curve is symmetrical to its ordinate of the central point of the curve. It means the size, shape and slope of the curve on one side of the curve is identical to the other side of the curve. If the curve is bisected then its right hand side completely matches to the left hand side. If the curve were folded among its vertical axis, the 2 halves would coincide. The height of the curve for a positive deviation of 3 units is the same as the height of the curve for the negative deviation of 3 units.
* The curve is asymptotic: The normal probability curve approaches the horizontal axis and extends from $-\infty$ to $+\infty$. Means the extreme ends of the curve tends to touch the baseline but never touch it. It is depicted in **Figure 10.20**.
* The mean, median and mode: The height of the normal curve is at its maximum at the mean. Hence, the mean and mode of the normal distribution coincide. Hence, normal distribution mean, median and mode are equal and fall at the middle point.

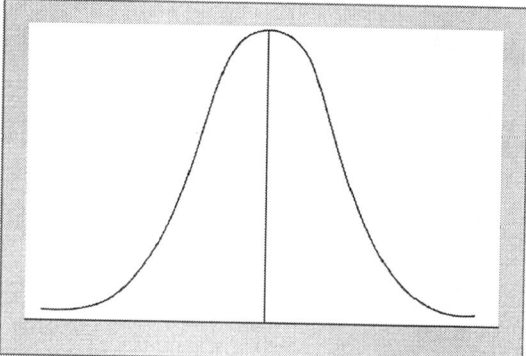

Fig. 10.20: Probability curve extending from $-\infty$ to $+\infty$.

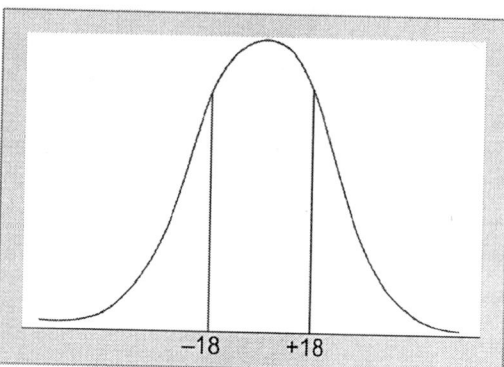

Fig. 10.21: Probability curve showing infinite difference.

- ❖ The points of inflection occur at ± 1 standard deviation unit: The points of influx in a normal probability curve occur at ± 1σ to unit above and below the mean. Thus, at this point the curve changes from convex to concave in relation to the horizontal axis.
- ❖ The total area of normal probability curve is divided into ± standard deviations: The total of normal probability curve is divided into six standard deviation units. From the center it is divided into three +ve standard deviation units and three –ve standard deviation units **(Fig. 10.21)**.

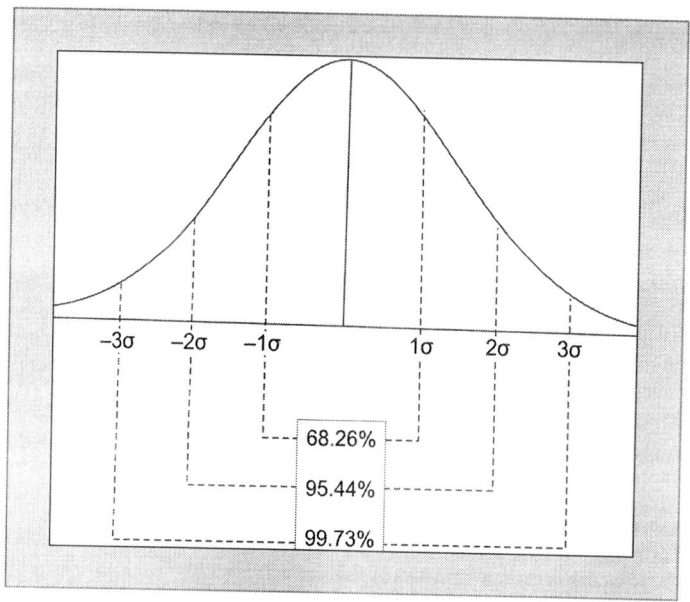

Fig. 10.22: Probability curve showing distribution of standard deviation.

Thus, ± 3σ of normal probability curve include different number of cases separately. Between ± 1σ lie the middle 2/3rd cases or 68.26%, between ± 2σ lie 95.44% cases and between ± 3σ lie 99.73% cases and beyond + 3σ only 0.37% cases fall **(Fig. 10.22)**.

- The Y ordinate represents the height of the normal probability curve. The Y ordinate of the normal probability curve represents the height of the curve. At the center the maximum ordinate occurs. The height of the curve at the mean or midpoint is denoted as Y_0.
- It is unimodal: The curve is having only one peak point. Because the maximum frequency occurs only at one point.
- The height of the curve symmetrically declines: The height of the curve decline to both the direction symmetrically from the central point. Means the $M + \sigma$ and $M - \sigma$ are equal if the distance from the mean is equal.
- The Mean of normal probability curve is μ and the standard deviation is σ: As the mean of the normal probability curve represent the population mean so it is represented by the μ (Meu). The standard deviation of the curve is represented by the Greek Letter, σ.
- The curve has its maximum height or ordinate at the starting point, i.e., the mean of the distribution. The first and the third quartile (Q_1 and Q_3) are at equal distance from Q_2 or median. The point of inflection (where the curvature changes its direction) is at point $\pm 1\ \sigma$, up and below the mean.
- As distinguished from binomial and Poisson distribution, where the variable is discrete and the variable distributed according to normal curve is a continuous one.

Importance of Normal Probability Curve

The normal distribution has long occupied central place in theory of statistics. The following importance is given below:
- The normal distribution has the remarkable property stated in the so-called central limit theorem. The central limit theorem gives the normal distribution its central place in theory of sampling. Since many important problems can be solved by the single pattern of sampling variability as a result, the work on statistical inferences is made simple.
- As *n* becomes large, the normal distribution serves as a good approximation of many discrete distribution. Whenever the exact discrete probability is laborious to obtain or impossible to calculate accurately.
- In a theoretical statistics, many problems can be solved under the assumption of a normal population.
- The distribution has numerous mathematical properties which make it popular and comparatively easy to manipulate.
- The normal distribution is used extensively in statistical quality control in setting of controlled limits.

Uses of Normal Probability Curve

- Normal probability curve is used to determine the percentage of cases in a normal distribution within given limits.
  The normal probability curve helps us to determine:
  - What percent of cases fall between two scores of a distribution.
  - What percent of scores lie above a particular score of a distribution.
  - What percent of scores lie below a particular score of a distribution.
- Normal probability curve is used to determine the value of a score whose percentile rank is given: By using normal probability curve table we can determine the raw score of the individual if the percentile rank is given.

- ❖ Normal probability curve is used to find the limits in a normal distribution which include a given percentage of cases: When a distribution is normally distributed and what we know about the distribution is mean and the standard deviation at that time by using the table area under normal probability curve we can determine the limits which include a given percentage of cases.
- ❖ It is used to compare two distributions in terms of overlapping: If scores of two groups on a particular variable are normally distributed. What we know about the group is the mean and standard deviation of both the groups. And we want to know how much the first group overlaps the second group or vice-versa at that time we can determine this by using the table area under NPC.
- ❖ Normal probability curve helps us in dividing a group into subgroups according to certain ability and assigning the grades: When we want to divide a large group in to certain subgroups according to some specified ability at that time we use the standard deviation units of a normal probability curve as units of scale.
- ❖ Normal probability curve helps to determine the relative difficulty of test items or problems: When it is known that what percentage of students successfully solved a problem we can determine the difficulty level of the item or problem by using table area under NPC.
- ❖ Normal probability curve is useful to normalize a frequency distribution: In order to normalize a frequency distribution we use normal probability curve. For the process of standardizing a psychological test this process is very much necessary.
- ❖ To test the significance of observations of experiments we use NPC: In an experiment we test the relationship among variables whether these are due to chance fluctuations or errors of sampling procedure or it is real relationship. This is done with the help of table area under NPC.
- ❖ Normal probability curve is used to generalize about population from the sample: We compute standard error of mean, standard error of standard deviation and other statistics to generalize about the population from which the sample are drawn. For this computation we use the table area under NPC.

Normal Probability Curve in Terms of Skewness

From the measures of variability, we can know that whether most of the items of the data are close to our away from these central tendencies. But these statistical means and measures of variation are not enough to draw sufficient inferences about the data. Another aspect of the data is to know its symmetry. Here by 'Graphic display' we have seen that a frequency may be symmetrical about mode or may not be. This symmetry is well-studied by the knowledge of the skewness. Skewness refers to lack of symmetry. A normal curve is a perfect symmetrical curve. In many distributions which deviate from the normal, the value of mean, median and mode are different and there is no symmetry between the two halves of the curve. Such distributions are said to be skewed. A uniform distribution would be the extreme case. It may happen that two distributions have the same mean and standard deviations.

Negative Skewness

A negatively skewed distribution rises slowly reaches its maximum and falls rapidly. In other words, the tail as well as the median are on the left-hand side. The curve is more inclined towards the left **(Fig. 10.23A)**.

Positive Skewness

A positively skewed distribution curve rises rapidly, reaches the maximum and falls slowly. In other words, the tail as well as median on the right-hand side. The curve is more inclined towards the right **(Fig. 10.23B)**.

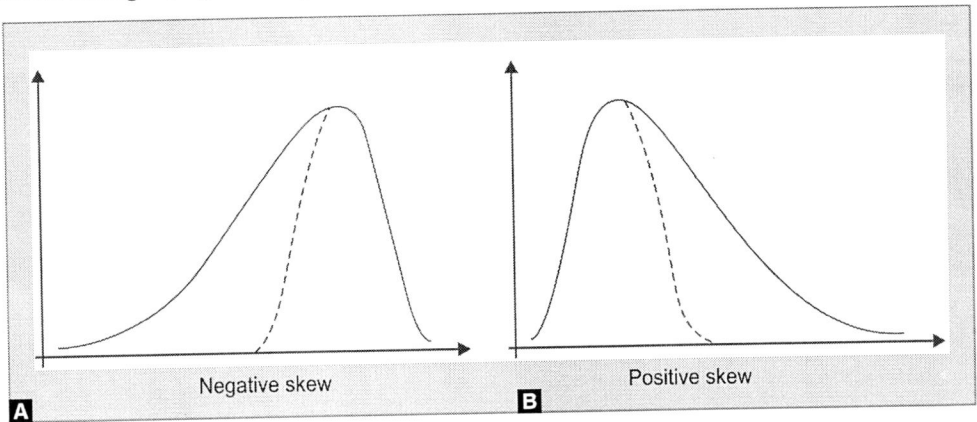

Figs. 10.23A and B: Skewed distribution curve.

Formula for skewness $Sk = 3(M-md)/\sigma$ (in terms of frequency distribution)
$Sk = [P90 + P10/2] - P50$ (in terms of percentile).

Kurtosis

A distribution, or data set, is symmetric if it looks the same to the left and right of the center point. Still one more aspect of the curve that we need to know is its flatness or otherwise its top. This is understood by what is known as 'Kurtosis.' Kurtosis is a measure of whether the data are heavy-tailed or light-tailed relative to a normal distribution. That is, data sets with high kurtosis tend to have heavy tails, or outliers. Data sets with low kurtosis tend to have light tails, or lack of outliers. When there are very few individuals whose scores are near to the average score for their group, the curve representing such a distribution becomes 'flattened' in the middle. On the other hand, when there are too many cases in the central area, the distribution curve becomes too 'peaked' in comparison with the normal curve. Both these characteristics of being flat or peaked, are used to describe the term kurtosis. **Figure 10.24** shows types of kurtosis.

Platykurtic

A frequency distribution is said to be platykurtic when the curve is flatter than the normal curve. platykurtic describes a statistical distribution with extremely dispersed points along the X-axis that results in a smaller peak (lower kurtosis) than curves typically seen in a normal distribution. Because this distribution has a low peak and corresponding thin tails, it is less clustered around the mean than are mesokurtic and leptokurtic distributions. The prefix of the term, 'platy', means broad, which fits the distribution's shape because it can be wide, broad or flat; distributions are deemed platykurtic when the excess kurtosis value is negative.

Leptokurtic

A frequency distribution is said to be leptokurtic when it is more peaked than the normal. Leptokurtic is a statistical distribution where the points along the X-axis are clustered, resulting

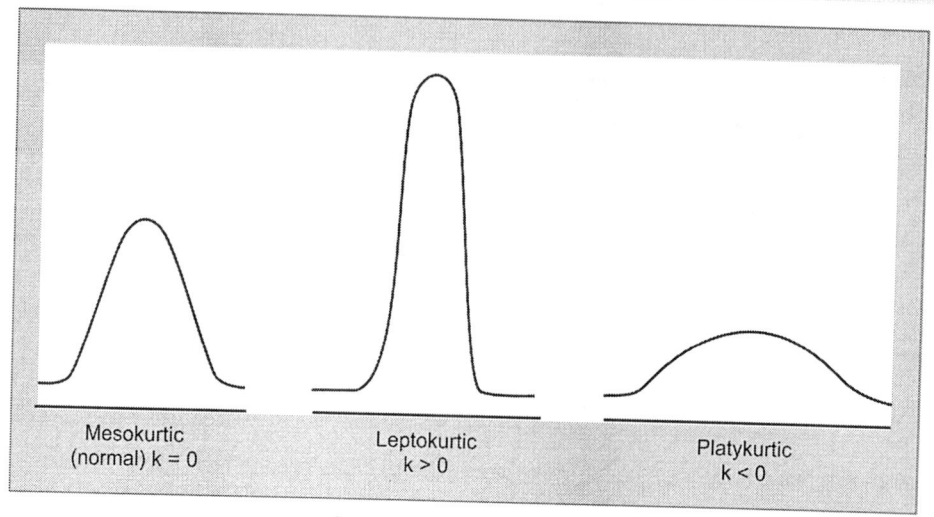

Fig. 10.24: Types of kurtosis.

in a higher peak, or higher kurtosis, than the curvature found in a normal distribution. This high peak and corresponding fat tails mean the distribution is more clustered around the mean than in a mesokurtic or platykurtic distribution and has a relatively smaller standard deviation. A distribution is leptokurtic when the kurtosis value is a large positive.

Mesokurtic

Mesokurtic is the distribution (frequency or graphical) whose kurtosis is similar to the kurtosis of the normally distributed data set. Kurtosis (Greek word meaning bulging) gives the measure of peakedness of a probability distribution of a random variable. A frequency distribution is said to be mesokurtic when it almost resembles the normal (neither too flat nor too peaked).

ANALYSIS OF QUALITATIVE DATA

Qualitative data refers to non-numeric information, such as interview transcripts, notes, video and audio recordings, images and text documents. Qualitative data analysis, is a search for general statements about relationships among categories of data. As qualitative data deals with descriptions, the major significance of qualitative data is the data can be observed but it is difficult to measure.

Qualitative data analysis is the range of processes and procedures whereby we move from the qualitative data that have been collected into some form of explanation, understanding or interpretation of the people and situations we are investigating. Here the idea is to examine the meaningful and symbolic content of qualitative data.

So qualitative data analysis is a time-consuming, detail-oriented, and seemingly overwhelming task which provides ways of discerning, examining, comparing, and interpreting meaningful patterns or themes. The most common analysis of qualitative data is based researcher interpretation. It is usually based on an interpretative philosophy. That is why the, expert or bystander observers examine the data, interpret it via forming an impression and report their impression in a structured and sometimes quantitative form. It deals in words and is guided by fewer universal rules and standardized procedures. It is also the range of processes and procedures whereby we move from the raw qualitative data into some form of explanation, understanding or interpretation of the people and situations we are investigating. The idea is to examine the meaningful and symbolic content of qualitative data. In contrast to quantitative analysis is an intensive and time-consuming activity that involves clustering together of related types of narrative information into a coherent scheme. Qualitative data analysis is a difficult procedure which needs researcher's expertize. Qualitative data analysis is the range of processes and procedures whereby we move from the qualitative data that have been collected into some form of explanation, understanding or interpretation of the people and situations.

Types of Qualitative Data Analysis

Qualitative data analysis can be divided into the following five categories:

1. **Content analysis:** This refers to the process of categorizing verbal or behavioral data to classify, summarize and tabulate the data. Content analysis is a widely used qualitative research technique. Rather than being a single method, current applications of content analysis show three distinct approaches, such as conventional, directed, and summative. All three approaches are used to interpret meaning from the content of text data and, hence, adhere to the naturalistic paradigm. The major differences among the approaches are coding schemes, origins of codes, and threats to trustworthiness. In conventional content analysis, coding categories are derived directly from the text data. With a directed approach, analysis starts with a theory or relevant research findings as guidance for initial codes. A summative content analysis involves counting and comparisons, usually of keywords or content, followed by the interpretation of the underlying context.
2. **Narrative analysis:** Narrative research is a term that subsumes a group of approaches that in turn rely on the written or spoken words or visual representation of individuals. This method involves the reformulation of stories presented by respondents taking into account context of each case and different experiences of each respondent. In other words, narrative analysis is the revision of primary qualitative data by researcher. Narrative methods otherwise called as "real world measures" that are appropriate when "real life problems" are investigated.
3. **Discourse analysis:** Discourse analysis is a qualitative method of analysis, which explores the meanings produced by language use and communication, the contexts and processes of these meanings and practices caused by these meanings. It is a method of analysis of naturally occurring talk and all types of written text.
4. **Framework analysis:** This is more advanced method that consists of several stages, such as familiarization, identifying a thematic framework, coding, charting, mapping and interpretation. Framework analysis is flexible during the analysis process in that it allows the user to either collect all the data and then analyze it or do data analysis during the collection process. In the analysis stage the gathered data is shifted, charted and sorted in accordance with key issues and themes.
5. **Grounded theory:** Grounded theory is a systematic methodology involving the construction of theories through methodical gathering and analysis of data. By collecting and analyzing qualitative data, the researcher can construct a new theory that is "grounded" in that data. As more data is collected, and re-reviewed, codes can be grouped into concepts, and then into categories. This method of qualitative data analysis starts with an analysis of a single case to formulate a theory. Then, additional cases are examined to see if they contribute to the theory.

Approaches in Analysis

Deductive approach: Using your research questions to group the data and then look for similarities and differences—Used when time and resources are limited—used when qualitative research is a smaller component of a larger quantitative study.

Inductive approach: Used when qualitative research is a major design of the inquiry—using emergent framework to group the data and then look for relationship.

Problem in Qualitative Data Analysis

Qualitative data analysis is very challenging task because of the following reasons:
- There are no universally accepted rules and methods for analysis of qualitative data. Therefore, validity of analyzed data is always a controversial issue.
- Volumes data is so large which may be a recording or several page narrations collected during qualitative studies which require a lots of hard work for drawing the meaningful conclusions.
- Qualitative data cannot be condensed too much like quantitative data because they may lose their richness of content and evidentiary value. Qualitative analysis requires powerful inductive skills (inducing universals from particulars) and creativity also.

Qualitative Data Analysis Process

Data analysis is the most complex and mysterious of all of the phases of a qualitative research. The analysis of qualitative data is carried out typically in active and inactive processes. Insights for qualitative analysis the researcher should completely familiar with whole data. Qualitative data analysis is a process of conjecture and verification of correction and modification of suggestion and defense. Qualitative data come in various forms. In many qualitative nursing studies, the database consists of interview transcripts from open-ended, focused, and exploratory interviews. However, there is no limit for qualitative database, and increasingly there are more and more creative use of such sources as recorded observations (both video and participatory), focus groups, texts and documents, multimedia or public domain sources, policy manuals, photographs, and lay autobiographical accounts. The data can be collect from several sources but it is noted that qualitative analysis is 'a process of fitting data together or making the invisible obvious linking and attributing consequences of antecedents'. There are four major process by which qualitative data analysis can done. They are as follows:
- **Comprehending:** Comprehend, means grasp mentally; understand or to perceive. In early analysis process, a qualitative researcher strives to make sense of the data and learn 'what is going on' by reading rereading the voluminous information collected in qualitative research. Once the researcher comprehends the topic in mind, the researcher is able to prepare a thorough and rich description of the phenomenon, which is completed only when a complete and accurate description has been written.
- **Synthesizing:** Synthesizing means to make something new by combining different things. In qualitative research, synthesizing involves a 'sifting' of the data, and putting pieces together to get new information. It also refers to the ability to put parts together to form a new whole. At this stage, the researcher gets a sense of what is typical and what is different about the phenomenon. At the end of the synthesis process, the researcher can make some generalized statements about the phenomenon and about the study participants.
- **Theorizing:** Theorizing means to think of or suggest ideas about what is possibly true or real: or to form or suggest a theory about something theorizing involves a systemic sorting of the data. During the theorizing process, the researcher develops alternative explanations of the phenomenon under study and then analyzes those explanations to determine their 'fit' with the data. The theorizing process continues to evolve until the best and most relevant explanation is obtained.
- **Recontextualizing:** The process of recontextualization involves the further development of the theory such that its applicability to other settings or groups is explored. In qualitative

inquiries, the ultimate goal of which is theory development, the theory must be re-contextualized and generalized.

Steps of Qualitative Data Analysis

In qualitative data analysis, data is obtained thorough loosely structured interviews with open-ended questions, focus group discussions (FGDs), observations and projective and participatory approaches. Irrespective of the purpose of the qualitative study and any of the above-mentioned techniques of data collection, the researcher ends up with a substantial number of pages of written text that needs to be analyzed. The procedures and outcome of the qualitative data analysis differ from those of quantitative data analysis which is described below:
- Organizing the data and identifying themes
- Order and reduce/code the data (data processing).
- Summarize the data in such a way that interpretation become easy, e.g., by preparing compilation sheet, descriptive narrates, flowcharts, diagrams, or matrices.
- Draw conclusions, relate these to the other data sets of the study, and decide how to integrate the data in the report.
- If required, develop strategies for further testing or confirming the qualitative data in order to prove their validity.

Organizing the Data and Identifying Themes

The best way to organize the data is to go back to the interview guide. Identify and differentiate between the actual theme what a researcher want from general data. The amount of data generated by one interview could answer an incredible number of questions. The researcher spend the rest time period trying to analyze all of that information. That is why it is important to go back to the original questions that the researcher want. During analyze data, a researcher always keeping in mind what he or she are trying to find out and why he or she wanted to do the interviews in the first place. After getting answer to original questions, he/she has to search other ideas and themes that have emerged from the data relate to your questions and in terms of future research considerations. Data should be organized in a way that is easy to look at, and that allows the researcher to go through each topic to pick out concepts and themes. One way to do this is to organize all the data from the transcript.

Ordering and Coding of Data

After identification of words/phrases used frequently, as well as ideas coming from how the interviewee has expressed himself/herself and from the stories that the subject has told to the researcher, he has to organize these ideas into codes or categories. During ordering or the coding of the qualitative data, research handles two types of data:
- Responses or answers acquired through open-ended questions.
- More elaborate narratives from loosely structured interviews or FGDs.
  Ordering and coding for the answers acquired through open-ended question involve following steps:
- A first, basic step in the analysis of answers to open-ended questions is to list the answers of a sample of 20–25 informants as they were provided (adding the questionnaire number in order to avoid losing the connection with the informants' other data).
- Next read the answers carefully, remembering the purpose of the question.

- *Make rough categories* of answers that seem to belong together and code them with respective keywords.
- List again all answers but now per code, so that you get some five to seven short lists.
- *Interpret* each list, and end up with some five to seven meaningful categories, each with a characteristics keyword, e.g., *pleasure, being sociable, giving status, giving self-confidence, addiction, defiance*. There may be a discussion on the need to split up some categories or combine others with few answers, e.g., answers 17 and 18. In that case there would be seven categories. The category defiance may have two answers; I do not see why I would give up smoking ! And why not ? The exclamation mark indicates defiance rather than lack of knowledge, with forms the motivation for the answer. Without this addition by the interviewer, these answers would have been difficult to code.

    Now a researcher can make a tentative interpretation according to the assumed willingness of informants to change their behavior. For those who smoke for pleasure or to socialize it might be most easy to give up smoking. Those who are addicted but tried to stop and those who feel they derive status from smoking might form a middle category, whereas for those who smoke to enhance their self-confidence and reduce stress or who are very defiant at the question why they smoke, it might be most difficult to stop.
- Now try a next batch of 2–25 answers and check if the labels work. It is quite possible that at this stage still some labels will be changed or that you decide to add new categories or combine others.
- Make a final list of labeled categories and code all data, including the data you have already processed with the abbreviated codes.

    Then discuss whether you will stick to your tentative interpretation of the data and what this means for the content of the messages to address different reasons for smoking. This content analysis is the most important purpose of the analysis. By counting the answers under each label, however, the researcher will gain insight as well in how common the different reasons are.

    Ordering and coding for the answers acquired through elaborated narratives involve the following steps:

    The data from interviews with key informants or focus group discussions (FGDs) is as a rule more bulky than answers to open-ended questions. The carefully transcribed field notes and tapes may consist of pages of narrative text. When analyzing the text we usually discover that, no matter how good our guidelines for the discussion were, the data contain valuable information but also a number of less-essential details. In addition, the data is usually not presented in the order we need for our analysis, since informants may jump from one topic to the other. To make the analysis easier, we have to order and reduce the data. Ordering is best done in relation to the objectives and the discussion topics. Again, it is best to systematically follow a number of steps.
- *Reread* research objectives and discussion topics.
- Carefully read a number of the interviews, focus group discussions, or narrative observations, which need to be analyzed. Number the material according to the broad discussion topic it pertains to; use a colored marker to highlight particularly illustrative remarks. Use the margins to define subtopics. Also be able to distinguished, varying from slight avoidance to complete expulsion. If stigma would be a topic in your discussion list, you would mark everything related to stigma within a margin, and add *keywords* such as self-stigma, spouse, in-laws, comm., in the margin, as well as keywords such as sleep(ing) sep(arately) or divorce indicating the severity of the stigma.

- List all keywords that belong to a certain topic in the subcategories that have been developed under, e.g., everything belonging to stigma could be subdivided and listed in the four major social settings in which stigma was found to manifest itself.
- Interpret the data, e.g., distinguish the major forms in which stigma manifests itself in these different social settings, try to make a ranking order of severity, and link it to other variables (such as degree of deformity, socioeconomic status) in order to understand differences in stigma.
- Then code all your qualitative data in this way. If necessary, adapt your coding scheme as you order, code, and interpret more data. In that case, you should again read and possibly recode the material you have already processed.

Summarizing Data in Compilation Sheets

After ordering the data we will have to summarize them. A useful first step is summarizing all data of each study unit per study population on separate compilation sheets. Like the master sheets for quantitative data, compilation sheets for qualitative data consist of a number of columns with the topics covered by the study as headings. These may be further subdivided in smaller themes that you identified and coded when ordering the data. Each interview, FGD, or observation gets a number and is successively entered in that sequence on the relevant compilation sheet. If there are different categories of informants within one study population.

Now you have an overview of all data per study population on one or more compilation sheet(s). If you read the columns, you have a list of answers of all group members on a certain (sub) topic. If you read horizontally, you can per informant relate different topics to each other or to personal characteristics of the informant. It also becomes easy to compare the answers of different groups on specific issues by comparing the compilation sheets.

You may notice that interpretation of data and labeling becomes indeed easy when using compilation sheets, as a researcher can visualize all aspects of his or her informants even if he or she looks at one aspect at a time for the whole study population.

The next step in summarizing may be the combining, contrasting, or further analysis of important topics through graphical displays, such as matrices, diagrams, flowcharts, and tables.

Further Summarizing of Data in Narrations, Matrices, Figures, and Quasi-Statistic Tables

Further summarization of data may be achieved through narrative analysis, matrices, figures and quasi-statistical tables.

Matrices: Matrices can be used for quantitative as well as qualitative data comparison. In qualitative data we may compare different groups or data sets on important variables, presented in keywords. A matrix is a chart that looks like a cross-table, but contains words (as well as, sometimes, numbers). In a focus group discussion on changing weaning practices, the researchers listed the answers of young mothers concerning the introduction of soft foods and those of mothers above childbearing age. They then summarized these answers in a matrix. This type of display made it easy for the researchers to conclude that:

- Younger mothers start giving soft foods, on average, 2.5 months earlier than the generation of their own mothers.
- Younger mothers use a larger variety of soft weaning foods than women in the preceding generations.

❖ Younger mothers give soft foods to their babies more frequently, but for the same reasons as their mothers did.

Matrices facilitate data analysis considerably. They are the most common form of graphic display of qualitative data. They can be used to order and compare information in many ways.

Diagrams: A diagram is a figure with boxes containing variables, and arrows indicating the relationships between these variables. When analyzing the problems you wanted to investigate during the development of your protocols, most groups developed a diagram. In a similar way, diagrams can be developed to summarize findings of a study. You might use a diagram to illustrate a crucial issue in your study, combining all available qualitative and quantitative data collected. Diagrams, like matrices, can be of great assistance in providing an overview of the data collected and in guiding data analysis.

Flowcharts: Flowcharts are special types of diagrams that express the logical sequence of actions or decisions. The preceding figure, indicating the successive steps in protocol development, is an example of a flowchart. Flowcharts are especially useful to summarize different flows of events that are mutually connected. A counseling team in Bulawayo, Zimbabwe. One central line presented the development of the disease over time, with crises and periods of relative well-being. Another line presented different forms of medical care sought, a third the flaws in economic status connected to the disease (e.g., loss of job, seeking employment elsewhere), a fourth the possible changes in social status such as divorce or remarriage, whereas a fifth line presented the patient's emotional status linked to events occurring in the four other fields. These flowcharts were extremely useful for comparison of data per informant and between different groups of informants (e.g., males/females, single/married). They highlighted the impact of the disease on the lives of different groups of patients and their way of coping with it.
Adapted from Meursing K (1997). A world of silence: Living with HIV in Matabeleand, Zimbabwe. Amsterdam: Royal Tropical Institute.

Quasi-statistical tables: In this technique of qualitative data analysis, the researcher using a quasi-statistical style typically begins with some preconceived ideas about the analysis and uses those ideas to sort the data. This approach is sometimes referred to as manifest content analysis. In this researcher review, the content of the narrative data searches for particular words or themes that have been specified in advance. The result of the search is information that can be analyzed statistically and hence the name quasi-statistic is given.

Narrative analysis: It is the study of an individual's speech. It is the most common approach of qualitative data analysis. In this approach, the stories of the respondents are narrated. The story is what a person shares about self. A searcher always tries to compare ideas presented by respondents about self. Narrative analysis could involve study of literature or diaries or folklore and autobiographies and compare them.

Integrating qualitative and quantitative data: Thus far we have discussed the analysis of qualitative data as a separate activity. However, if a research team has collected qualitative as well as quantitative data, which is the case in most health science research studies, it would be foolish not to look at them in combination, as this can inspire to deeper and more rewarding analysis.

Drawing and Verifying Conclusions

Drawing and verifying conclusions is the essence of data analysis. It is not an isolated activity, however. When we start summarizing our data in compilation sheets, flowcharts, matrices, or diagrams, we continuously draw conclusions, and modify or reject quite a number of them as we proceed. Writing helps generate new ideas as well. Therefore, writing should start as early as possible, right from the onset of data processing and analysis, even if only for ourselves. No creative insights should get lost.

Note: Collection, processing, analysis, and reporting of qualitative data are closely interwined, and not (as is the case with quantitative data) distinct successive steps. It may often be necessary to go back to the original field notes and verify conclusions, collect additional data if available data appear controversial, and get feedback from all parties concerned.

* **Reporting the data:** Basically, there are two ways of reporting qualitative data that form part of a study in which different research techniques were used. One way is summarizing the major qualitative results in a separate section of the findings, with examples and quotations, following the objectives that guided the collection of this particular data together with the results of other, more quantitative data collection tools and would subsequently be reflected in the summary of the findings and the recommendations.

  Another possibility is to fully integrate different data sets in the chapter of findings, ordered according to the objectives of the entire study. If quantitative and qualitative data have been analyzed and sometimes even collected in an integrated way, it would also be logical to present them in an integrated fashion. Attention should be paid that no valuable data gets lost. Therefore, a rough draft of all important findings is required in any case, after which it can be decided to present the data either in separate sections or chopped up for integration with other data.

Establishing the Validity of Qualitative Data

Data generated after the qualitative study may often generate questions concerning its validity. Therefore, to establish the validity of the qualitative data following strategies must be applied.

* **Check for representativeness of data:** Although in qualitative research informants have usually not been selected randomly, they must have been selected systematically, according to previously established rules. Check whether you have indeed interviewed all categories of informants needed to get a complete picture of your topic (not relying excessively on talkative authorities). Make sure that you do not generalize from unrepresentative events.
* **Check for bias:** Due to observer bias or the influence of the researcher on the research situation, the results can be drastically affected.
* **Cross-check data with evidence from other, independent sources:** These sources may be different independent informants, different research techniques employed to investigate the same topic or results from other, similar studies. The data should confirm or at least not contradict each other. Actively cross-checking data, looking for independent evidence or counter-evidence, is one of the most important ways to enhance the validity of researcher data.
* **Compare and contrast data:** Comparison will often have been built into the research design through including different categories of informants. If we want to be sure.
* **Use extreme (groups of) informants to the maximum:** In the discussion of study design and sampling we stated that it may be useful to look for categories of informants that represent the extremes on a certain variable.
* **Carry out additional research to test the findings of your study:** The results of your study may be so intriguing that you decide to do a follow-up study afterwards. Such a study may be undertaken for several reasons.
  * To replicate certain findings.
  * To rule out (or identify) possible intervening variables.
  * To rule out rival explanations by investigating them.

- To look for negative evidence.
  Additional studies undertaken for one or more of these reasons may serves to make the results of your original study more convincing.
- **Get feedback from your informants:** Qualitative researcher needs to involve all parties concerned at the various stages of the research. This is important not only for ethical reasons or because it will improve the chances that the results will be implemented, but also because it will improve the quality of your study design, of data, and of the conclusions drawn from these data. Suggestions and additional information collected during feedback sessions will invariably increase the quality of your research report.

Computer Analysis of Qualitative Data

With the ever-increasing importance of computers in research, strategies for analyzing qualitative data by computer have been are being developed. There are several possibilities, ranging from simple word-processing programs to highly sophisticated Qualitative Data Management Software including possibilities for statistical testing of associations. As numbers are usually small in Health Sciences Research and content analysis, which can be done manually, is most likely more important than testing of associations, we will not elaborate these techniques here. Rather we refer the interested students to Anthropology or Psychology departments at universities that have experience with programs such as Qualitan or SPSS-1.

SUMMARY

- Analysis and interpretation of data is the most important phase of the research process, which involves the computation of the certain measures along with searching for patterns of relationship that exists among data groups. Analysis is the process of organizing and synthesizing the data so as to answer research questions and test hypothesis.
- Analysis of quantitative data deals with information collected during research study, which can be quantified, and statistical calculations can be computed. Quantitative data is presented in a numerical format, collected in a standardized manner.
- Data preparation involves checking or logging the data in which can be done just after data collection, checking the data for accuracy by comparing with original raw data, entering the data into the computer, transforming the data, and developing and documenting a database structure that integrates the various measures.
- Descriptive statistics involves the measures to condense data, measures of central tendency, measures of dispersion and measures of relationship.
- Measures to condense data is an appropriate presentation of data which involves organization of data in such a manner that meaningful conclusions and inferences can drawn to answer the research question. Quantitative data are generally condensed and presented through tables, charts, graphs and diagram.
- One of the most important objectives of statistical analysis is to get one single value that describe the characteristics of the entire mass of unwieldy data. Such a value is called central value or average otherwise known as central tendency.
- Two distributions of statistical data may be symmetrical and have common means, medians and modes and identical frequencies in the modal class. Yet with these points in common they may differ widely in the scatter or in their values about the measures of central tendencies. In statistics, dispersion (also called variability, scatter, or spread) denotes how stretched or squeezed a distribution. In conducting research the researcher has to find out

the relationship between different variables which can be measured by correlation and regression analysis.

- A chi-squared test, also referred to as c2 test (or chi-square test), is any statistical hypothesis test in which the sampling distribution of the test statistic is a chi-square distribution when the null hypothesis is true. Chi-squared tests are often constructed from a sum of squared errors, or through the sample variance.
- Theoretical test done on T-distribution was done by WS Gosset in the early 1900. One sample t-test is a statistical procedure used to examine the mean difference between the sample and the known value of the population mean.
- In paired sample hypothesis testing, a sample from the population is chosen and two measurements for each element in the sample are taken. Each set of measurements is considered a sample.
- Analysis of variance (ANOVA) is a collection of statistical models used to analyze the differences among group means and their associated procedure. It is a statistical measure that analyzes the variance of two or more comparable series or sample through the F-test technique to ascertain whether the difference in mean values is significant or not and whether the different samples under study are drawn from same universe or from different universe is the same or not.

QUESTIONS TO TEST YOUR KNOWLEDGE

Q1. What do you mean by data analysis? Write down the steps of quantitative data analysis.
(2 + 8)

Q2. Enumerate different types of tables, charts and graphs used for presentation of data.
(15)

Q3. Describe the concept of central tendency. Explain about geometric mean with suitable example.
(5 + 10)

Q4. What do you mean by measures of dispersion? Enumerate different types of measures of dispersion.
(3 + 12)

Q5. Explain about various types of correlation with examples.
(10)

Q6. Write short notes among the following:
(5 × 6)
   a. Normal probability curve
   b. Mode
   c. Correlation coefficient
   d. Chi-squared test
   e. ANOVA
   f. Pared t-test

7. Multiple choice questions:
(1 × 18)
   I. Which correlation is the strongest?
      a. +.10
      b. -.95
      c. +.90
      d. -1.00
   II. Which one of these is NOT normally associated with qualititative data?
      a. Words
      b. Narrative
      c. Bar diagramme
      d. Images
   III. A _____ is a range of numbers inferred from the sample that has a certain probability of including the population parameter over the long run.
      a. Hypothesis
      b. Lower limit
      c. Confidence interval
      d. Probability limit

IV. One use of a regression line:
   a. to determine if any x-values are outliers.
   b. to determine if any y-values are outliers.
   c. to determine if a change in x causes a change in y.
   d. to estimate the change in y for a one-unit change in x.

V. During analysis the process of marking segments of data with symbols, descriptive words, or category names is known as:
   a. Concurring
   b. Coding
   c. Coloring
   d. Segmenting

VI. A procedure that is used to determine the sample size needed to prevent a Type II error is:
   a. Sample calculation
   b. Sample analysis
   c. Power Analysis
   d. Error analysis

VII. When a researcher accepts the null hypothesis that is false, he commits what type of error?
   a. Type I
   b. Type II
   c. Type III
   d. Type IV

VIII. When a researcher wishes to do a measure of central tendency, he will most likely use which of the following descriptive statistics?
   a. Mode
   b. Median
   c. Mean
   d. All of the above

IX. The standard deviation is:
   a. The square root of the variance
   b. A measure of variability
   c. An approximate indicator of how numbers vary from the mean
   d. All of the above

X. The most frequently occurring number in a set of values is called the:
   a. Mean
   b. Median
   c. Mode
   d. Range

XI. Which of the following is NOT a common measure of central tendency?
   a. Mode
   b. Range
   c. Median
   d. Mean

XII. _____ are used when you want to visually examine the relationship between two quantitative variables.
   a. Bar graphs
   b. Pie graphs
   c. Line graphs
   d. Scatterplots

XIII. The median is:
   a. The middle point
   b. The highest number
   c. The average
   d. Affected by extreme scores

XIV. The area under normal curve between the point x- 3σ and x+ σ is:
   a. 66.26% of total area under the curve
   b. 95.44% of total area under the curve
   c. 99.74% of total area under the curve
   d. 99.26% of total area under the curve

XV. Which of the following would indicate that a probability curve is not bell-shaped?
   a. The range is equal to 5 standard deviations.
   b. The range is larger than the interquartile range.
   c. The mean is much smaller than the median.
   d. There are no outliers.

XVI. The coefficient value between two variable is 1.25 which indicate that there is a:
   a. Positive relationship
   b. Negative relationship
   c. No relationship
   d. Wrong calculation

XVII. In a frequency distribution curve when mean >median>mode it is a:
 a. Positive skewed distribution curve
 b. Negative skewed distribution curve
 c. Normal skewed distribution curve
 d. No skewness

ANSWERS

I. d	II. c	III. c	IV. d	V. b
VI. a	VII. b	VIII. d	IX. d	X. c
XI. b	XII. d	XIII. a	XIV. c	XV. c
XVI. d	XVII. a			

Chapter 11

Research Critique

Learning Objectives

After completion of this chapter, the students will be able to:
- Explain the concept, importance, purposes and principles of research critique.
- Describe the critique skills required to critique research studies.
- Identify the basic steps of critique process.
- Critique the quantitative research studies by following steps.
- Critique qualitative research studies by following recommended standards.
- Enumerate about rigors, auditability, theoretical connectedness, heuristic relevance and what to be avoid during critique.

INTRODUCTION TO THE CONCEPT OF RESEARCH CRITIQUE

After collecting and analyzing the data, the researcher has to accomplish the task of drawing inferences followed by report writing. This has to be done very carefully, otherwise misleading conclusions may be drawn and the whole purpose of doing research may get vitiated. It is only through interpretation that the researcher can expose relations and processes that underlie his findings. Nursing practice can be based on evidence-based practice and that evidence must be solid. An evidence or a research result can only considered as solid if research reports are critically appraised. Consumers sometimes think that if a report was accepted for publication, the study must be sound. Unfortunately, this is not true. Moreover every research has limitations and weaknesses. Although disciplined research is the best possible means of answering many questions still no single study can provide conclusive evidence. Rather, evidence is accumulated through the conduct— and evaluation—of several studies addressing the same or a similar research question. The strength and weakness of these studies can be identified when it is evaluated.

Research critique refers to planned, systematic and careful evaluation of a research work. It based on some prespecified standard criteria to judge the strength and weakness of work. It requires critical thinking and intellectual skills, and involves a careful examination of all aspects of study to judge the merits, limitation, meaning and significance based on previous research experience. Research critique is a thoughtful, objective, and balanced consideration on the quality of the study by a professional analysis of its weaknesses and strengths. A critique may be done for a variety of purposes like acting as an expert reviewer to assess whether this research paper should be published or providing helpful comments on a work before it is submitted for publication or sometimes, as a learning experience for emerging scholars to practice their developing research skills.

A critique emphasizes the aspects of the research like problem statement and its importance whether it is relevant, need for the study, hypothesis, research design, the elements of the research design and evaluates how well the author has carried out these elements, etc. It also covers the data analysis whether that has been properly carried out and interpreted, discussions by comparing with other reports recommendations and bibliography.

DEFINITIONS

* A research critique is a careful appraisal of the strengths and weaknesses of the study.
* An intellectual research critique is a careful, complete examination of a study to judge its strengths, weaknesses, logical links, meaning and significance.
* The process of objectivity and critically evaluating a research report's content for scientific merit and application to practice, theory or education.
* Critiquing is a systematic process for evaluating research studies and the results reported.
* 'Systematic, unbiased, careful examination of all aspects of a study to judge the merits, limitations, meaning and significance based on previous research experience and knowledge of the topic'. —*Burns N and Grove S, 2005*
* Critical appraisal has been defined as the '...application of rules of evidence to a study to assess the validity of the data, completeness of reporting, methods and procedures, conclusions, compliance with ethical standards, etc'.

IMPORTANCE OF RESEARCH CRITIQUE

* To broaden understanding for use in practice.
* For implementing an evidence-based nursing practice.
* Encourages nurses to participate in clinical inquiry and provide evidence for use in practice.

PURPOSES OF CRITIQUE

* To assess students' methodological and analytical skills (identify limitations and strengths).
* Seasoned researcher to help journal editions.
* Written critique is a guide to researcher.
* To advance nursing knowledge and profession. Critiques should offer guidance about ways in which study results may have been compromised, and should provide guidance about alternative research strategies to address the research question.
* To evaluate the critiques/methodological skill and understanding of the students.
* To improve the scientific flaws of the research. Critiquing individual studies plays a role in assembling evidence into integrative reviews of the literature on a topic.

PRINCIPLES OF RESEARCH CRITIQUE (FIG. 11.1)

Some principles should be kept in mind while appraising a research work:

* **Be objective:** During critiquing of research the researcher should be objective in nature by making comments on specific to the work he/she is reviewing irrespective of name, job and related information of author. First, she or he should convey a sincere interest and understanding of the article. Never ridicule or demean the project or researcher.
* **Be constructive:** The critical appraisal of research should be oriented to improve the research process rather than criticizing it negatively. The

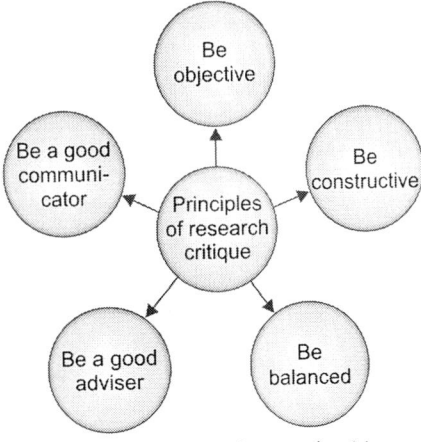

Fig. 11.1: Principles of research critique.

export should start commenting on positive points of the report first than should take about weak points and scope for improvement in research study. When pointing out a study's weaknesses include explanations that justify your comments.

- ❖ **Be balanced:** The report should be considered in a balanced way, identify in inadequacies as well as adequacies. The evaluator should not focus on a particular aspect of research report like talking about only adequacies and inadequacies. All reports have some positive features and as a researcher he/she must be sure to find and note them. During critiquing must justify his/her criticisms with offering a rationale for concerns.
- ❖ **Be a good adviser:** Critique should be an advisory in nature. Just identifying problems is not the end. Suggest alternatives, indicating how a different approach would have solved a method-logic problem is the role of an evaluator. Make sure the recommendations are practical. The evaluator should avoid excessive nit-picking and fault-finding on trivial details and should advise the scope of improvement in weak areas and suggest alternatives to make things more trustworthy.
- ❖ **Be sensitive:** Always an evaluator should be sensitive in handling negative comments. He/she should be sensitive towards the researcher's feeling. Do not be condescending or sarcastic towards researcher's work. The negative comment can be represent in a constructive way.
- ❖ **Be a good communicator:** An evaluator should be always a good communicator by choosing clear concise statements to communicate observations or critique report. He/she should avoid ambiguity and should not use patronizing or condemning language or unnecessary flattery merely to boost researcher's self-esteem. She/he should be always aware of her or his own negative attitudes toward the subject matter or the task.

FOUR KEY ASPECTS OF CRITIQUE

1. Understanding the purpose and problem, while determining if the design and methodology are consistent with the purpose.
2. Determining if the methodology is properly applied.
3. Assessing if outcomes and conclusions are believable and supported by findings.
4. Reflecting on overall quality, strengths, and limitations.

CRITIQUE SKILLS

For critiquing the research the researcher must have the research critique skill. A critique identifies the central problem or issue, defines the central claim, looks at the specific questions, notes experimental and theoretical approaches, and reviews the results and their significance. Critiquing skill can be assessed by assessing the researcher's critical thinking, logical reasoning, knowledge of research methodology, attention to details and recognition of strengths and weaknesses of the researches (**Fig. 11.2**).

Critical Thinking

Critical thinking is clear, reasoned thinking involving critique. The national council for excellence in critical thinking defines critical thinking as the intellectually disciplined process of actively and skillfully conceptualizing, applying, analyzing, synthesizing, and/or evaluating information gathered from, or generated by, observation, experience, reflection, reasoning, or communication, as a guide to belief and action.

Logical Reasoning

Logical reasoning is a given a precondition or premise, a conclusion or logical consequence and a rule or material conditional that implies the conclusion given the precondition. Logical reasoning can explained as deductive reasoning determines whether the truth of a conclusion can be determined for that rule, based solely on the truth of the premises or inductive reasoning as opposed to deductive reasoning attempts to support a determination of the rule. It hypothesizes a rule after numerous examples are taken to be a conclusion that follows from a precondition in terms of such a rule.

Knowledge of Research Methodology

Research methodology is a way to systematically solve the problem which depict, how scientifically the study is conducted. A researcher must have in-depth knowledge on research methodology (both qualitative and quantitative research) to evaluate or critique research. Without in-depth knowledge it is difficult for a researcher to enter to the study. She or he should also be sound practically in conducting research.

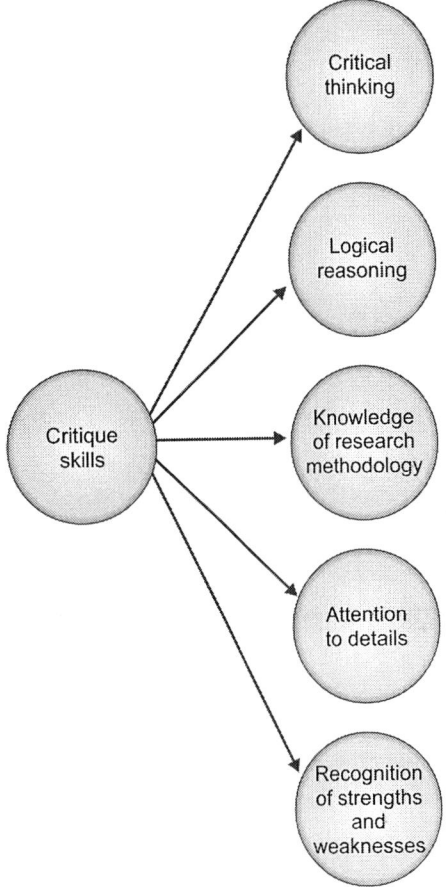

Fig. 11.2: Types of critique skills.

Attention to Details

During critiquing research the researcher has to focus on his/her attention to the whole study not only the important or interesting aspect. He/she has to go through details from the introduction to bibliography. Sometimes in the busy schedule the researcher has only make her/his attention to the main highlight points of the research, but during that she/he may be overcome some important aspects. As in research every aspect is an important one, the researcher should not exclude anything and go through details.

Recognition of Strengths and Weaknesses

Critical appraisal is a systematic process used to identify the strengths and weaknesses of a research article in order to assess the usefulness and validity of research findings. The most important components of a critical appraisal are an evaluation of the appropriateness of the study design for the research question and a careful assessment of the key methodological features of this design. Other factors that also should be considered include the suitability of the statistical methods used and their subsequent interpretation, potential conflicts of interest and the relevance of the research to one's own practice.

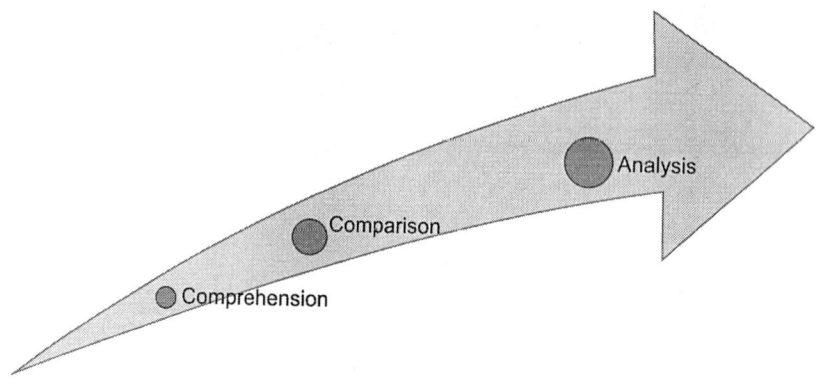

Fig.11.3: Critique process for quantitative studies.

CRITIQUE PROCESS FOR QUANTITATIVE STUDIES

The critique process is different in both qualitative and quantitative research. A researcher will follow some basic steps for all quantitative researches, they are as follows **(Fig.11.3)**:

Comprehension

Comprehension means the ability to grasp the meaning of material by interpreting it. It is the first step of research critique process. First the researcher will read the article carefully identify terms he/she does not understand and determine their meaning in a dictionary. Highlight difficult and important aspects each step of the research process.

Comparison

In this step the researcher will compare the research, which he/she is critiquing with an ideal research. This requires knowledge of what each step of the research process should be like. The ideal is compared with the real. Examine the extent to which the researcher followed the rules for an ideal study.

Analysis

A systematic examination and evaluation of data or information, by breaking it into its component parts to uncover their interrelationships. Herein research critiquing in the step of analysis the researcher will observe whether the study is significant, gave proper result, shows logical links connecting one study element with another.

STEPS FOR CRITIQUING QUANTITATIVE RESEARCH STUDIES

A research study needs to follow the steps in the process in a logical manner. There should also be a clear link between the steps beginning with the purpose of the study and following through the literature review, the theoretical framework, the research question, the methodology section, the data analysis, and the findings. In critiquing the steps in the research process a number of questions need to be asked. However, these questions are seeking more than a simple 'yes' or 'no' answer. The questions are posed to stimulate the reviewer to consider the implications of what the researcher has done.

Writing Style

Research reports should be well-written, grammatically correct, concise and well-organized. The use of jargon should be avoided where possible. The style should be such that it attracts the reader to read on. During critique the evaluator will search the answer for the following questions:
- Is the paper well-organized?
- Is the narrative wordy and redundant?
- Are there irrelevant sections that can be deleted?
- Are there errors in spelling or grammar? If so identify them.

Author(s)

The author(s') qualifications and job title can be a useful indicator into the researcher(s') knowledge of the area under investigation and ability to ask the appropriate questions. Conversely a research study should be evaluated on its own merits and not assumed to be valid and reliable simply based on the author(s') qualifications. The evaluator will assess whether the researcher(s') qualifications/position indicate a degree of knowledge in this particular field of conducting research.

Report Title

The title should be between 10 and 15 words long and should clearly identify for the reader the purpose of the study. Titles that are too long or too short can be confusing or misleading. It should succinctly suggesting key variables and study population. The evaluator has to find out whether the title clear, accurate and unambiguous or not.

Abstract

The abstract should provide a succinct overview of the research and should include information regarding the purpose of the study, method, sample size and selection. It provides a snapshot of the study. From the snapshot, decide how relevant the source is for the purposes, in terms of topic, population, and methodology. Evaluator may ask the question to himself during critiquing the abstract as does the abstract clearly concisely summarizes main features of the report (problem, method, result and conclusion)?

Research Problem

A research problem is often first presented to the reader in the introduction to the study. Depending on what is to be investigated some authors will refer to it as the purpose of the study. In either case the statement should at least broadly indicate to the reader what is to be studied. Broad problems are often multifaceted and will need to become narrower and more focused before they can be researched. In this the literature review can play a major role during critiquing the evaluator will judge the significances of research problem which already done.

He/she will evaluate what problem existed (in the setting, in terms of a lack of research, a need for further research, etc.) that the researcher(s) attempted to address.

Literature Review

The primary purpose of the literature review is to define or develop the research question while also identifying an appropriate method of data collection. It should also help to identify any gaps in the literature relating to the problem and to suggest how those gaps might be filled. The literature review should demonstrate an appropriate depth and breadth of reading around the topic in question. The majority of studies included should be of recent origin and ideally less than five-year-old. Another important consideration is the type and source of literature presented. Primary empirical data from the original source is more favorable than a secondary source or anecdotal information where the author relies on personal evidence or opinion that is not founded on research. The researcher during critique will observed whether:

- Review begins with an introduction which identifies the key words used to conduct the search and information about which databases were used.
- Well-organized and included in a form of summary.
- The themes that emerged from the literature should then be presented and discussed.
- The data is reviewed critically, highlighting both the strengths and limitations of the study and be compared and contrasted with the findings of other studies.
- The review must identify important gaps in the literature.

Theoretical Framework

Following the identification of the research problem and the review of the literature the researcher should present the theoretical framework. Theoretical frameworks are a concept that novice and experienced researchers find confusing. It is initially important to note that not all research studies use a defined theoretical framework. A theoretical framework can be a conceptual model that is used as a guide for the study or themes from the literature that are conceptually mapped and used to set boundaries for the research.

A sound framework also identifies the various concepts being studied and the relationship between those concepts. Such relationships should have been identified in the literature. The research study should then build on this theory through empirical observation. Some theoretical frameworks may include a hypothesis. Theoretical frameworks tend to be better developed in experimental and quasi-experimental studies and often poorly developed or nonexistent in descriptive studies. The theoretical framework should be clearly identified and explained to the reader. The researcher will evaluate:

- Has a conceptual or theoretical framework been identified?
- Is the framework adequately described?
- Is the framework appropriate?

Aims and Objectives, Research Question and Research Hypothesis

The purpose of the aims and objectives of a study, the research question and the research hypothesis is to form a link between the initially stated purpose of the study or research problem and how the study will be undertaken. They should be clearly stated and be congruent with the data presented in the literature review. The use of these items is dependent on the type of research being performed. Some descriptive studies may not identify any of these items but simply refer to the purpose of the study or the research problem, others will include either aims and objectives or research questions. Correlational designs, study the relationships that exist between two or more variables and accordingly use either a research question or hypothesis. Experimental and quasi-experimental studies should clearly state a hypothesis identifying the variables to be manipulated, the population that is being studied and the predicted outcome. The following questions can be asked like:

- Have aims and objectives, a research question or hypothesis been identified?

- If so are they clearly stated?
- Do they reflect the information presented in the literature review?

Ethical Considerations

Beauchamp and Childress (2001) identify four fundamental moral principles: (i) autonomy, (ii) nonmaleficence, (iii) beneficence, and (iv) justice. Autonomy infers that an individual has the right to freely decide to participate in a research study without fear of coercion and with a full knowledge of what is being investigated. Nonmaleficence implies an intention of not harming and preventing harm occurring to participants both of a physical and psychological nature. Beneficence is interpreted as the research benefiting the participant and society as a whole. Justice is concerned with all participants being treated as equals and no one group of individuals receiving preferential treatment because, e.g., of their position in society. The latter pair are often linked and imply that the researcher has a duty to respect the confidentiality and/or the anonymity of participants and nonparticipating subjects. Ethical committees or institutional review boards have to give approval before research can be undertaken. Their role is to determine that ethical principles are being applied and that the rights of the individual are being adhered to.

The researcher will check:
- Were the participants fully informed about the nature of the research?
- Was the autonomy/confidentiality of the participants guaranteed?
- Were the participants protected from harm?
- Was ethical permission granted for the study?

Operational Definitions

In a research study the researcher needs to ensure that the reader understands what is meant by the terms and concepts that are used in the research. To ensure this any concepts or terms referred to should be clearly defined. The researcher will check:
- Are all the terms, theories and concepts mentioned in the study defined.
- Whether that are defined operationally which is different from dictionary definition.

Research Design

There are several types of quantitative studies that can be structured under the headings of true experimental, quasi-experimental and nonexperimental designs. Although it is outside the remit of this article, within each of these categories there are a range of designs that will impact on how the data collection and data analysis phases of the study are undertaken. However, Robson (2002) states these designs are similar in many respects as most are concerned with patterns of group behavior, averages, tendencies and properties. For critiquing research design the following questions can answer.
- What type of design is used?
- Does the design seem to flow from the proposed research problem, theoretical framework, literature review, and hypothesis?
- What type(s) of data collection method(s) is/are used in the study?
- Are the data collection procedures similar for all subjects?
- How have the rights of subjects been protected?
- What indications are given that informed consent of the subjects has been ensured?

Sample and Sample Size

The degree to which a sample reflects the population it was drawn from is known as representativeness and in quantitative research this is a decisive factor in determining the adequacy of a study. In order to select a sample that is likely to be representative and thus identify findings that are probably generalizable to the target population a probability sample should be used. The size of the sample is also important in quantitative research as small samples are at risk of being overly representative of small subgroups within the target population. For example, if, in a sample of general nurses, it was noticed that 40% of the respondents were males, then males would appear to be over-represented in the sample, thereby creating a sampling error. The risk of sampling errors decrease as larger sample sizes are used. In selecting the sample the researcher should clearly identify who the target population are and what criteria were used to include or exclude participants. During critiquing of the sample and sampling technique the evaluator should observe the following:

- How was the sample selected?
- What type of sampling method is used? Is it appropriate to the design?
- Does the sample reflect the population as identified in the problem or purpose statement?
- Is the sample size appropriate?
- To what population may the findings be generalized? What are the limitations in generalizability?

Data Collection Method

The next element to consider after the research design is the data collection method. In a quantitative study any number of strategies can be adopted when collecting data and these can include interviews, questionnaires, attitude scales or observational tools. Questionnaires are the most commonly used data gathering instruments and consist mainly of closed questions with a choice of fixed answers.

Postal questionnaires are administered via the mail and have the value of perceived anonymity. Questionnaires can also be administered in face-to-face interviews or in some instances over the telephone.

Instrument Design

After identifying the appropriate data gathering method the next step that needs to be considered is the design of the instrument. Researchers have the choice of using a previously designed instrument or developing one for the study and this choice should be clearly declared for the reader. Designing an instrument is a protracted and sometimes difficult process, but the overall aim is that the final questions will be clearly linked to the research questions and will elicit accurate information and will help achieve the goals of the research. This, however, needs to be demonstrated by the researcher if a previously designed instrument is selected the researcher should clearly establish that chosen instrument is the most appropriate. This is achieved by outlining how the instrument has measured the concepts under study. Previously designed instruments are often in the form of standardized tests or scales that have been developed for the purpose of measuring a range of views, perceptions, attitudes, opinions or even abilities. There are a multitude of tests and scales available, therefore the researcher is expected to provide the appropriate evidence in relation to the validity and reliability of the instrument.

The evaluator who is critiquing the research should observe:
- ❖ Has the data gathering instrument been described?
- ❖ Is the instrument appropriate?
- ❖ How was it developed?
- ❖ Do the instruments or tools directly measure the variables of interest?
- ❖ Does the researcher describe clearly how meaning or scores are derived from the instruments?
- ❖ Were reliability and validity testing undertaken and the results discussed?
- ❖ Was a pilot study undertaken?

Validity and Reliability

One of the most important features of any instrument is that it measures the concept being studied in an unwavering and consistent way. These are addressed under the broad headings of validity and reliability respectively. In general, validity is described as the ability of the instrument to measure what it is supposed to measure and reliability the instrument's ability to consistently and accurately measure the concept under study (Wood et al, 2006). For the most part, if a well-established 'off-the-shelf' instrument has been used and not adapted in any way, the validity and reliability will have been determined already and the researcher should outline what this is. However, if the instrument has been adapted in any way or is being used for a new population then previous validity and reliability will not apply. In these circumstances the researcher should indicate how the reliability and validity of the adapted instrument was established if the chosen instrument is clear and unambiguous and to ensure that the proposed study has been conceptually well-planned a miniversion of the main study, referred to as a pilot study, should be undertaken before the main study. Samples used in the pilot study are generally omitted from the main study. Following the pilot study the researcher may adjust definitions, alter the research question, address changes to the measuring instrument or even alter the sampling strategy. Having described the research design, the researcher should outline in clear, logical steps the process by which the data was collected. All steps should be fully described and easy to follow.

Analysis and Results

Data analysis in quantitative research studies is often seen as a daunting process. Much of this is associated with apparently complex language and the notion of statistical tests. The researcher should clearly identify what statistical tests were undertaken, why these tests were used and what were the results. A rule of thumb is that studies that are descriptive in design only use descriptive statistics, correlational studies, quasi-experimental and experimental studies use inferential statistics. The latter is subdivided into tests to measure relationships and differences between variables. Inferential statistical tests are used to identify if a relationship or difference between variables is statistically significant. Statistical significance helps the researcher to rule out one important threat to validity and that is the result could be due to chance rather than to real differences in the population. Quantitative studies usually identify the lowest level of significance as $Ps0.05$ (P = probability). To enhance readability researchers frequently present their findings and data analysis section under the headings of the research questions. This can help the reviewer determine if the results that are presented clearly answer the research questions. Tables, charts and graphs may

be used to summarize the results and should be accurate, clearly identified and enhance the presentation of result. The percentage of the sample who participated in the study is an important element in considering the generalizability of the results. At least 50% of the sample is needed to participate if a response bias is to be avoided:
- What level of measurement is used to measure each of the major variables?
- What descriptive or inferential statistics are reported?
- Were these descriptive or inferential statistics appropriate to the level of measurement for each variable? Are the inferential statistics used appropriate to the intent of the hypotheses?
- Does the author report the level of significance set for the study? If so, what is it?
- If tables or figures are used, do they supplement and economize the text and precise titles?

Discussion/Conclusion/Recommendations

The discussion of the findings should logically from the data and should be related back to the literature review thus placing the study in context. If the hypothesis was deemed to have been supported by the findings, the researcher should develop this in the discussion. If a theoretical or conceptual framework was used in the study then the relationship with the findings should be explored. Any interpretations or inferences drawn should be clearly identified as such and consistent with the results.

The significance of the findings should be stated but these should be considered within the overall strengths and limitations of the study. In this section some consideration should be given to whether or not the findings of the study were generalizable, also referred to as external validity. Not all studies make a claim to generalizability but the researcher should have undertaken an assessment of the key factors in the design, sampling and analysis of the study to support any such claim. Finally the researcher should have explored the clinical significance and relevance of the study. Applying findings in practice should be suggested with caution and will obviously depend on the nature and purpose of the study.

In addition, the researcher should make relevant and meaningful suggestions for future research in the area. During critiquing of the research study the evaluator should focus on following points:
- Are the findings linked back to the literature review?
- If a hypothesis was identified was it supported?
- Are the results interpreted in the context of the problem/purpose, hypothesis, and theoretical framework/literature reviewed?
- What relevance for nursing practice does the investigator identify, if any?
- What generalizations are made?
- What recommendations for future research are stated or implied?
- Are there other studies with similar findings?
- What risks/benefits are involved for patients if the research findings would be used in practice?

References

The research study should conclude with an accurate list of all the books; journal articles, reports and other media that were referred to in the work. The referenced material is also a useful source of further information on the subject being studied.
- Were all the books, journals and other media alluded to in the study accurately referenced?
- Were a standardized system of writing report is followed during writing bibliography?

QUALITATIVE RESEARCH CRITIQUE

For critiquing qualitative studies there are some standards by which we can evaluate qualitative studies. That's are **(Fig. 11.4)**:
- Standard I : Descriptive vividness
- Standard II : Methodological congruence
- Standard III : Analytical precision
- Standard IV : Theoretical connectedness
- Standard V : Heuristic relevance

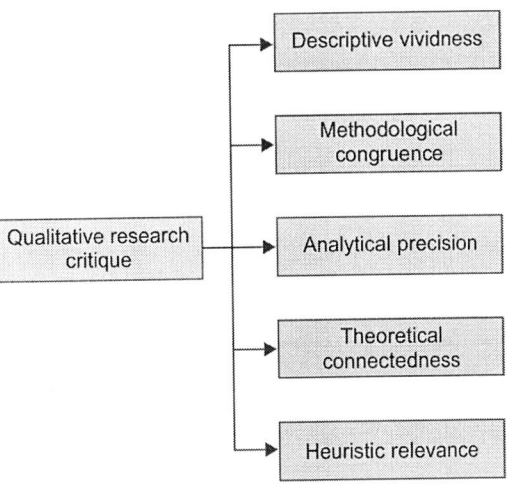

Fig. 11.4: Qualitative research critique process

Standard I: Descriptive Vividness

Descriptive vividness means clarity in description. Description of site, subjects, experience of collecting the data, and thinking of the researcher during the process, need to be presented so clearly that the reader has a sense of personally experiencing the event. The descriptive vividness of the study can be analysis by asking following questions during evaluating the research study:
- Is essential descriptive information included?
- Is there clarity in the description of the study?
- Is there credibility in the description of the study?
- Is there adequate length of time spent at the site to gain the familiarity necessary for vivid description?
- Does the researcher validate findings with the study participants?
- Is the descriptive narrative written clearly?

Threats to Descriptive Vividness

- Failure to include essential descriptive information
- Lack of clarity and/or depth of the description
- Inadequate skills in writing descriptive narrative
- Reluctance to reveal self in the written material

Standard II: Methodological Congruence

Methodological congruence depict that the methodological approach used by the researchers was consistent with the philosophical basis throughout the study. Methodological congruence has four dimensions.
1. Rigor in documentation
2. Procedural rigor
3. Ethical rigor
4. Auditability

Rigor in Documentation

Documentation is an important part in qualitative studies. Rigor in documentation means the strictness in documentation. The rigor in documentation include:

- Clear, concise presentation by the researcher of the study elements.
- The reviewer examines the study elements for completeness and clarity. The study element includes:

Abstract

Clearly concisely summarizes the main features of the study.

Introduction

Problem stated unambiguously and significant to nursing.
- Phenomenon is identified.
- Philosophical base of study is made explicit.
- Purpose and type of qualitative study is stated.
- Study questions or aims are identified.
- Assumptions are identified.

Literature Review

- Adequately summarizes the existing body of knowledge related to problem.
- Provide a solid basis for the study.

Conceptual Underpinning

Key concepts are adequately defined conceptually.

Statements of Methods

- Research design and tradition
- Access to site, sample, and population
- Sampling technique
- Researcher's role and interview structure
- Data collection procedure

Data Analysis

- Coding and data analysis methods sufficiently described
- Findings effectively summarized.

Discussion

- Interpretation of finding with contest of prior studies
- Implication in practice and recommendation for future research mentioned
- Conclusion drawn
- The reviewer identifies any threats to rigor in documentation.

Threats to Rigor in Documentation

Failure to present all elements or steps of the study accurately or clearly.

Procedural Rigor

Procedural rigor can applied during data collection procedure because data collection procedure in qualitative studies is a very difficult task for the researcher. Here the researcher has to collect data by focus group discussion or unstructured interview schedule or observation technique so the researcher needs to make clear the steps taken to ensure that data were accurately recorded and that the data obtained are representative of the data as a whole. During critique the researcher has to get answer all the following questions like:

- Did the researcher tap the participant's experience versus her or his theoretical knowledge of the phenomenon?
- Did the researcher describe steps taken to ensure that the participant did not misrepresent herself or himself, or misinform the researcher?
- Did the researcher describe steps taken to deter the informant from substituting supposition about an event rather than recalling the actual experience?
- Did the researcher eliminate the potential for 'elite bias' by placing equal weight on high-status or elite informant data and low-status or less articulate informant data?
- Did the researcher describe steps taken to avoid influence or distortion of the events observed by her or his presence? (like the Hawthorne effect)
- Were sufficient data gathered?
- Was sufficient time spent gathering data?
- Were the approaches for gaining access to the site or participants appropriate?
- Was the selection of participants appropriate?

Threats to Procedural Rigor

- The researcher asked the wrong questions. The questions need to tap the subjects' experiences, not their theoretical knowledge of the phenomenon.
- The questions included terminology from the theoretical orientation of the researcher.
- The presence of the researcher distorted the event being observed.
- The researcher's involvement with the subject-participants distorted the data.
- Atypical events were interpreted as typical.
- The informants lacked credibility.
- An insufficient amount of data were gathered.
- An insufficient length of time was spent in data gathering.
- The approaches for gaining access to the site and/or subjects were inappropriate.
- The researcher failed to keep in-depth field notes.

Ethical Rigor

Ethical rigor requires recognition and discussion by the researcher of the ethical implications related to the conduct of the study. The reviewer will check the written consent is obtained from subjects and documented and also evaluate the confidentiality of data maintained. The appropriate handling of confidential data is based on three dimensions: (i) the respect to people and their autonomy and freedom to maintain privacy and secrecy, (ii) the concept that secrets can be shared as each person choose, and (iii) the understanding that the promise of confidentiality acknowledge each person's desire and right to share information. The report must indicate that the researcher took action to ensure that the rights of subjects were protected during the study. The reviewer examines the data gathering process and identifies potential threats to ethical rigor. The reviewer examines:

- Were participants informed of their rights?
- Was informed consent obtained from the participants and documented?
- Were mechanisms developed and implemented to protect participants' rights?

Threats to Ethical Rigor
- ❖ The researcher failed to inform the subjects of their rights.
- ❖ The researcher failed to obtain consent from the subjects.
- ❖ The researcher failed to ensure the protection of the subjects' rights.

Auditability

Auditability is established by the reader being able to follow the steps of the research form the research questions, to the data collection, to the data, and then to the findings (categories, themes, model). By the steps for interpretation and synthesis and data examples provided, the reader should be able to follow the researcher's thinking. Here the researcher has to develop a decision trail for that, the researcher must report all the decisions involved in the transformation of data to the theoretical schema. A second researcher, using the original data and the decision trail, should be able to arrive at conclusions similar to those of the original researcher. The reviewer examines the decision trail for threats to auditability.

- ❖ Was the description of the data collection process adequate?
- ❖ Were the records of the raw data sufficient to allow judgments to be made?
- ❖ Did the researcher describe the decision rules for arriving at ratings or judgments?
- ❖ Could other researchers arrive at similar conclusions after applying the decision rules to the data?
- ❖ Did the researcher record the nature of the decisions, the data on which they were based, and the reasoning that entered into the decisions?

Threats to Auditability
- ❖ The description of the data collection process was inadequate.
- ❖ The researcher failed to develop or identify the decision rules for arriving at ratings or judgments.
- ❖ The researcher failed to record the nature of the decisions, data upon which they were based, and reasoning that entered into the decisions.
- ❖ The evidence for conclusions was not presented.
- ❖ Other researchers were unable to arrive at similar conclusions after applying the decision rules to the data.

Standard III: Analytical Precision

Analytical precision requires that the researcher make intense efforts to identify and record the decision-making processes through which data transformations are made and they can make accurate analysis. Premature patterning may occur before the researcher can logically fit all of the data within the emerging schema. The consequence may be a poor fit between data and theoretical schema.

When critiquing a study, the reviewer examines the decision-making processes and the theoretical schema to detect threats to analytical precision. The interpretive statements should match with the findings. The reviewer will ask the following to check the analytical precision:

- ❖ Did the interpretive theoretical statements correspond with the findings?
- ❖ Did the set of themes, categories, or theoretical statements depict or describe a whole picture?
- ❖ Can the hypotheses or propositions developed during the study be verified by data?

- Were the hypotheses or propositions presented in the research report?
- Are the study conclusions based on the data gathered?

Threats to Analytical Precision

- The interpretive statements do not correspond with findings.
- The categories, themes, or common elements are not logical.
- The inclusion and exclusion criteria for categories, themes, or common elements are not consistently followed.

Standard IV: Theoretical Connectedness

Every research is based on some theory. During critiquing research the reviewer will observe the theoretical schema which should be clearly expressed, logically consistent, reflective of the data and compatible with the knowledge base of nursing. The theoretical concepts adequately defined and/or validated. The reviewer can assess the following aspects to assess the theoretical connectedness:

- Are the theoretical concepts adequately defined and/or validated by data?
- Are the relationships among the concepts clearly expressed?
- Are the proposed relationships among the concepts validated by data?
- Does the theory developed during the study yield a comprehensive picture of the phenomenon under study?
- Is a conceptual framework or map derived from the data?
- Is there a clear connection made between the data and the (nursing) frameworks?

Threats to Theoretical Connectedness

- The concepts are inadequately refined.
- The concepts are not validated by data.
- The relationships between concepts are not clearly expressed.
- The proposed relationships among concepts are not validated by data.

Standard V: Heuristic Relevance

Heuristic relevance reflects the reader's capacity to recognize the phenomenon described in the study, its theoretical significance, its applicability to nursing practice situations, and its influence on future research activities. Here the reviewer observe the significance and intuitive recognition of the researcher when individuals are confronted with the theoretical schema derived from the data, it has meaning within their personal knowledge base.

- Is the phenomenon described well?
- Would other researchers recognize or be familiar with the phenomenon?
- Is the description of the phenomenon consistent with common meanings or experiences?
- Did the researcher examine the existing body of knowledge?
- Was the process studied related to nursing and health?
- Was the relationship exist with the existing body of knowledge?
- Did the researcher examine the existing body of knowledge?
- Was the process studied related to nursing and health? (Do we need this?)

Threats to Intuitive Recognition

* The reader is unable to recognize the phenomenon.
* The description is not consistent with common meanings.
* Theoretical connectedness is lacking.
* Threats to relationship to existing body of knowledge.
* The researcher failed to examine the existing body of knowledge.
* The process studied was not related to nursing and health.
* There is a lack of correspondence with the existing knowledge base in nursing.

WHAT TO BE AVOID DURING CRITIQUE?

* It is not legitimate to criticize the research paper for something beyond its purpose. Do not complain that an author did not include something unless that something is a necessary part of a research article.
* Do not require the unobtainable. We all would like perfect data and ideal measures for variables, but neither usually exists in reality. It is legitimate to criticize data or measures if better ones are readily available. Otherwise do not complain if the author has done the best she can with imperfect data.
* Do not make an abundance of broad and general statements of the type. 'This research was well done with an interesting question and good data.' This means nothing. You must be concrete, describing specific strengths and weaknesses. Clearly state your reasons for concluding that the author has either done a good or less-than-good job on one or more parts of the elements of research.
* Do not turn in sloppy research. Making nothing but positive comments on a fellow student's paper is of no value whatsoever. We are here to learn. Definitely praise items where the author was particularly creative, industrious, or ingenious. But also comment (politely, but firmly) on weaknesses so the author can address them before turning a paper in for a grade or as a journal submission.

SUMMARY

* Research critique refers to planned, systematic and careful evaluation of a research work. It based on some prespecified standard criteria to judge the strength and weakness of work. An intellectual research critique is a careful, complete examination of a study to judge its strengths, weaknesses, logical links, meaning and significance.
* Some principles should be kept in mind while appraising a research work are objectivity, constructively, be a good advisor, sensitivity, be balance always and be a good communicator.
* For critiquing the research the researcher must have the research critique skill. Critiquing skill can be assessed by assessing the researcher's critical thinking, logical reasoning, knowledge of research methodology, attention to details and recognition of strengths and weaknesses of the researches.
* Researcher will follow some basic steps for all quantitative researches like comprehension, comparison and analysis. When critiquing quantitative researches each step of research process starting from abstract to bibliography and annexure will be reviewed properly.
* For critiquing qualitative studies there are some standards by which we can evaluate qualitative studies. That's are: Standard I: Descriptive vividness, Standard II: Methodological

congruence, Standard III: Analytical precision, Standard IV: Theoretical connectedness and Standard V: Heuristic relevance.

- Descriptive vividness means clarity in description. Methodological congruence depict that the methodological approach used by the researchers was consistent with the philosophical basis throughout the study.
- Analytical precision requires that the researcher make intense efforts to identify and record the decision-making processes through which data transformations are made and they can make accurate analysis.
- Every research is based on some theory. During critiquing research the reviewer will observe the theoretical schema which should be clearly expressed, logically consistent, reflective of the data and compatible with the knowledge base of nursing.
- Heuristic relevance reflects the reader's capacity to recognize the phenomenon described in the study, its theoretical significance, its applicability to nursing practice situations, and its influence on future research activities.

QUESTIONS TO TEST YOUR KNOWLEDGE

Q1. What do you mean by research critique? Explain its principles. Enumerate the critique skills. (3 + 4 + 3)

Q2. What are the basic steps for critiquing quantitative researches? Explain as a nurse researcher how you will critique a quantitative research study? (3 + 12 = 15)

Q3. Enumerate the standard for critiquing qualitative research studies. (15)

Q4. Multiple choice questions: (1 x 10)

   I. A planned, systematic and careful evaluation of a research work is called:
     a. Research critique
     b. Research report
     c. Research proposal
     d. Research methodology

   II. Which of the following critique skill is the ability to grasp the meaning of material by interpreting it:
     a. Comparison
     b. Comprehension
     c. Interpretation
     d. Analysis

   III. Descriptive vividness is a standard to critique:
     a. Experimental studies
     b. Descriptive studies
     c. Any research studies
     d. Qualitative research studies

   IV. Rigor in documentation means:
     a. Elaborative documentation
     b. Strictness in documentation
     c. Concisely documentation
     d. Problem stated unambiguously

   V. Procedural rigor can applied during:
     a. Selection of research problem
     b. Selection of best methodology
     c. During data collection procedure
     d. During validation of tools

   VI. Auditability is established by the:
     a. Reader's point of view
     b. Evaluator's point of view
     c. Researcher's point of view
     d. None of the above

   VII. When critiquing a study, the reviewer examines the _____ to detect threats to analytical precision.
     a. Decision making process and theoretical schema
     b. Data collection methods and procedures
     c. Selection of samples and data collection procedure
     d. Data collection procedure and sampling technique

VIII. Which of the followings reflects the reader's capacity to recognize the phenomenon described in the study?
   a. Theoretical connectedness
   b. Heuristic relevance
   c. Descriptive vividness
   d. Methodological congruence

IX. The researcher failed to ensure the protection of the subjects' rights is an example of threat to:
   a. Procedural rigor
   b. Rigor in documentation
   c. Ethical rigor
   d. Auditability

X. The researcher asked the wrong questions during data collection is an example of threat to:
   a. Procedural rigor
   b. Rigor in documentation
   c. Ethical rigor
   d. Auditability

ANSWERS

| I. a | II. b | III. d | IV. b | V. c |
| VI. a | VII. a | VIII. b | IX. c | X. a |

Chapter 12

Communication and Utilization of Research

Learning Objectives

After completion of this chapter, the students will be able to:
- Describe about the steps for communicating the research.
- Explain the process of writing a research report.
- Enumerate the types of research report.
- Explain the guidelines for writing research report.
- Write a research report by following steps.
- Publish article in journal by following IMRAD formula.
- Utilizes of research findings in different activities.
- Identify the barriers in utilization of nursing research.
- Explain the strategies of facilitate utilization of nursing research.
- Describe the concept, purposes and elements research proposal.
- Develop and present a research proposal for any project.
- Enumerate application and uses of computer in nursing research.

INTRODUCTION

Research is a public enterprise. Whenever an individual undertakes a research project, the commitment includes the responsibility to communicate the completed project to others. A research project cannot be considered complete and there are no values until its results are effectively communicated with its users and consumers. The findings of the research study must be shared which is essential to guide nursing practice, nursing education and nursing administration. Without publication, the findings cannot be followed by any reviewer which means no utilization of research. Disseminating research results contributes to the base of evidence for nursing practice, and is a professional responsibility. Therefore, communication with the research findings is one of the essential and final steps of the research process. Communication with the research findings is essential which carried out through the dissemination of the empirical research evidences generated through research study. The dissemination of the research findings is achieved through either written or the oral means. In written means of communication, researcher writes a detailed description of the whole research process, which may be done in the form of theses, dissertations, research articles, scientific papers, etc., while oral communication with the research findings are achieved through the presentation of the final results and effects of the research process of a group of people in a professional scientific conference on either oral scientific paper or the poster presentation. The accumulation of new scientific knowledge is essential to guide nursing practice, nursing education and nursing administration.

Why Communicate Research Results?

❖ It is essential for utilization.
❖ It allows for other nurses to critique.
❖ It stimulates others to replicate or develop similar studies.
❖ Disseminating research results contributes to the base of evidence for nursing practice.
❖ It provides rewards for the researcher.
  - Recognition
  - Advancement
  - Psychological boost
  - Financial compensation

STEPS FOR COMMUNICATING THE RESEARCH

In order to share or report the research findings, researcher has to follow some criteria, which are as follows:

Selecting Proper Channel for Communicating

To determine the appropriate communication channel, the researcher has to identify the people he/she wants to communicate with, research how the people obtain information. The researcher has to consider the complexity of the message to communicate, calculate the cost of communicating and decide whether he/she wants the communication to be interactive. The choice of channel is not simple; for a communicating the result. The choice of channel may be student-related theses and dissertations which are only useful for that group of students who read in same library, if thesis is donated to the library however, professional academicians generally need publication of research articles in professional journals, books which is more valid can be referred by all the professionals, or oral research presentations in conference through papers or slides. Most conferences also give researchers the option of presenting findings in poster sessions in which results are summarized on a poster.

Identifying the Consumers

The researcher has to identify his/her target audience. Who can be benefitted by the research study, researchers must know in advance to whom they want to communicate their research findings, such as nursing research findings to clinical bedside nurses, nurse educators, nurse administrators, healthcare professionals, or even the general public. This will help in choosing the right method, mode, and content of research to be communicated.

Developing an Effective Plan for Writing a Research Report

A plan for writing a research includes the following aspects:

Decide on Authorship

Researchers have to decide among themselves as to who will be the leading author and the contributing authors or first author or second author and so on. Authorship is an explicit way of assigning responsibility and giving credit for intellectual work. Authorship practices should be judged by how honestly they reflect actual contributions to the final product. The International

Committee of Medical Journal Editors (ICMJE) recommends that authorship should be based on the following four criteria:
1. Substantial contributions to the conception or design of the work; or the acquisition, analysis, or interpretation of data for the work.
2. Drafting the work or revising it critically for important intellectual content.
3. Final approval of the version to be published.
4. Agreement to be accountable for all aspects of the work in ensuring that questions related to the accuracy or integrity of any part of the work are appropriately investigated and resolved.

Deciding about the Content

The research report should be presented in the order of the research process, beginning with the problem of the study and ending with conclusions, implications, and recommendations for future studies. The major part of the research report is written in the past tense because the study has already occurred. Hypotheses and conclusions are written in the present tense, and the implications and recommendations are directed towards the future. Detail about the content or how to write the research report will be discussed later. Researchers also have to decide, how many pages are required to communicate the findings of the research effectively because it may varies according to the type of the journal.

Preparing Outline of Report

It is important that if there are multiple authors of a report, each one has responsibility for different sections of manuscript. The advantage of having an outline is that it can be incorporated into a timeline that sets goals for completing the manuscript. Assemble the material needed to begin a draft and finally start preparing a report with outlined timeline.

Selection of a Medium

In selecting a medium for publication or presentation, some important factors must be kept in mind whether it is a journal or published in the internet site or it will be presented in the conference/workshop. After selecting a medium the researcher has to follow the regulation for publication/presentation.

WRITING A RESEARCH REPORT

A research report is the ultimate outcome of the research process. It gives the detailed and accurate accounts of the conduct of disciplined studies accomplished to solve problems or to reveal new knowledge. Research report writing is the oral or written presentation of the evidence and the findings in such detail and form as to be readily understood and accessed by the reader and as to enable him to verify the validity of the conclusions. According to American Marketing Society, its purpose is to convey to interested persons the whole result of study in sufficient detail and to enable each reader to comprehend the data and to determine himself the validity of the conclusions. It is covers, disseminations, presents the conclusions for the information and knowledge to others, to check the validity of the generalizations, to encourage others to carry on research on the same or allied problem.

A research process cannot be considered complete until its report has been written and disseminated. Writing a report highlights the research project and helps in the dissemination of the research findings. Dissemination of research findings serves scientific, professional, and public functions. An effective dissemination of scientific information leads to an overall improvement in knowledge and practice among healthcare providers.

Characteristics of Good Research Report

Research reports are an effective means of communicating the research findings to the readers and interested audience. A well-written research report is one which effectively, efficiently, and widely disseminates the research information among its users. A good research report has following characteristics:

- A research report must have the characteristics of conciseness, clarity, honesty, completeness and accuracy.
- A research report must be long enough to cover the subject content and short enough to maintain interest among its users and consumers. Sometimes the size is depends upon the way the researcher communicate. If it is like a form of thesis when the researcher is submitting it to the universities or academic institution as a part of their curriculum to fulfil their higher degree course. Here the report should be in detail, but if it is presented in workshop or published in journal it should be in brief and only to touch the major aspects. The reviewer can contact to the researcher for clarification.
- It should be complete in nature and cover all aspects.
- It must be written and presented logically, systemic in steps by following research process.
- It should be free from technical jargon, abbreviation and ambiguous terminology.
- It should be written in an objective manner and presented in such a way which depicts the systemic way of fulfilment of objective.
- Use of relevant table, diagram, and figures can make the report effective for other.
- Presentation of the research report must be lucid and visually attractive, so that it can be interesting to its users.
- Research report must reflect its originality.

TYPES OF REPORT

There are mainly three types of report.
1. Technical report
2. Popular report
3. Oral presentation or verbal report

Technical Report

Technical report is used whenever a full written report of the study is required for record keeping or for public dissemination. In this main emphasis is on:
- The methods employed.
- Assumptions made in the course of the study.
- The detailed presentation of the findings their limitations and supporting data, e.g., thesis and dissertation.

Popular Report

It is used if the research results have policy implications. The popular report is the one which gives emphasis on simplicity and attractiveness. The simplification is sought through clear writing and liberal use of charts and diagrams. Attractive layout with large print, many subheadings, and cartoons are the characteristics of a popular report. For example, policy made by government (health policy, e.g., prevention of HIV and prevention of TB).

Oral Presentation or Verbal Report

Oral reports are useful method for the disseminating of knowledge among the users. The oral reports are generally written and presented to a group of professionals at conferences, which can be either read out or presented through poster or computer slide presentation. For example, class presentation and case study presentation.

GUIDELINES FOR WRITING RESEARCH REPORT

Develop Thinking

There is a high positive correlation between good thinking and effective writing. Research is not merely the accumulation, evaluation and assimilation of facts; it is a process of rebuilding facts into a meaningful whole. This demands patent deep and alert thinking which alone results in clear writing of the report.

Divide Narration

Divide narrative into paragraphs and use of informative headlines whenever necessary. Paragraphing is an important feature of any report. It serves to break the text to readable units linking one paragraph to another is an essential technique for maintaining continuing.

Minimize the Use of Technical Language or Jargon

Most disciplines are criticized for their use of technical jargon. They stress here that range of possible readers can be increased by use of simple straightforward language. Clarity; conciseness and simplicity are critical attributes of any kind of good writing. But they are particularly important in technical writing. A technical vocabulary may be an important facilitator of communicating among those who share it, but may serve as a barrier of when communicating with others. If there is a popular word that is equivalent to a technical one, the popular word should be used. It is more important than the report avoids the use of jargon.

Use Visual Aids

In the form of tables and figures to illustrate the principle finding of the study. It is important that such illustration be used to emphasize points made in the text rather than to replace them.

Be Objective

The report should be unbiased and objective justified by fact. As a general rule long excerpts from works of others should be avoided. Too many quotations of reference of others written either creates an impression of showmanship or that the teacher has done very little work of his own.

Treat Data Confidentiality

Confidentiality is not an issue if individuals have voluntary provided data with full awareness that these will be revealed to others. But where the researcher has promised to the respondents to protect that anonymity, the same should be written in such a way as to preclude the possibility of respondents' identification.

Revise and Rewrite

Revising is a part of writing. Few writers are so expert that they produce what they are on first try. Quite often, the writer will discover, on examining the completed work that there are serious flaws in the arrangement of material calling for transpositions or the works needs to be shortened or faulty sentences need to be restructured and so on. This should not dishearten the report writer. He should remember that this is a common occurrence in all writing and even among the best writers.

STEPS IN WRITING REPORT

Logical Analysis of the Subject Matter

It is the first step which is primarily concerned with the development of a subject. This involves careful reading of the assignment task as outlined in syllabi. Analyze the task should answer following question.
- What is purpose of research?
- Who is the audience?
- Word limit?
- Expected format of report, etc.

Preparation of the Final Outline

It is the next step in writing the research report. 'Outlines are the framework upon which works are constructed. They are an aid to the logical organization of the material and a remainder of the points to be stressed in report.' A researcher should prepare an outline to organize the work. Preparation of outlines helps to discards the irrelevant information and save time.

Preparation of the Rough Draft

This step is of utmost importance for the researchers as it involves actually writing down what they have done in the context of their research studies. The researchers write down the procedures adopted by them in collecting the material for their study along with various limitations, the techniques of analysis adopted by them, the broad findings and generalizations, and the various suggestions they want to offer regarding the problems encountered. In the drafting stage the researcher has to prepare the draft for research.

Draft the Body

This step contains placement of introduction, literature review, methodology, result, discussion, conclusion and recommendations.

Draft of the Supplementary Information

In this step, the researcher should organize reference, bibliography and appendices.

Draft Preliminary Informations

Once the main body and supplementary materials is been organized, the preliminary material like cover page, table of contents, acknowledgments and abstract should be written and placed at proper place.

Rewriting and Polishing the Rough Draft

This step happens to be the most difficult part of all formal writing. The careful revision makes the difference between a mediocre and a good piece of writing. While rewriting and polishing, one should check the report for weaknesses in logical development or presentation. The researcher should check the mechanics of writing grammar, spelling, and usage.

Preparation of Final Bibliography

Next in the order comes the task of the preparation of the final bibliography. It is a list of books, journal articles, papers presented, etc., that have contributed or are in some way pertinent to the research which has been done. The bibliography should be arranged alphabetically and may be divided into two parts; the first part may contain the names of books and journals, and the second part may contain the names of magazines and newspaper articles.

Writing the Final Draft

This constitutes the last step. The final draft should be written in a concise and objective style and in simple language, avoiding vague expressions such as 'it seems', 'there may be', etc. While writing the final draft researcher must avoid abstract terminology. It must be remembered that every report should be an attempt to solve some intellectual problem and must contribute to the solution of a problem and must add to the knowledge of both the researcher and the reader. The final draft of report must include citation and bibliography. Before handing report be sure to proofread it for any typing errors.

FORMAT OF A THESIS OR DISSERTATION

Thesis is also a type of research report which describe details about research. It is especially written in academic purpose. Generally in nursing during completion of BSc nursing, MSc nursing or PhD nursing course the student nurse has to develop a thesis and present to his/her university and college library. The thesis may be concise and presented in the seminar/ workshop or given for publication in journal later. Although writing styles often vary from thesis-to-thesis and university-to-university, the most widely accepted and generalized thesis formats may be composed with all necessary information.

Broadly the thesis can be divided into different sections/subsections with appropriate headings for easy understanding of the thesis. A description of the layout and format of a scientific thesis or dissertation, with all its parts and subparts, is given below.

Preliminary Pages

This section includes:

Cover Page

The cover page will be providing all the basic information. Collectively, these can be grouped under 'cover page', which can also become the front page of the thesis. It generally contains information like title of the thesis, author name, followed by previous qualification if applicable, department, why thesis published like 'Thesis submitted for the partial fulfillment of the requirement for the degree in Master of Sciences in Nursing of the Berhampur University, Odisha University, name of the Supervisor, month and year of submission of the thesis, etc.,

Certification and Declaration

After cover page the dissertation paper consists of the certification by guide, co-guide, certification by the head of the institution followed by declaration by the author himself. An example of certification is given below.

Certificate by guide

This is to certify that the study 'effectiveness of video-assisted teaching module regarding prevention of malnutrition among under-fives on knowledge of the mothers in a selected rural community, Odisha was carried out by Santilata Panda, MSc Nursing, 2nd year student in Community Health Nursing Specialty, College of Nursing, Berhampur, Odisha, under my guidance.

Signature of guide

Acknowledgment

Acknowledgment is the statements of acknowledging something or someone. An acknowledgment for a thesis is designed to 'tip researcher's hat' to people who were the most helpful in helping the researcher complete the project which must include the citation of the words of gratitude and appreciation for the people who have contributed in compilation of the research task including supervisor, co-supervisor, Principal/HOD, other faculty members, ethical committee, other authorities who have facilitated the access of the data collection sources, study participants, friends, family members, and other people who have directly and indirectly facilitated the conduction of the research study. It is usually specific—naming the person and the type of help a researcher received.

Index/Table of Contents

This must include the sequence of the contents placed in the research report (thesis/dissertation) along with the page numbers. The table of contents should not contain listings for the pages that precede it, but it must list all parts of the thesis or dissertation that follow it. It must list all appendices and a references section. It includes page numbers for all the items but may or may not assign separate chapter numbers. This subsection facilitates the reader to have easy access of the desired information from the research report without wasting time.

List of Tables

This includes a list of the headings of tables in a sequence as they have placed in the thesis/dissertation. This subsection facilitates the easy location of the information and data as per the need of the reader.

List of the Figures

This includes a list of headings of figures in a sequence as they have placed in the thesis/dissertation. This subsection facilitates the easy location of the information and data as per the need of the reader.

List of the Abbreviations

This includes the description and details of the abbreviations used in the thesis/dissertation. This subsection provides reader information about the abbreviations in advance, so that a smooth reading can be facilitated.

Main Text

This section includes:

Chapter I

Chapter I must include about the introduction, significance or need of the study, statement of the problem, and purpose of the study, delimitation, hypothesis operational definitions and conceptual framework/theoretical framework.

- **Introduction:** The introduction started with a suitable quotation to draw the attention of the readers. Then it simply explain the concept what the researcher is going to study. The primary goal of the introductory paragraphs is to attract the attention of the readers and to get them interested in the subject. It sets the stage for the paper and places the topic in perspective. The introduction is not much differing from need for study. It often contains dramatic and general statements about the need for the study and uses dramatic illustrations or quotes to set the tone. When writing the introduction, the author(s) must think from readers' perspectives, i.e., would the target audience continue reading the test after first chapter?
- **Significance or need of the study:** This section lays the foundation on which the research study is based. In need for study the researcher has to specify why he/she selected the same study? What are the importance? The researcher has to justify each and every aspects. For example, in a problem statement 'effectiveness of structure teaching program on knowledge of adolescent girls regarding prevention of anemia' here he/she has to justify why he/she selected adolescent girls, what is its significance, why selected anemia on knowledge of adolescent girls, why selected structure teaching program, why not any other methods. The researcher has to write the justification of each and every part of the problem statement. So overall need for study explains the way in which your study relates to the larger issues and uses a persuasive rationale to justify this study. It makes the purpose worth pursuing.
- **Research problem or questions:** This section includes the statement of the research problem or research question. For example, 'effectiveness of SIM on knowledge of staff nurses regarding infection prevention in labor room.'
  Objectives: This section includes the statements of the action and outcome which the researcher wants to achieve during research activity. For example:
  - To assess the prevalence of pin site infection among patients with external skeletal fixation.
  - To determine the relationship of pin site infection with selected biophysiological characteristics of the patients with external skeletal fixation.

- **Hypotheses and assumption:** Each research is based on a hypothesis and assumptions, Assumptions are basically beliefs and ideas that we hold to be true based on which the research can be started and hypothesis are the predictions which researchers have to test through their research findings.
- **Scope and delimitation:** All research studies also have limitations and a finite scope. Limitations are often imposed by time and budget constraints. Precisely list the limitations of the study. Describe the extent to which you believe the limitations degrade the quality of the research.
- **Operational definitions:** This section involves the operationally defined terms used in the research study in the manner, where researcher is going to study the variables.
- **Conceptual framework:** This section involves the description and diagrammatic presentation of the conceptual framework/theoretical framework developed for the research study. Theoretical framework can adopted directly from the theory.

Chapter II: Literature Review

The literature review tells the reader what other researchers have discovered about the paper's topic or tells the reader about other research that is relevant to the topic. It should shape the way readers think about a topic—it educates readers about what the community of scholars says about a topic and its surrounding issues. Generally, the literature review has its own voice. The sources of information are not extensively quoted or 'copied and pasted.' Instead, the author puts facts and ideas into his/her own words while pointing out where the information came from. The literature review must consists of citations which consist of authors' last names and the year of publication. One finds complete information on sources by looking up last names and dates in alphabetized references—so there is no need to put all that information in the site of reference.

This chapter is important because it shows what previous researchers have explored and discovered about the phenomenon under study. It is usually quite long and primarily depends upon how much research has previously been done in the area you are planning to investigate. If you are planning to explore a relatively new area, the literature review should cite similar areas of study or studies that lead up to the current research. Never say that your area is so new that no research exists. It is one of the key elements that proposal readers look at when deciding whether or not to approve a proposal.

Chapter III: Methodology (Materials and Methods)

This section includes the following elements:
- Design of the research study
- Descriptions of variables
- Research setting
- Target population
- Sampling technique and sample size
- Development and description of research instruments
- Validity and reliability of research tool(s)
- Procedure and time frame of data collection
- Pilot study
- Feasibility of the study
- Ethical considerations
- Analysis plan

Chapter IV: Analysis and Interpretation of Data

Analysis and interpretation of data is the most important phase of the research report, which involves the computation of the certain measures along with searching for patterns of relationship that exists among data groups. This section presents the description of the study sample and analysis and interpretation of the data through descriptive and inferential statistics and data are usually presented through tables, graphs, etc.

Chapter V: Discussion, Summary, Conclusion and Recommendations

The discussion includes the explanation of findings with the present context, where the researcher presents his/her finding through critical analysis along with comparison with other similar research findings. In discussion the researcher states where his study is in comparison to other literature review. This section also presents the verdict on whether your findings support existing theories. Explain the results and present possible reasons why the results might have turned out the way they did. Lastly summaries the thesis, give conclusion, implication and recommendations. Implications means application how the thesis or the finding of the study can be useful in nursing practice, education and administration. Recommendations means what can be done further. The researcher should state what type of study further can done to get better findings. So the researcher give recommendations regarding further studies. He/she can write the **limitations here**.

End Matter

References

References may be written in American Psychological Association (APA), Campbell, or Vancouver style. However, in health sciences Vancouver style of references is commonly used. Details of Vancouver style of references is commonly used. Details of Vancouver style are discussed separately in this chapter, which may be referred to for more information.

Bibliography

It is a list of all the materials that have been consulted while conducting a research study or writing an academic article, paper or book based on research. References, on the other hand, are those that have been directly referred to and referenced in your research report, article or book.

Appendix/Annexure

At the end of the report, appendices should be written to account for all the technical data, such as research instruments, sample information, mathematical derivations, etc.

WRITING THE REFERENCES/BIBLIOGRAPHY

Difference between References and Bibliography

Most people are not aware of the differences between bibliography and references. They often mistake the two to be the same. However, they are different and used in different contexts in each essay, article or book.

Bibliography is listing of all the materials that have been consulted while writing an article or a book. References, on the other hand, are those that have been referred to or referenced in your article or book.

You might have consulted a lot of books, essays, and websites for writing something. Though you might have referred to these materials while preparing a rough draft, the contents of these may or may not have been included in the actual text. A list of all such materials is known as bibliography. References are a list of those materials that are directly included in your actual text.

While all the items in references are cited directly in the text, all the items of bibliography may not be cited directly in the text. While references can be used to support your statement or argument or used to supplement your findings, a bibliography does not have such roles. As such references are used for establishing something in a more authoritative way. Readers could refer your references and evaluate the correctness of your statement. Meanwhile, a bibliography does not support your arguments directly as it is not cited, and the reader cannot clearly establish where a particular item of the bibliography is referred in your study.

A bibliography will contain all research materials, including books, magazines, periodicals, websites and scientific papers, what a researcher have referred, read and which readers might find valuable to know about even though he/she did not specifically cite them within the body of his/her writing. The bibliography option gives the opportunity to show how much background reading you did to inform your writing. References contain source of material like quotes or texts which has been actually used when writing an essay or book. So the reference list only those sources are included which have been mentioned in, in-text citation.

Both bibliography and references appear at the end of the book or article, but if both are available, bibliography comes after the reference list. A bibliography may contain all the items that have appeared in the reference list, plus some additional works.

Both bibliography and references are arranged alphabetically. But a reference list can also be arranged in numeric style, which means arranging the references chronologically according to the numbers in the text.

While writing a bibliography, you should have to include the authors, last and first name, year of publication, name of the book or journal, place of publication, and name of publishers. In case of websites, organizations as authors, or other such sources, additional information should be provided for the convenience of the readers. Therefore, to sum up the differences between bibliography and references are as follows:

- Bibliography is listing of all the materials that have been consulted while writing an article, essay or book. References, on the other hand, are those that have been directly referred to or referred in your article or book.
- Items of a bibliography are not directly included in the text. References are those that are directly cited in your actual text.
- Both bibliography and references list are arranged alphabetically. A reference list can only follow the number as per in-text citation if it only follows Vancouver style.

STYLE OF WRITING REFERENCE/BIBLIOGRAPHY

Though there are various standard styles of writing reference still it differs in terms of formatting, use of punctuation and the order of information among these styles. Such differences occur at both the levels of referencing, i.e., in-text citation, and reference/bibliography list. Some of the standard methods used for citing the source of work are called as referencing styles or citation styles. These are as follows:
- Harvard
- Vancouver
- APA (American Psychological Association) Referencing Style

- MLA ((Modern Language Association) Referencing Style
- Chicago/Turabian Referencing Style

There are other styles that are not that common but are still required at some places:
- ACS (American Chemical Society)
- AGLC (Australian Guide to Legal Citation)
- AMA (American Medical Association)
- CSE/CBE (Council of Science Editors/Council of Biology Editors)
- IEEE (Institute of Electrical and Electronics Engineers)

The reference style depends upon the type of research conducted or essay written belongs to which specialization. Moreover, the publishers or the academic institutions decide their citing styles. In nursing two more common writing style of reference/bibliography are APA style and Vancouver style of writing.

Regardless of what citation style is being used, there are key pieces of information that need to be collected in order to create the citation.

For books and/or journals:
- Author name
- Title of publication
- Article title (if using a journal)
- Date of publication
- Place of publication
- Publisher
- Volume and issue number of a journal, magazine or encyclopedia
- Page number(s)

For websites:
- Author and/or editor name
- Title of the website
- Company or organization that owns or posts to the website
- URL (website address)
- Date of access

APA Referencing Style

American Psychological Association, commonly known as APA referencing is very similar to that of Harvard referencing style. Where Harvard is most commonly used in UK and Australia, APA is more popular in USA.

APA style throughout the text requires the double line spacing, worthy to mention it is required also for the reference section.

Brief History

- This style of referencing came forth in 1929 in the form of "Publication Manual of the American Psychological Association".
- With the passage of time the manual kept on having revisions and edition. So far 6th editions of the manual have been published.
- The latest edition came to the publication in 2009.

It is mostly used in the various fields of social sciences. It is also used in some other fields, such as business, education and nursing.

General Rules for in-text Citation

In reference in-text citation only the last name (surname) of the author is used; author's name and year of publication are separated by a comma (,). For example: (Ghaznavi, 2003)

However, if there are more than one authors with the same family name, their initials are recommended to use in the in-text citation to avoid the confusion.

It is also allowed to write the author's name out of the bracket. For example: Pravakaran K.(2003, p 40) observes ....

Punctuation marks such as comma or full stop are used after the citation and not before them.

General Rules for Reference/Bibliography List

- Detailed references are listed on a separate page at the end of the document.
- The title 'References' is given to the list, placed in center and in bold font.
- Only those sources are to be listed that has been cited in your work.
- There is a use of double line spacing between each entry.
- Each reference carries hanging indent, i.e., the first line of each reference is flushed to the left margin, remaining lines are indented.
- Author's name and the year are separated by a comma.
- Year of publication is put in parenthesis after author.
- Each reference ends up with a full stop (.).
- The list is arranged in an alphabetical order with reference to the first author's surname or the first significant word of the title (if the reference has begun with it in case of the absence of author's name).
- If more than one sources have the same first author but the later authors are different, the references are listed first by the first author's name then arranged alphabetically by the subsequent author/s name.
- If there are sources whose authors' surnames are same but the initials are different, the references are listed first by the first author's surname and then by chronologically by the initials of first name.
- If you have used the sources of the same author/s with different years of publication, the references are listed first by the first author's name then chronologically by publication year.
- If there are sources of the same author/s with the same year of publication, the references are listed first by the first author's name then by the small letters put after the year.
- If a title or a corporate author has been used instead of author's name, the reference is listed under the first important word and not under A, An or The.
- If the first word of a reference is a numeric digit and not an alphabet, the reference is listed before the references having alphabetical start.
- Page number is required to mention only when a part of work (such as article from a journal or newspaper, a chapter from an edited book, etc.,) is used; if the whole work is considered here is no need to mention the page number.
- If there is reference to a single page an abbreviation p. is used, and if there are multiple pages pp. is used.
- Titles of a bigger source such as a book or journal are italicized.
- Titles which are a part of a bigger work such as a chapter of a book, article in a journal or newspaper are enclosed in double quotation marks without being italicized.
- If you want to mention sources that have been utilized in the hunt of knowledge but are not cited in your document, they can be mentioned under the heading of "Bibliography" on a separate page.

- ❖ The name of an author is written in a way: last name is written first and afterwards initials of the first name/s are written; comma is put after surname and a full stop is put after each initial. For example, the name of the author Bijayalaskhmi Dash will be written as Dash B.L. If two authors publishing one article than in the in-text citation only the surnames of the two authors will be used separated by 'and' In the reference list both the surname and initials of the two authors are used separated by 'and'.
- ❖ In-text citation and reference list entry for three to five authors in the in-text citation only the surnames will be written separated by comas (,) only before last surname and will be inserted. For example (Dash, Panigrahi and Ratha 2019). But in reference/bibliography list both the surname and initials of all the authors are used, last two separated by 'and' and the remaining by comma (,). For example, Dash B.L, Panigrahi.S and Ratha. P (2019). In-text citation and reference list entry for six (6) or more authors after writing the surnsme of first author we have to put For example, Dash et al., 2019 but in the reference list write the names of first six and the last author. Last two names are separated by "........," and the remaining by commas.

Examples of Bibliography writing following APA Style

- ❖ Basavanthappa BT, 2001, *Nursing Administration*, 3rd edition. J.P Brothers publications, New Delhi, pp.92-97.
- ❖ Vati. J, 2013, *Principles and Practice of Nursing Management and Administration*, 1st edition. J.P Brothers publications New Delhi, pp. 345-380p.
- ❖ Yadav.R,J. and Singh.P., (2002) "Knowledge Attitude and Practice of Mothers about Breast Feeding", *Indian Journal of Community Medicine*, Vol.X.X. pp. 527-531.
- ❖ Bharati. S. et al.,(2008) "Determinants of Nutritional Status of Preschool Children in India" Journal of Biosocial Science Cambridge University. pp. 127-131.

VANCOUVER REFERENCING STYLE

The Vancouver Style or Uniform Requirements Style, is based on an American National Standards Institute (ANSI) standard adapted by the National Library of Medicine (NLM) for databases such as Medline. It was developed in Vancouver in 1978 by editors of medical journals who now meet annually as the International Committee of Medical Journal Editors Communication and Utilization of Research. This meeting that time actually formed for Uniform Requirements for Manuscripts Submitted to Biomedical Journals (ICMJE). Over 500 medical journals [including prestigious journals such as British Medical Journal (BMJ)], Canadian Medical Association Journal (CMAJ), and Journal of American Medical Association (JAMA) use this style.

Citation within the Text

This Vancouver style uses the note system of referencing. Using this style, in-text citation is done with a numeric digit and then detailed references are provided at the end of the document on a separate page.

General Rules for in-text Citation

- ❖ A number each citation has given in superscript whatever information is provided like.[1,2]
- ❖ Number to each source is given in the sequence as it appears in your document.
- ❖ If you cite the same source again in your document use the same number that you have used previously for the source in your work.

- Name of author may sometime be used in your text when it is used in between the sentence but it must follow a number, for example, According to Sharma et al.,[5]
- Either square [ ] or curved brackets ( ) can be used as long as it is consistent.
- Reference numbers should be inserted to the left or inside of colons and semi-colons.
- Reference numbers are generally placed outside or after full stops and commas
- Whatever format is chosen, it is important that the punctuation is consistently applied to the whole document.

General Rules for Reference/Bibliography List

- Detailed references are listed on a separate page at the end of the document.
- The title 'References' is given to the list for only those sources are to be listed that has been cited in between the test. Each reference ends up with a full stop (.).
- The list is arranged in the same order as the references are used in your work.
- Each entry is preceded by the numeric digit used for it in the text.
- Titles of a bigger source such as a book or journal are italicized.
- Titles which are a part of a bigger work such as a chapter of a book, article in a journal or newspaper are neither italicized nor enclosed in any quotation marks.
- If you want to mention sources that have been utilized in the hunt of knowledge but are not cited in your document, they can be mentioned under the heading of "Bibliography" on a separate page.
- The year will be written at the end if there is no other volume and if it is a book. If it is a journal the year will be written followed by month volume issue.
- If you are writing the exact words of an author without doing paraphrasing, it is called as quotation. In this case it is essential to mention the page number. But even though it is not direct extract from the books we are writing page number for our easy reference.

The Writing Style Based on Different Authors

- *If single author than the writing style will be:*
  Author(s): Family name and initials (no more than 2 initials with no spaces between initials). Title of book. Edition of book if later than 1st ed. Place of publication: Publisher name; Year of publication. Page no.
  Example: Basavanthappa BT. Nursing research and statics, 3rd ed. New Delhi: Jaypee Brothers Medicals Publishers (P) Ltd, 2014. Page no- 280
- *For two to six authors the bibliography writing style will be:*
  Author(s): Family name and initials (no more than 2 initials with no spaces between initials) multiple authors separated by a comma. Title of book. Edition of book if later than 1st ed. Place of publication: Publisher name; Year of publication.
  Example: Denise. F.P., Beck. C.T., Nursing Research principle and method. 7th ed. New Delhi: Wolter Kluwer India; page no 605 -621.
- *If more than six authors are the author then writing style will be:*
  Author(s): Family name and initials (no more than 2 initials and no space between initials), Multiple authors separated by a comma. After the 6th author add "et al." Title of book. Edition of book if later than 1st ed. Place of publication: Publisher name; Year of publication.
- Example: Hofmeyr GJ, Neilson JP, Alfirevic Z, Crowther CA, Gulmezoglu AM, Hodnett ED, et al. A Cochrane pocketbook: Pregnancy and childbirth. Chichester, England: John Wiley and Sons; 2008.

- *If author is not available in the source,* use the name of a corporate author; name of an organization, a company or a publisher. Owning a document in case of the absence of any specific author/s is called as corporate author. If it is a book than begin a reference with the title of the book if no person or organization can be identified as the author and no editors or translators are given. Do not use anonymous.
- *If it is a book than* Title of book. Edition of book if later than 1st ed. Place of publication: Publisher name; Year of publication. Example: A guide for women with early breast cancer. Sydney: National Breast Cancer; 2003.
  For a report:
  Example: Attaining Millennium Development Goals in India Role of Public Policy and Service Delivery, The World Bank, Washington DC. 2004
- *Different editions of same author/authors*
  Author(s): Family name and initials, multiple authors separated by a comma. Title of book. Edition of book if later than 1st ed. Place of publication: Publisher name; Year of publication. Note: Include the edition number after the book title for all editions except the first edition. Abbreviate edition to 'ed.'
  Sharma S. K. Nursing research and statistics. 2nd .3rd.ed. New Delhi: Elsevier India Private Limited; 2014
- *Chapter in an edited book*
  Author(s) of chapter: Family name and initials, Title of chapter. In: Editor(s) of book - Family name and initials, editors. Title of book. edition (if not first). Place of publication: Publisher name; Year of publication. p. [page numbers of chapter].
  Example: Rowlands TE, Haine LS. Acute limb ischaemia. In: Donnelly R, London NJM, editors. ABC of arterial and venous disease. 2nd ed. West Sussex: Blackwell Publishing; 2009. p. 123-140.
- *Chapter from an electronic book*
  Author(s) of book: Family name and initials. Title of book [Internet]. # edition. Place of Publication: Publisher Name; Year of Publication. Chapter [chapter number], Chapter title. [cited date - year, month abbreviated, day]. Available from: URL
  Darwin C. On the origin of species by means of natural selection or the preservation of favoured races in the struggle for life [Internet]. London: John Murray; 1859. Chapter 5, Laws of variation. [cited 2010 Apr 22]. Available from: http://www.talkorigins.org/faqs/origin/chapter5.html
- *Electronic book from a full text database*
  Elements of the citation Author(s) of book: Family name and initials. Title of book [Internet]. # edition. [type of medium - eBook]. Place of Publication: Publisher Name; Year of Publication [cited date - year, month abbreviated, day]. Available from: [name of database].
  Example: Macdonald S. editor. Maye's midwifery 14th ed. [eBook]. Edinburgh: Bailliere Tindall; 2011 [cited 2012 Aug 26]. Available from: Ebrary.

PUBLICATION OF ARTICLE IN JOURNAL

For publishing article in journal a researcher has to follow all the same steps what he/she has to do for communicating his/her research report by any means like selecting proper channel, identifying the consumers by knowing the audience, deciding on authorship, deciding on content, assembling materials and writing effectively the content. Before writing begins only there should be especially a clear idea of the journal to which a manuscript will be submitted.

Each journals differ in their goals, types of manuscript sought, and readership. All journals issue goal statements, as well as guidelines for preparing and submitting a manuscript is published in journals themselves and on their websites which the researcher must follow. Journals differ in prestige, acceptance rates, issues per year, word limits and reference styles. Several of these characteristics are usually taken into account in selecting a journal. Prestige is often assessed in terms of a journal's *impact factor*. It is sometimes useful to send a query letter to a journal to ask the editor whether there is interest in a manuscript. The query letter should briefly describe the topic and methods, title and a tentative submission date. The query letter is essential to know about articles it's requirement, the editors want more articles on not for publication.

Preparing the Manuscript

Once a journal has been selected, the information included in the journal's instructions to authors should be carefully reviewed. These instructions typically give authors such information as maximum page length, what font and margins are permissible, what type of abstract is desired, what reference style should be used, and how to submit the manuscript. In most cases, manuscripts now must be submitted online. Manuscript for journals must be no more than 15-20 pages, doubled spaced, not counting references and tables. Greatest spaces should be allocated to methods and results. Care should be taken in using and preparing citations only published work can be cited. The reference style of American Psychological Associations (2010) is the style used by many journals.

Content of Journal Articles

Many quantitative and qualitative journal articles follow a conventional organization called the IMRAD format.
  This format involves organizing material into four main sections:
1. Introduction
2. Method
3. Results
4. Discussion
  These sections, respectively address the following questions:
* Why was the study done? what question (problem) was studied?(I)
* How was the study done?(M)
* What was learned or what are the findings? (R)
* What does it mean?(D)

The format for publication is:
Front matter
1. Title
2. Authors
3. Abstract

Article body
1. Introduction
2. Material and methods
3. Results
4. Discussion

End matter
1. Acknowledgments
2. References

Title

Full title of the paper, which should be concise, informative, and generally not exceeding more than 15 words. Generally in thesis we are writing full problem statement like 'A study to assess the effectiveness of structure teaching program on knowledge of mothers of under five children regarding prevention of malnutrition among under fives in Suapanji Sahi Ankoli Berhampur' but when it published in the journal it should be like 'effectiveness of structure teaching program on knowledge of mothers regarding prevention of malnutrition.' Length of titles must be reduced by omitting unnecessary terms such as 'A study of...............,' 'report of...............,' 'An investigation to examine the effect of............. and the same meaning repetitive term also be avoided. The title should be presented in capital letters, only the initial letters of principal words are capitalized.

Types of Title

- **Declarative titles:** Declarative titles state the main findings or conclusions (e.g., a three-month weight loss program increases self-esteem in adolescent girls).
- **Descriptive titles** describe the subject of the article but do not reveal the main conclusions (e.g., the effects of family support on patients with dementia).
- **Interrogative titles:** Introduce the subject in the form of a question (e.g., does cognitive training improve performance on pattern recognition tasks?).

Each of these three types is useful and you should choose a format depending on what kind of information a researcher want to convey to his audience. Declarative titles are generally used in research articles and they convey the largest amount of information. They are also good if you want to emphasize the technical side of the research. Interrogative titles, on the other hand, are less common and they are more suitable for literature review articles. But out of the three, descriptive titles seem to be most common type in journals.

Authors

Title of the articles is followed by the name of the authors in the form that publication should be provided. The degree of affiliation and full official address should be given on a separate sheet at the end of the paper. One of the authors should be designed to receive correspondence, who must take responsibility of keeping the other authors informed of the progress of paper.

Abstract

The abstract is a brief description of the study placed at the beginning of the article in a single paragraphs summarizing the study's main features. It answers, in about 100–200 words, the following:
- What were the research questions?
- What methods did the researcher use to address the questions?
- What did the researcher find?
- What are the implications for nursing practice?

Some journals have structured abstracts with specific headings, e.g., abstracts in *Nursing Research* organize study information under the following headings:
- Background
- Objectives
- Method
- Results
- Conclusions

Journal abstracts sometimes written as unstructured paragraph of 100–200 words, with or without subheadings. If the subheading are not mentioned also the abstract should be described by following same subheadings.

Keywords

It is often necessary to include keywords that will be used in indexes to help others locate your study. Substantive, methodologic, and theoretical terms can be used as keywords.

Introduction

The introduction communicates the research problem and its context.
This section usually describes:
- The central phenomena, concepts, or variables under study.
- The current state of evidence based on a literature review.
- The theoretical or conceptual framework.
- The study purpose research questions, or hypotheses to be tested.
- The study's significance.

The introduction sets the stage for a description of what the researcher did and what was learned.

Method Section

The method section describes the methods used to answer the research questions. Difference between the qualitative and quantitative research report is discussed in **Table 12.1**.

Table 12.1: Difference between the qualitative and quantitative research report.

Quantitative research report	
In a quantitative study the method section usually describes: • The research design • The sampling plan • Methods of data collection and instruments used • Study procedures • Analytic procedures and methods	In qualitative study the method section have the same issues but with different emphases: • Provide more information about the research setting and study context • Less information on sampling • Less discussion about data collection methods • More information on data collection procedures
Result section	
In quantitative study the researchers typically report: • The names of statistical tests used • The value of the calculated statistic • The significance	• In qualitative study the researchers organize findings according to the major themes, processes or categories identified in the data • Often have several subsections, also present the researcher's emerging theory about the phenomenon under study.

Discussion Section

In the discussion section, researchers draw conclusions about what the results mean, and how the evidence can be used in practice. The researcher has to give comparison of other studies.

In this stage the researcher can identify and reviews study limitations and find out the implications of the limitations for the integrity of the results.

Limitations can be point out by sample deficiencies, design problems, weakness in data collection, and so forth. A discussion section that presents these limitations demonstrates to readers that the author was aware of these limitations and probably took them into account in interpreting the findings.

Acknowledgments

People who helped with the research but whose contribution does not qualify them for authorship are sometimes acknowledged in the report.

This might include statistical consultants, data collectors, or people who reviewed the manuscript.

Acknowledgments should also give credit to organizations that made the project possible, such as funding agencies or organizations that helped with subject recruitment.

References

Each report concludes with a list of references cited in the text, using a reference style specified by those reviewing the manuscript.

Checklist

A few journals, such as the international journal of nursing studies, require the completion of an author checklist that requires authors to state their compliance with various requirements, such as total word count, declaration of keywords, and so on.

Style of Research Journal Articles

Four factors contribute to this impression:
1. Compactness
2. Jargon
3. Objectivity
4. Statistical information

Compactness

When publishing any article in journal compactness is the major characteristics a researcher should follow. Generally journal space is limited, so authors compress a lot of information into a short space. Interesting, personalized aspects of the study cannot be reported. In qualitative studies, only a handful of supporting quotes can be included.

Jargon

The authors of research reports generally use terms that may seem esoteric but it should be avoided technical jargon, abbreviation be an important facilitator of communicating among those who share it, but may serve as a barrier of when communicating with others. If there is a popular word that is equivalent to a technical one, the popular word should be used.

Objectivity

Generally quantitative research report which are published in journal should be objectivity in nature. In quantitative research design, based on the objectives research hypothesis developed which are proved in research.

Statistical Information

The statistical information in the journal should be clear. Numbers and statistical symbols can intimidate readers who do not have statistical training.

Submission of a manuscript: When the manuscript is ready for journal submission, a cover letter should be drafted. The cover letter should state the title of the paper, name and contact information of the corresponding author (usually the lead author).

The letter may include assurance that:
- The paper is original and has not been published or submitted elsewhere.
- All authors have read and approved the manuscript.
- There are no conflicts of interest.

Many journals also require a signed copyright transfer form, which transfers all copyright ownership of the manuscript to the journal and warrants that all authors signing the form participated sufficiently in the research to justify authorship.

In submitting an article online, it is usually necessary to upload several files with different parts of your manuscript.
- The title page, should be in the first file.
- The next file usually contains the abstract, main text, and the reference list.
- Tables and figures submitted separately, one file at a time.
- If there are two tables and one figure, these would be submitted in three files.
- At the end of the submission process, a PDF file that contains all the various elements is created for your review prior to submission.

Manuscript review: Most of nursing journals have a policy of independent, anonymous (blind) peer reviews by two or more experts in the field. Journals which follow such policies are refereed journals and are in general more prestigious than nonrefereed journals. When submitting a manuscript to a refereed journal, authors' names should not appear anywhere except on the title page.

Peer reviewers make recommendations to the editors about whether to accept the manuscript for publication, accept it contingent on revisions, or reject it. The information about the editors with reviewers decision together and comments are informed to the author(s).

When resubmitting a revised manuscript to the same journal, each reviewers recommendation should be addressed, either by making the requested change, or by explaining in the cover letter accompanying the resubmission the rationale for not revising. It can take a long time between the submission of the original manuscript and the publication of a journal article. If a manuscript is rejected, it should be inform to the author about the cause of rejection. When it is submitted to another journal the reviewers' comments should be taken into consideration. Manuscript need to be reviewed by several experts before final acceptance.

Five major criteria for the manuscript to be accepted for publication:
1. The importance, timelines, relevance and prevalence of the problem addressed.
2. The quality of writing style (i.e., well-written, clear, straightforward, easier to follow, logical).
3. The study design applied (appropriate, rigorous, comprehensive).

4. The degree to which the literature review was thoughtful, focused and up to date.
5. The use of sufficiently large sample.

Five reasons for rejection of article:
1. Inappropriate, incomplete and insufficiently described statistics.
2. Over interpretation of results.
3. Use of inappropriate, suboptimal or insufficiently described population or instruments.
4. Small or biased samples.
5. Text that is poorly written or difficult to follow.

Electronic publication: Electronic publications cover the rapidly increasing area of publications that require a computer to be used to access the information that they contain. They can be documents distributed free of charge or obtained by purchase. They are supplied in two forms, (i) offline publications and (ii) online publications. Some electronic publications are not supplied on physical carriers and need to be copied into the libraries' access system and be stored on hard disk stacks, tape streamers or other data storage systems; others are supplied on physical carriers and can be stored on shelves. This chapter will, therefore, be looking not at the physical carriers—they have been covered in the preceding chapters—but at the specific problems of acquiring, selecting, storing and accessing this group of documents. Most journals that publish in hard copy format now also have online capabilities. Such mechanisms expand journal's circulation, make findings accessible for worldwide. Some researchers or research team develop their own web page with information about their studies.

Offline publications: An offline publication is an electronic document which is bibliographically identifiable, which is stored in machine readable form on an electronic storage medium. CD-ROM, diskettes or floppy disks and magnetic tapes are examples. Offline monograph, e.g., a CD-ROM encyclopedia. Offline serial, e.g., a CD-ROM journal.

Online publications: An online publication (or resource) is an electronic document which is bibliographically identifiable, which is stored in machine readable form on an electronic storage medium and which is available online.

For example:
- An electronic journal, a worldwide web page or an online database
- Online monograph, e.g., a dictionary on the web.
- Online serial, e.g., an electronic journal on the web.
- Online resource, e.g., an organization's home page.

Advantages
- Dissemination can occur more rapidly.
- Cutting down on publication lag time.
- Accessible to worldwide audience.
- Can include audio and video supplements not possible in hard copy journals.

Drawbacks

There are many opportunities to publish results on internet without a peer review process.

UTILIZATION OF RESEARCH FINDINGS

From the beginning, nursing has been recognized as both an art and a science. Florence Nightingale's book, *Notes on Nursing*, provided the information necessary for those who nursed others back to health. At the time of its first publication, nursing schools did not exist, there was no distinct body of nursing science, nor were there recognizable nursing practices. And yet, the fundamentals laid forth by Nightingale remain timeless. She combined basic concepts of care using principles of ventilation and warming, environment, noise, nutrition, bedding, light and cleanliness, with scientific strategies, such as observation, data collection and statistical analysis. Nightingale was not only the first nurse to conduct research, but also the first to disseminate research findings and implement research-based practice.

Today, 140 years later, the need for research-based practice is still widely accepted. But unfortunately, many current nursing interventions are based on tradition rather than science. Some traditional procedures seem very logical and helpful when considered at face value, but a review of the scientific literature reveals that intervention is not only ineffective, but also potentially harmful. One such example is the common practice of instilling saline into the trachea prior to deep suctioning. Though it seems logical that saline would help to liquefy tracheal secretions and facilitate removal of secretions, most research studies have not supported this act. In today's cost- and time-conscious healthcare environment, nurses cannot afford to spend time on unnecessary or ineffective procedures. At a time when nurses are now asked to take care of more complicated illnesses and demanding patients, striving for decreased lengths of stay, the nurse must work smarter, not only harder.

Therefore, it is not a novel idea that nurses need to engage in research, and integrate research findings into practice. In spite of this, the actual utilization of research and practice has yet to be realized. The gap that exists between research and practice has been termed the research-practice gap. Although many different reasons are put forward for the research-practice gap, there is agreement that ways should be found to strengthen the role of research in nursing and to overcome the factors inhibiting this role.

Despite barriers that may be present, each nurse must recognize the value of research-based clinical practice and identify strategies that will minimize barriers and facilitate the change process. Each nurse can help to create an environment that supports and encourages evidence-based practice. Consulting with nurse researchers, communicating and collaborating with peers, and attending research conferences can facilitate research utilization in practice settings.

Barriers in Utilization of Nursing Research

A major barrier to research utilization is the absence of published research on specific clinical issues. In addition, published research may have limitations (e.g., sample size or design) that restrict the ability to generalize results to clinical practice settings. Nurses may lack experience reading and critiquing research reports and may have difficulty interpreting study designs and statistical findings. These factors are compounded by the fact that many research projects never are published or presented, making their findings inaccessible to staff nurses. Some of the main constrains to the use of nursing research findings are as follows:

- Nurses lack time to actively participate in conducting and implementing research.
- They lack to the resources to read current research findings.
- Nurses do not understand the importance of research.
- Research is a minute and difficult component of undergraduate nursing programs.
- Healthcare system in our own scenario pays little attention to research on nursing issues.
- Lack of access to research literature for the bedside clinical nurses.
- Investigators' lack of preservation of research from a clinical perspective, and their use of research jargon can make it difficult for staff nurses to understand or interpret study results.

- Published research may have few clinical applications, and staff nurses may not read nursing research journals.
- Research reports most often are presented to audiences of researches; therefore, pertinent clinical findings may not reach nurses who can practically use these new ideas in patient care.
- Voda et al. found that lack of research utilization is basically due to:
  - Failure to directly involve the clinical nurses in research projects.
  - Researchers not directly being involved with patient care.
  - Nurses failing to read research articles.

Funk, Champagne, Wiese, and Tornquist, (1991) identified the barriers to research utilization under four categories as discussed below.

Factors related to Nurses

- Nurses have a lack of time, motivation, confidence, research knowledge, money and resources.
- Nurses do not see the value of research for practice.
- They see little benefit for self from research.
- They are inflexible and unwilling to change/try new ideas.
- There is not a documented need to change practice.
- Nurses lack confidence in new research findings.
- Nurses do not feel capable of evaluating the quality of the research.
- Nurses lack time and resources to stay in touch with knowledgeable colleagues with whom to discuss the research.
- Nurses are unaware about the importance of the research.

Nursing Research Factors

- The research has methodological inadequacies.
- The conclusions drawn from the research are not justified.
- The research has not been replicated.
- The literature reports conflicting results.
- The nurses are uncertain whether to believe the results of the research.
- Research reports/articles are not published fast enough.
- Nursing research generally lack the appropriate clinical applicable recommendations.

Organizational Factors

- Organizations fail to provide access to journals and research resources.
- Organizations lack the funding to support new research findings.
- Administration does not allow implementation of the research findings.
- Physicians will not cooperate with implementation of new research findings.
- There is insufficient time on the job to implement new ideas.
- Other staff is not supportive of implementation.
- The facilities are inadequate for implementation.
- Nurses do not feel that they have enough authority to change patient care procedures.
- The nurses do not have time to read research literature and participate in research activities.
- The nurses feel results are not generalized to their setting.

Communication Factors

- Lack of collaboration between researchers and clinicians.
- Lack of presentation of research findings to nurses in clinical setting.
- Lack of publication in clinical nursing journals.
- Lack understandable research publications.
- Overwhelming amount of contradicting information in medical and nursing journals as well as in textbooks.
- Implications for practice are not made clear.
- Research reports/articles are not readily available.
- The research is not reported clearly and readably.
- Statistical analyzes are not understandable.
- The relevant literature is not complied in one place.
- The research is not relevant to the nurse's practice.

Strategies to Facilitate Utilization of Nursing Research

The most crucial factor in facilitating research utilization is the identification of clinically relevant problems and issues. Other facilitating factors include environments in which individuals are committed to critical thinking and to the research utilization process. Nursing administrators who provide adequate resources (e.g., personnel, money and time) help promote research utilization. Staff nurses in these environments benefit from having increased understanding of research and research utilization.

Nurses administrators facilitate research utilization when they clearly communicate to staff nurses the value of research utilization and provide incentives for this process to occur. By negotiating linkages between practice setting and academia, nurse administrators can support collaboration between clinical nurses and expert researchers. Nurse administrators can work with medical librarians to facilitate staff nurses' access to the nursing literature by negotiating flexible library hours and computerized literature searches using the Internet.

The barriers to research-based practice are multidimensional, so the process to implement effective strategies to overcome these barriers will require a combined effort from nurses in education, research, administration and clinical practice. Strategies for each of these areas are presented below.

Nurse Educators

Nurse educators are crucial role models in providing a foundation for research-based practice. They must have the ability to foster an appreciation for research and make it interesting for the nursing students. When nurse educators refer to research findings regularly in their lectures, include research-based publications in their reference lists, and continually refer students to research articles, the students will soon get the message that research is an important foundation for practice. Research should not be limited to only a single course, but rather be a constant emphasis. Clinical seminars should also include a discussion on research-based articles appropriate to that specific clinical rotation each week postconferences. Students should be encouraged to seek the latest research findings in their field so they can possess the most current practice.

Undergraduate students should complete their program with the ability to criticize and debate current research studies rather than writing a research proposal for a study they will not conduct.

Since many masters' programs now focus on nurse practitioner education, graduate students can benefit from participation in research utilization projects. Nursing students must see that change occurs, but only if the need for change is identified. It allows reflecting the skills they need to use after graduation. Research-based clinical practices that will solve problems, while making work procedures more efficient and therefore less costly, are good reasons for change. To sum up educators must:

- Use research findings to support lectures and teachings.
- Incorporate research findings in clinical assignments.
- Strive to make research exciting so that students can be motivated to conduct research activity.

Nurse Researchers

Dissemination methods used by researchers in publications and presentations often inhibit rather than support research-based practice. The clinical nurse often finds the language and the results difficult to interpret and apply to the patient. For patients to benefit from research-based practice, researchers must make an elaborate effort to include information that specifically addresses practical clinical applications of their findings. In addition, rapid dissemination of research results is important. Presenting findings at regional and national meetings will help accomplish this goal. Disseminating the information in the literature is critical.

The research community also needs to increase the emphasis on similar studies to strengthen the foundation for research-based practice and minimize the conflicting views. Currently, clinicians are confused when reading conflicting information in journals. This causes uncertainty about the validity of the studies and their applicability for practice. Clearer and more useful reports are key issues for overcoming barriers to research-based practice. To sum up researchers must practice some following measures:

- Focus their research activity on current clinical problems.
- Disseminate research results as early as possible.
- Present research findings locally, regionally and nationally.
- Publish the research findings in clinical as well as scientific journals.
- Clearly delineate practice implications of results.

Nurse Administrators

The organization should establish the expectation of research-based practice. The culture of research should be pervasive in the organization. If nurses are allowed to continually question current practices, then the expectation will exist for the present and future nurses to do so.

The structure of the healthcare organization should support research-based practice. Establishing a department of nursing research immediately indicates the institution's level of commitment to research. Having an expert consultant or expert nurse researcher will provide the necessary support for inexperienced researchers to engage in various aspects of the research process. Nurses should also hold positions on internal review boards. Collaborative research projects should be encouraged so that each discipline's perspective can be considered when developing a plan of care. Job descriptions should address this important aspect of the health care team member's duties. To sum up nursing administrators must follow some of the measures given below:

- Establish a research-friendly culture.
- Encourage clinicians to question traditions.

- Reward risk-taking and innovation.
- Require research basis for practice changes.
- Incorporate research role in job descriptions.
- Provide research resources, such as medical and nursing literature, internet access, consultants, etc.
- Encourage and support continuing education, conference participation and publishing.
- Encourage role model research collaboration.

Nurse Clinicians

Nurses should be encouraged to update their research skills. This can be accomplished by seeking advanced nursing degrees or the organization can work to provide education regarding research utilization. Institutions can send key nurses to conferences which provide practice updates, or bring in researchers to share their findings with nurses, as well as other members of the interdisciplinary team. This can increase acceptance by physicians and other healthcare providers of nursing research findings. Libraries with journals that focus on research-based practices should be accessible to nurses who work in clinical areas. The more opportunity the nurse has to read research articles, the greater the chance that research findings will be adopted.

An additional way to make findings accessible is to encourage nurses to publish their findings in professional journals. Many clinical journals are now emphasizing research-based practice. Clinical nurses need time to think critically about their patients and the nursing interventions they are administering. The institution should provide time to use library resources, and time to access online services. This recognition of time needed to access the research will result in a reduction of ineffective nursing interventions which actually cost the institution time and money to sum up nurse clinicians must take initiative for the following measures:

- Question practice traditions.
- Stay updated with literature.
- Commit to continuous learning, such as continuing education, joining professional organizations and pursuing advanced degrees.
- Collaborate with researchers to rely clinical issues and questions.
- Support research conduct in the clinical setting.
- Take the risks to make changes and improve practice.

When barriers to research utilization are identified, nurse administrators, clinicians and researchers can design and implement specific strategies to overcome these obstacles. These strategies may be specific to staff members, facilities or situations. For example, one facility may find it helpful to offer incentives (e.g., pay increases within a clinical ladder program), whereas another facility may support research utilization activities by forming a nursing research committee. Other strategies include providing staff nurses with time to read research reports and having experts available to help staff nurses interpret and critique research findings.

DEVELOPMENT AND PRESENTING A RESEARCH PROPOSAL

Writing a proposal for a research project program is a problem of persuasion. A research proposal is a document proposing a research project, generally in the sciences or academia, and generally constitutes a request for sponsorship of that research. Proposals are evaluated on the cost and potential impact of the proposed research, and on the soundness of the proposed plan for carrying it out. It can be written in the educational institutions like nursing colleges specifically for postgraduate degrees for getting approval of universities to conduct a research. The research proposal outlines the process from beginning to end and may be used to request financing for the project, certification for performing certain parts of research of the experiment, or as a required task before beginning a college dissertation. It is a briefly written plan for research which contain an outline of the research idea, and that can be communicated to the faculty, university or the funding agency, so that an approved project can be implemented. It is a request for support of sponsored research, instruction, or extension projects. In academic carrier when research is conducting for partial fulfilment of any study program the research proposals develops to assess the quality and originality of the ideas and skills in critical thinking and the feasibility of the research project which can be submitted to the universities for approval. The research proposal is the document that finally establishes that there is a niche for the chosen area of study and that the research design is feasible. Development of the research proposal starts when the research problem is sufficiently specified to begin work and the researcher is satisfied that the problem is feasible. Research proposal serves strong foundation for the actual research study, which is conducted after a due approval by the experts from faculty or funding agency.

Research proposal can convince members of the scientific community that the research is significant and feasible. It can clearly state why the problem selected and what is its significance and what problems can arises in conducting such types of research. In academic institution, the research proposal is commonly known as *synopsis*.

Definition of Research Proposal

A research proposal is an outline of the research idea, which help in communicating this idea to faculty or the funding agency, so that an approved project can be implemented.

A research proposal is a comprehensive summary plan of what you intend to do, how it will be done, and why it is important.

Meaning of Research Proposal

A research proposal is a written document proposing a research project specifying what the investigator proposes to study. Proposals serve to communicate the research problem, is significance, and planned procedure for solving the problem to the interested party. That 'party' may be a funding agency, a faculty advisor, or institutional officers depending upon the circumstances.

Document that is typically written by a scientist or academic which describes the ideas for an investigation on a certain topic. The research proposal outlines the process from beginning to end and may be used to request financing for the project, certification for performing certain parts of research of the experiment, or as a required task before beginning a college dissertation.

A research proposal is a comprehensive summary of what you intend to do, how it will be done, and why it is important. Some of the agencies view written research proposal as an actual commitment on the part of the researcher that the study will proceed as originally outlined. Research proposal may answer the following questions.

- ❖ What does a researcher want to do? How much will it cost? How much time will it take?
- ❖ How does the proposed project relate to the sponsor's interests?
- ❖ Why the researcher select that? What is its significance?
- ❖ What difference will the project make to your students, your field, your patients, the state, the nation, the world, or whatever the appropriate categories are?
- ❖ What has already been done in the area of the research?

- What is the plan methodology?
- How will the results be evaluated or analyzed?

These questions will be answered in different ways and receive different emphases depending on the nature of the proposed project and on the agency to which the proposal is being submitted. Most agencies provide detailed instructions or guidelines concerning the preparation of proposals.

Purposes of Proposal

A clean, well thought-out, proposal forms the backbone for the thesis itself. A good thesis proposal hinges on a good idea. Getting a good idea hinges on familiarity with the topic which can be possible by longer preparatory period of reading, observation, discussion, and incubation.

- Research proposal provide an opportunity to the researcher and the experts to think through project carefully, and clarify and define what exactly to study.
- It serves as a blueprint and guiding path for the researcher to carry out the research project. Research proposal describe what to do, why it should be done, how to do it and what is the expectation of result.
- Being clear about the research from the beginning will help the researcher to complete his/her thesis in a timely fashion.
- Research proposal helps the researcher to communicate to the supervisor, faculty, department, and funding agency about the study planning, so that the desired suggestions and support to carry out the research project can be obtained.
- Proposal also helps the department to make a right decision about allotment of guide for the candidate pursing a particular project.
- It also gives an opportunity to receive feedback from supervisor and others in the academic community as well as possible funders.
- Research proposal also serves as a contract between researcher, guide and university.
- Research proposal also can be used to seek ethical approval from the institutional, regional or national-level research ethical committee.
- Research proposals are generally submitted to a scholarship committee or other funding agency to seek the financial grants for implementation of the research project.
- Have thought about the issues involved and are able to provide more than a broad description of the topic which are planning for research.

Type of Proposals

Solicited Proposals

Submitted in response to a specific solicitation issued by a sponsor. Such solicitations, typically called request for proposals (RFP), or request for quotations (RFQ), are usually specific in their requirements regarding format and technical content, and may stipulate certain award terms and conditions. Broad agency announcements (BAAs) are not considered formal solicitations.

Unsolicited Proposals

Submitted to a sponsor that has not issued a specific solicitation but is believed by the investigator to have an interest in the subject.

Preproposals

Requested when a sponsor wishes to minimize an applicant's effort in preparing a full proposal. Preproposals are usually in the form of a letter of intent or brief abstract. After the preproposal is reviewed, the sponsor notifies the investigator if a full proposal is warranted.

Continuation or Noncompeting Proposals

Confirm the original proposal and funding requirements of a multiyear project for which the sponsor has already provided funding for an initial period (normally one year). Continued support is usually contingent on satisfactory work progress and the availability of funds.

Renewal or Competing Proposals

Are requests for continued support for an existing project that is about to terminate and from the sponsor's viewpoint, generally have the same status as an unsolicited proposal.

Golden Rules for Proposal Writing

In academic carrier proposal writing is important for completing graduation and postgraduation degrees. The proposal is, in effect, an intellectual scholastic (not legal) contract between a researcher and his/her committee. It specifies what one will do, how to do it, and how will interpret the results. In specifying what will be done it also gives criteria for determining whether it is done. In approving the proposal, the research committee gives their best judgment that the approach to the research is reasonable and likely to yield the anticipated results. They are implicitly agreeing that they will accept the result as adequate for the purpose of granting a degree. Research proposals communicate a research problem and proposed methods of solving it. A written document, specifying what the investigator proposes to study and written before beginning the research. The content and organization are broadly similar to that for a research report, but proposals are written in the future tense, (i.e., indicating what the researcher will do) and obviously do not include results and conclusion.

Contents

Be clear, objective, succinct and realistic in your objectives. The objective in writing a proposal is to describe what one will do, why it should be done, how the researcher will do it and what he/she expects will result. Being clear about these things from the beginning will help a researcher complete his/her thesis in a timely fashion. Need for study should be justifying why the problem is selected and how will the research benefit the wider society or contribute to the research community. The content should be a complete plan.

Style

- If space allows, provide a 'punchy' project title
- Structure your text—if allowed use section headings
- Present the information in short paragraphs rather than a solid block of text
- Write short sentences with future tense.

Process

- ❖ Identify prospective supervisors and discuss your idea with them.
- ❖ Avoid blanket general e-mails to several prospective supervisors.
- ❖ Allow plenty of time.
- ❖ Get feedback from your prospective supervisor. Be prepared to take their comments on board.
- ❖ If applying to an external funding agency, remember that the reviewer may not be an expert in your field of research.
- ❖ Stick to the guidelines and remember the deadline.

IMPORTANCE OF A PROPOSAL BEFORE CONDUCTING A RESEARCH

Writing the research proposal is very important before actual conducting of any research. Because research is a teamwork and you have opinion of others if it is in written form. Research proposal is used for finalization of a research plan after presentation and discussion before research committee or board. It is also necessary to submit for applying grants to any agency. Once developed, it serves as a plan for conducting the research. In reality, as best (1983) puts it, no worthwhile research can result in the absence of a well-designed proposal. By formulating a research proposal, researcher wants to show that the problem propose to investigate is significant enough, the method plan to use is suitable and feasible, and the results are likely to prove fruitful and will make an original contribution. In short, through research proposal researcher wants to convince the other peoples (reader or audience) regarding selected problem. Proposals help the researcher to estimate the size of a project. Do not make the project too big.

FORMAT OF RESEARCH PROPOSAL

Different funding agencies or colleges may have different guidelines/format requirements. Where this is the case, the principal investigator should prepare the proposal in the required format, provided that the format used gives all or most of the details as contained in the guidelines of the particular institute.

Before an attempt is made to start with a research project, a research proposal should be complied. For the beginner researcher, this is usually the most difficult part. It is, however, the most important aspect of the research project and should be considered carefully by the researcher. This does not only require subject knowledge, but also insight into the problem that is going to be investigated, so as to give logical structure to research study. The research proposal can be envisaged as the process (step-by-step guidelines) to plan and to give structure to the prospective research with the final aim of increasing the validity of the research. It is therefore a written submission to spell out in a logical format the nature of the design and the means and strategies that are going to be used.

A research proposal usually consists of the following elements.

Title Page

The title page of the research proposal provides the first impression for the audience of researcher's proposal. It consists of research title, about the author and about the institution.

Title

The title must be complete, specific, precise and it should provide the focus of researcher's investigation. It should be also accurate, descriptive and comprehensive. The researcher must be sure that the title gives a glimpse of the nature of the proposed investigation and includes the key ideas. It should not be more than two to three lines long, and should indicate what one intends to do or find out. 'Effectiveness of diet therapy on management of malnutrition among SAM child in nutrition rehabilitation center Bhubaneswar'.

The title or statement of problem is usually only formulated after the research problem and subproblems have been stated which follows all the steps we consider in developing problem statement like decide on the general area of study or investigation by identifying area of interest, explore the phenomena by following review and narrow the topic to a specific problem than review the topic to determine present level of knowledge and evaluate the research problem for feasibility and finally formulating the statement of research problem. As the title of a proposal is the problem statement of a research in precise form it should be include:

- What is researched?
- The place of research
- The objective
- The research design
- The population among study will be conducted.

About Investigators

Problem statement must allow the investigator to describe the problem systematically, to reflect on its importance, its priority in the country and in the local area, and to point out why the proposed research on the problem should be undertaken.

With the title of the research project, the first cover title page of the proposal should also consists, the investigators' detail, details about the guides and co-guides if any, and detail about the institution under which a research project will be conducted. The investigator detail includes:

- Full names of all the investigators with their qualification, designations and their institutional/departmental affiliations.
- The principal/main investigator (responsible for the work) should be the first one. If there are coinvestigators, these should be indicated as appropriate with their qualifications, academic titles and institutional affiliations.
- Brief up-to-date curriculum vitae of each of the investigators and coinvestigators should be provided.

Institution where the research project will be conducted: The researcher(s) has/have to mention the name of the institution in which the research project will be conducted. For examples:

- The World Health Organization
- The Govt. College of Nursing, Berhampur, MKCG Medical College Campus, Odisha
- Indian Nursing Council

The Real Content of Research Proposal

Introduction

A well-written introduction is the most efficient way to hook the reader and set the context of the researcher's proposed research. In introduction we use to define the research problem, define the groups whom we chosen and write the major consequence of the research problem. For writing major consequence the researcher should undergone literature review and write the recent data. It should not be more than one or two paragraph.

Need for Study (Rationale/Justification for the Research Project)

In need for study the researcher has to write why such problem is selected. For example, if researcher selected a problem statement like 'effectiveness of structure teaching program on knowledge of adolescence girls regarding prevention of anemia she/he has to justify why she/he has taken adolescent girls with anemia. What is the mortality and morbidity of anemia among adolescent girls, why anemia is more common among adolescent girls and its consequence among adolescent girls, etc.? Lastly she/he has to justify what is her/his own view, what she/he faced in her/his clinical life and why she/he select such a problem statement. A review of the relevant recent literature (majority being in the past 5–10 years at most) must be done. Locally available information published or unpublished may be included (i.e., the potential significance to healthcare delivery, or otherwise). It should not be more than one page.

Objectives of the Study

- **Broad general objectives:** The general objectives of the study state what the researcher expects to achieve by the study in general terms means after completion of the study, i.e., the main issues that are being looked at/for are laid down in the broad objectives. For example, in previous problem statement the research objective is 'to assess the effectiveness of structure teaching program on knowledge of adolescence girls regarding prevention of anemia.'
- **Specific objectives:** General objectives can break into small logically connected parts to form specific objectives. Specific objectives are narrow goals. The specific issues that are being looked at/for can be included in specific objectives. These must be measurable, either qualitatively or quantitatively, and form a guide to the research methodology, data analysis, and presentation of results. For example, 'to prepare a high reliable tool.'

Formulating Hypothesis

Hypothesis is a tentative prediction or explanation about the relationship between variables. A hypothesis is not a question, but rather it is a statement about the relationship between two or more variables. Hypotheses enables the researcher to objectively investigate new areas of discovery. Thus, it provides a powerful tool for the advancement of knowledge. Hypothesis provides clear relevance of data and specific goals to the researchers. Hypothesis in research proposal can be formulated after the researcher gained a thorough knowledge about the research project. The researcher can develop null or alternative hypothesis based on the review.

Operational Definitions

This section involves the operationally defined terms used in the research study in the manner, where researcher is going to study the variables. Generally the terms used in the problem statement and methodology should be operationally defined in research proposal.

Methodology

The research proposal also consists of research design approach, population, sample, sampling technique, location of the study where the study will be carried out, ethical consideration, the design of the tool, data collection plan, tentative date for data collection, method for data collection and plan for data analysis. Every aspects of the purposed research will be explained in the future tense. The proposal will also state the delimitations (the researcher's boundaries) and limitations (the constraints the researcher will face during conducting the research).

- ❖ **Research design and approach:** The selection of a research strategy is the core of research design and approach, and is probably the single most important decision the investigator has to make. As proposal is the planning stage the choice of research design whether descriptive, experimental or any form of qualitative research a combination of these will be decided in this stage. We are describing it research approach when it spell out broad strategy like qualitative approach, experimental approach but when we will discuss about design it become some specific like pretest post-test control group design it is called as research design.
- ❖ **Location of study/study setting:** Where the study is going to be conducted. All the areas in/at which the survey/study will be carried out must be indicated. For example, "A study to assess the knowledge of mothers of infant regarding weaning in a selected urban area Ankoli," Berhampur, Ganjam, Odisha. Here the place is Ankoli which is coming under Berhampur City in Ganjam district of Odisha state.
- ❖ **Study population:** Who are to be included in the study or from which group going to draw, e.g., in the above problem statement mothers of infant of Ankoli is the assessable population from which sample has been drawn.
- ❖ **Study period:** The entire period of the study including preparation of the proposal, submission and approval, training (where necessary), pretesting (of the questionnaire), data collection, data analysis, report preparation, and dissemination of the finding. If the study is in phases, each must be specified and the time for each given.
- ❖ **Sample:** Under this heading details about sample, i.e., sample size and how it has been arrived at/worked out. Its justification, sampling technique for selection, inclusion and exclusion criteria must be included. Selection of sample size must be depends upon the type of study will be conducted. In sampling technique we are giving importance on random sampling technique but sometime based on the situation nonrandom sampling technique can be selected.
- ❖ **Data collection:** As the proposal is the planning of the research detail about data collection like data collection method and procedure, tools used for data collection, how to obtain validity and reliability of the tool must be included, the tentative period for data collection, what data will be collected, who will collect data, scoring process everything will be included. For example, for the proposal to conduct a study on "compare the quality of life among tuberculosis new cases, TB retreatment and TB with 'HIV' with a view to develop counselling guideline" data collection heading should describe in following manner. "A structured interview schedule will be used to collect the data which will be two parts. Part-I will describe about demographic characteristics, such as age, sex, educational status, religion, type of family, occupation, per capita income, marital status, category of TB, and contact history with TB patient. Part-II will be a five point rating scale consisting of 34 items based on the six domains of, level of independence, social relationship, environmental status, personal belief/spiritual wellbeing QOL, i.e., physical wellbeing, psychological wellbeing. Data will be collected from 02.03.2015 to 6.04.2015 in 180 TB clients (TB New-60, TB retreatment-60 and TB with HIV-60) from indoor, TB and chest OPD and ART center of MKCG. Medical College and Hospital, Berhampur"
- ❖ **Plan for data analyses:** The data analysis plan must be included in proposal like what statistics will be used, what the researcher predict the result will be. For example, for a study on "effectiveness of need based teaching on Maternal and Child Health (MCH) service

of ASHA in the state of Odisha" the plan for data analysis must be written in following manner. "The collected data will be planned to be organized, tabulated and analyzed by using descriptive statistics such as mean, mean percentage and standard deviations and inferential statistics includes 't' test and chi-square test. Paired 't' test will be used to find out the difference in knowledge and practice between pre and post-test. Chi-square test to find out the association between the post-test knowledge and practice score of the ASHAs with their demographic variables".

Budgetary Estimates

The budgetary estimates are more emphasized when some funding agency providing funding for conducting research. The budget plan should include all items, that should be estimated in monetary term. It includes all the estimated spending throughout the research like the wages of the persons who involved in the research and the money for hospitality of research participants also. Under each heading the money is estimated lastly it will be made subtotal and total. The justification for each budget should be mention. A Gantt chart can be drawn to specify the activities which will be carried in which time.

Bibliography

The proposal must be end with bibliography. The bibliography may follow any one style of writing (Vancouver or APA style) and the citation on each extract must be mention.

A research proposal is a written document specifying what a researcher intends to study. Major components of a research proposal includes front matter such as a cover page an abstract, statement of the problem, back ground and significance of the problem, specific objectives, methods and work plan or schedule, proposal written for funding usually also include section on personnel and facilities and a budget.

SAMPLE OF A RESEARCH PROPOSAL

1.	Name of the candidate and address	Miss. Renuka Acharya 1st year MSc Nursing
2.	Name of the institute	College of Nursing Berhampur MKCG Medical College Campus Dist. Ganjam. Odisha
3.	Course of the study and subject	1st Year MSc Nursing (Community Health Nursing)
4.	Title of the study	Effectiveness of need based structured teaching program on maternal and child health services of ASHA

Introduction

Mothers and children not only constitute a large group but they are also vulnerable or special group comprised of 71.4% of population of the developing countries, (NRHM 2010 Roy Shree and Sahu Biswamitra 2012). Globally, there are 430 maternal deaths for every 100,000 live births. In developing countries the figure is 480 maternal deaths for every 100,000 live births

(738/100,000)(Darshan K. et al., 2011 Adewoye kr et al., 2013). Every year, in India, 28 million pregnancies take place with 67,000 maternal deaths, 11 million women left with chronic ill health, and 1 million neonatal deaths. The maternal mortality rate in India is 408 per 100,000 live births. This means that around 1,25,000 women die each year due to pregnancy related causes( ). The maternal mortality rate also varies from state to state. The maternal rate is highest in Odisha (738/100,000) when compared to other states in India (Nandan D, Kushwah SS and Dubey DK, 2009; Neelanjana Pandey, 2012).

MCH service is important to communities, families and the nation due to its profound effects on the health of women, immediate survival of the newborn and long-term well-being of children, particularly girls and the well-being of families. ASHA would act as a bridge between the ANM and posted under NRHM and the village and be accountable to the Panchayat. The ASHA functions includes encouraging acceptance of neonatal care and immunization, use of weight charts for children up to the age of 6 years, nutrition, health education related to hygiene and infectious diseases, simple curative care, identification of pregnant women and children at risk and collection of information on births, deaths, eligible couples etc. (Tran TK et al., 2012, Roy Shree and Sahu Biswamitra, 2013).

Need for Study

India has a long history of programmatic efforts to improve the health of mothers and children and has made significant gains in the fifty years since independence. Despite these gains, maternal and child deaths constitute a significant burden of disease. According to WHO estimates, India contributes about 2.4 million of the 10.8 global child deaths and 25% of 529,000 global maternal deaths (Darshan K et al., 2011).

Further, neonatal mortality in India is about 36/1000 live births and neonatal mortality accounts for 50% of deaths of all children under five. Three quarters of all neonatal deaths occurring the first week of life, and about 20% take place in the first 24 hours (Nirupam Bajpai and Ravindra H 2011 K4Health 2010).

This is also the period when most maternal deaths take place. Thus, the provision of maternal and newborn care through a continuum of care approach, ensuring care during critical periods of delivery and postnatal period. Most maternal deaths and pregnancy complications can be prevented by quality antenatal, natal and postnatal care. Current utilization of any antenatal care services in India is only 77% (72% in rural and 91% in urban areas). Despite the efforts, utilization of MCH services by the rural community has not reached the desired level (Smitha Kochukuttan, 2013).

Around 9.2 million children die every year before reaching their fifth birthday. Most of these deaths occur in developing countries in which leading causes are: acute lower respiratory infections (mostly pneumonia:19% of all deaths in under fives), diarrheal (17%), malaria (8%), measles (4%), HIV/AIDS (3%), neonatal deaths—mainly preterm births, birth asphyxia, infections (37%) and injuries (3%). Poor or delayed "health care seeking" contributes to 70% of child deaths. Most deaths among under-five are still attributable to just a handful of conditions and are avoidable through existing interventions. (Shashank KJ, et al., 2013; Sushama S et al., 2012).

The National Rural Health Mission (NRHM) was launched in India by the Hon'ble Prime Minister on12th April 2005. The Mission attempts to achieve a huge variety goals through a set of core strategies by the appointment of Accredited Social Health Activist (ASHA). Activity of ASHA is one of the key components in the National Rural Health Mission, which felt to be significant in reducing maternal and infant mortality and morbidity as well as control of specific diseases, and improvement of nutrition status of children and mothers and to achieve health related millennium development goals identifying.

Different studies conducted to assess the performance of ASHA services reveal that the training provided are in adequate comparing their responsibilities and recommended for the need of continues teaching program (Nandan D, Kushwah SS, Dubey DK, 2009 Shree R, Biswamitra S, 2013; Adewoye KR et al., 2013; Bhargavi C, N Sharma).

Thakre SS et al., 2011, conducted a study on effectiveness of the training course of ASHA on Infant Feeding Practices at a Rural Teaching Hospital, and found that the training on the knowledge, attitude and practices of breastfeeding was found to be effective. The difference in the pre and the post-test score of the participants was found to be statistically significant.

Investigator in her community practice also observed that ASHAs have lack of knowledge and practice in different aspects of MCH care. Thus it is felt that an effective teaching program can help to improve the performance of the ASHA. It is felt that a need based program will be more effective because there is uniqueness of each community and a need based program can be easy to operate and will be more effective and successful. Thus the investigator is fascinated to conduct a study on effectiveness of need based teaching program on MCH care service of ASHA in the state of South Odisha.

Objectives

- Identify learning needs and practices of MCH services among ASHA in South Odisha.
- Prepare a need based structured teaching program on MCH services by ASHA
- Compare pre and post-test knowledge and practice scores of MCH services by ASHA in South Odisha.
- Find out association between post-test knowledge and practice scores of MCH service by ASHA.
- Find out significant difference between pre and post-test knowledge and practice scores of MCH services among ASHA.
- Find out significant association between post-test knowledge and post-test practices of MCH services among ASHA.
- Find out significant association between post-test knowledge and practices of MCH services with the selected demographic variables of ASHA.

Operational Definitions

Effectiveness: Operationalized as the significant difference between pre-test and post-test knowledge and practice scores of ASHAs.

Knowledge: Correct responses of ASHAs towards a structured questionnaire on MCH services.

Practices: Practice refers to the correct responses of ASHAs to the practice items related to MCH services as measured by the checklist.

MCH care service: It refers to services by ASHA related to antenatal care, postnatal care, neonatal care, infant care, care of under-fives and family planning.

ASHA (Accredited Social Health Activist): Refers to community health workers instituted by the government of India's Ministry of Health and Family Welfare as part of the National Rural Health Mission for betterment of MCH care.

Need based teaching: The teaching materials prepared for ASHA on MCH care according to their learning needs as identified through knowledge questionnaire, felt needs and observation checklist for practice. It includes antenatal and postnatal care of mothers, care of newborn and under-fives, identification and timely referral of high risk mothers and children and services related to family planning.

Structured teaching program: It refers to the teaching package which is to be delivered in two teaching and one practical session of one hour each in sequence to the ASHA.

Delimitation

The study will limited to the ASHAs of South Odisha who will be:
- Willing to participate in the study.
- Able to speak, read write Odia.
- Present during the period of data collection.
- Have completed the NRHM training and working as ASHA worker for at least one year in a given area

Hypotheses

- Ho_1: There will be no significant difference between pre and post-test knowledge and practice scores of ASHA workers regarding MCH services.
- Ho_2: There will be no significant association between post-test knowledge and practice scores of ASHA workers MCH services with their selected demographic variables.
- Ho_3: There will be no significant association between post-test knowledge and practices MCH services of ASHA workers.

Research Design and Approach

Study will be carried out in two phases.
- **Phase I:** A simple descriptive study to assess the existing knowledge and practices and identify felt needs of ASHAs regarding MCH services.
- **Phase II:** Quasi-experimental, design where pre and post-test with control group with experimental approach will be used to evaluate the effectiveness of need based teaching on knowledge and practices of the ASHAs regarding MCH care.

Phase -II O_1 - --- O_3

O_2 - X - O_4

$O_4 - O_3$ = Effectiveness

The symbols used are:

O_1 = Pretest knowledge and practice scores of ASHA in control group regarding MCH services

O_2 = Pretest knowledge and practice scores of ASHA in experimental group regarding MCH services

X = Implementation of need based structured teaching programme for ASHAs in experimental group regarding MCH of care

O_3 = Post-test knowledge and practice scores of ASHAs in control group regarding MCH services

O_4 = Post-test knowledge and practice scores of ASHAs in experimental group regarding MCH

E = Effectiveness

Setting of population

Study will be conducted in the south region of Odisha

Population
All the ASHAs of south Odisha state are population for the present study.
Sampling Technique:
Sample
All the ASHAs of Southern region of Odisha will be the sample for the present study.
Sample Size
The sample comprised of 100 ASHAs for Phase I and 150 control and 150 experimental group ASHAs for Phase II
Sampling Technique
Multistage random sampling will be selected to select the samples for the study.
Tools and instruments
The tools will be used for the present study are:
- Structured questionnaires for assessing the knowledge
- Check list for assessing the practice
- Need based structured teaching programme

Scoring Process

Each item for knowledge section has four options with only one most appropriate answer. For the correct response to each item the score will be "one" and for wrong response "zero". Check list to be used to assess practices. It has two positions. Correct practice will score one and for wrong score is zero. The level of knowledge and practice will be classified as poor, average, good, very good and excellent based on the percentage of the scores obtained.

Validity and Reliability of the Tool

The content validity of the tools will be established. The tools will be given to at least ten experts in various fields, such as, community health nursing, pediatric nursing, community medicine and biostatistics and their opinions and suggestions will be taken to modify the tools. The research consultant and guide will be consulted to finalizing the tools. Validity of the teaching module will be established based on the suggestions of the experts.

Reliability of the questionnaire will be tested by implementing same tool 25 ASHAs in other than the sample area. Split-half method (Spearman Brown's correlation coefficient formula) and test retest method will be used and coefficient and correlation will be considered to find out the reliability of the checklist and structured teaching module.

The approved tools will be translated to Oriya and retranslated to English to find out the correctness of the tool.

Data Collection Procedure

The data will be collected by the investigator herself first by pretest. The researcher will assess the knowledge and practice of ASHAs and identify the needs in which area the ASHA have gap in knowledge and practice. Then the researcher will develop a need based teaching program and provide teaching to ASHAs. After 15 day of pretest post-test will be carried out based on their knowledge and practice. The data will be collected after obtaining written permission from the CDPO, and verbal permission from the ASHAs.

Plan for Data Analyses

The collected data will be planned to be organized, tabulated and analyzed by using descriptive statistics, such as mean, mean percentage and standard deviations and inferential statistics includes 't' test and chi-square test. Paired 't' test will be used to find out the difference in knowledge and practice between pre and post-test. Chi-square test to find out the association between the post-test knowledge and practice score of the ASHAs with their demographic variables.

Bibliography

1. Sushama S, et al. Effectiveness of the Training Course of ASHA on Infant Feeding Practices at a Rural Teaching Hospital: A Cross Sectional Study. Journal of Clinical and Diagnostic Research. 2012 August, Vol-6(6): 1038.
2. Shashank KJ, et. al. A study to evaluate working profile of accredited Social health activist (ASHA) and to assess their knowledge about infant health care. Int J Cur Res Rev. 2013; 5(12): 97-103.
3. Darshan K, et al. A cross sectional study of the knowledge, attitude and practice of ASHA workers regarding child health (under five years of age) in Surendranagar district health line ISSN 2229-337X 2011 July-December Volume 2 Issue 2.
4. Government of India, NRHM-ASHA (2005) Module Guidelines, Ministry of Health and Family Welfare, New Delhi.
5. Prasot RM, et al. Factors influencing overall performance of ASHAs in MCH care services under NRHM In rural Lucknow. Indian J Prev Soc Med. 2012; 43(3): 249-454.
6. Bajpai N, Ravindra H. Dholakia Improving The Performance Of Accredited Social Health Activists In India. Working Paper No. 1 May 2011 working papers series Columbia Global Centers | South Asia, Columbia University. p. 10-63.
7. Wang H, et al. Performance-based Payment System for ASHAs in India What Does International Experience Tell Us? Technical Report, March 2012 Vistaar Project USAID.
8. Evaluation Study of National Rural Health Mission (NRHM) In 7 States Programme Evaluation Organisation Planning Commission Government of India New Delhi-110001 February 2011.
9. Manish K, et al. Indian Journal of Community Medicine. 2010; 35(3): 414-19.

COMPUTER IN NURSING RESEARCH

Always computers used to solve the problems faced by the mankind. Since the time of invention, the size of the computers has drastically reduced from a room size to the size, that can be accommodated in a human palm. Previously, the people use to think the word computer means "something which computes or a machine for performing calculations automatically". But, today computer means not merely a "calculator". It does vast variety of jobs with tremendous speed and efficiency. Today people use computers in almost every walk of life. Computers have become a subject of nursing curriculum also. Nursing practice, education, administration and research in every field the computer is tremendously used. Use of computer in research is so extensive. Advances in computer-based technology have become an important aspect of nursing research. With emphasis on innovation in research by funding agencies, including the National Institutes of Health, nurse researchers are attracted to innovative computer technologies. It is difficult to conceive today a scientific research project without a computer. In-depth and extensive studies cannot be carried out without the use of computer, particularly those involving complex computations and data analysis. Computer in nursing research is used at all stages of study from the proposal stage to the presentation of findings. A brief description about major uses of computer in nursing research is given below. A funded research study becomes a logistical challenge for most researchers in managing the steps of the process, maintaining the integrity of the procedures, managing the information and paper flow, and keeping confidential and secure the data collection and storage, which culminates in analyzing and reporting the results. The computer can involves throughout the whole process.

Research Problem, Purpose, Main Question, or Hypothesis

The internet and electronic research databases provide access to a large portion of the existing quantitative and qualitative literature. This provides foundational data, theory and research findings to help shape the research purpose and investigate about the selected problem in depth. By examining the literature, one can begin to identify the gaps in the literature which can help you to formulate your primary research question(s) and/or hypotheses. Nowadays the internet and electronic research databases forms a major source of research problems. Thousands of research articles, proposals and presented research reports are available and easily accessible at the site. Students prefer to search at the website rather than searching in books and journals because it is easy to search at website.

Literature Review

Literature review is not just a step on conducting research. It can started from the selection of problem statement to discussion, recommendation and writing of bibliography. Internet is the best source for searching literature. Large amount of full text research papers and articles are available through these electronic research databases. The bibliographic references are stored in the electronic databases of the world wide webs. Access to these databases is usually achieved through academic and health organizations or through personal or group subscriptions. Examples include CINAL. Academic Search Premier, EBS, MEDLIN, PsyhINFO and JSTOR. There are also some open-access databases available on the internet such as the Directory of Open Access Journals (DAJ, available at http://www.doaj.org). In the latest computers, references can be written automatically in different styles like APA, MLA, etc. This also saves time of researcher. He needs not to visit libraries and wastes his time by searching the studies in different journals.

Conceptual Framework

Visual display software can be used to create a visual representation in the form of concept maps, flowcharts, or visual models of your research conceptual framework (either qualitative or quantitative). This helps you to accomplish three results:
1. To visually represent your main concepts and subconcepts to organize and guide the research process planning.
2. To visually explain your research proposal to reviewers and funding agencies.
3. To illustrate the conceptual framework that emerges from your data, especially in qualitative research.

Research Design

Selection of appropriate research designs may be achieved by the help of computer. Computer programs, new technologies and the internet can be used both to facilitate research design planning and data collection, as well as provide the context for a research study. Word processing, spreadsheets and database programs can all be applied to plan the study.

Sampling

In random sampling cryptographically secure random number generators such as *Fortuna or Yarrow* can be used to generate true random number selection to facilitate an unbiased random sample selection for experimental and quasi-experimental studies. Computers can also be used for the estimation of the sample size.

Research Instruments and Data Collection

Computer programs, the Internet and other technologies can also be used to both create and/or implement a research instrument in both quantitative and qualitative research. In addition, the use of computers to facilitate interviews is becoming quite common, through the use of chat rooms, forum-like settings, 'talking' computers that use Flash-based, narrative-led interviews and web video-recorded sessions. Researchers find these types of interviews very suitable when exploring sensitive issues, such as violence, sexual behavior, maltreatment and interpersonal interactions. The collection of patient physiologic parameters has easy by using computer. Research surveys and questionnaires, traditional administered in paper and pencil forms, can be programmed into a computer application either in a microcomputer or on a website accessed through the internet. Scientists and technologists from a variety of disciplines are identifying the domain of data and information that is transferable across situations, sites, or circumstances that can be captured electronically for a wide array of analyzes to learn how the health system impacts the patients it serves.

Legal and Ethical Considerations

Computer may help in taking informed consent. All research, including computer-assisted or-focused research must include the means to provide enough information to research participants to agree to give informed consent before being involved in the study. The actual consent form can be created on a computer using a word-processing program. It can also be included as a downloadable file through e-mail or the internet. A key consideration of all research studies is the issue of participant confidentiality and security of all collected data, both demographic and study related. When computers are used to collect the data, this issue becomes even more critical, since potential illegal access to the information becomes more likely. Therefore, this must be handled more sensitively.

Data Analysis Methods

One of the most profound influences that technology has had on research is in data analysis applications. Literally hundreds of hours can be saved by using the appropriate analysis software in both quantitative and qualitative research. More rigorous testing can be achieved through a huge reduction in analyst error. In quantities studies, SPSS (http://www.spss.com/spss) has become very popular tool for data analysis. This software has been considered the premier parametric and nonparametric data analysis software for several decades. Once available only by mainframe computers, PC version are now available. Example of statistics that can easily be calculated are descriptive statistics, chi-square, correlation, t-tests and analysis of variance (ANOVA). Not only analysis of the data, the analyzed data can be presented by tabulation, graph and charts which can be easily prepared in computer. Most statistical packages including SPSS, SAS and STATA, and even spreadsheets, such as excel, provide the user with tools for simple to complex graphical translation of numeric information thus allowing the researcher to display, store, and communicate aggregated data in meaningful ways.

- In qualitative studies data can also be analyzed using some of the selected software, such as:
- **QSR'S N6 and Nvitro:** QSR an Australian company offers two elite qualitative analysis software packages particularly suited to analyzing phenomenological, action, grounded theory and mixed methods data. They may be accessed at: (http://www.qsrinternational.com/products/product overview/product-overview.htm).
- *WEFTQDA* **(http://www.pressure.to/qda):** This open-source qualitative analysis tool works much like N6 above, but in a simpler, more straight forward manner. It is free to use and allows the research to organize narrative and interview data into themes, matrixes frequency counts and to apply Boolean queries.
- **AtlasTi (http://www.atlasti.com):** This 'knowledge workbench' software is excellent for analyzing text, video, audio and other multimedia qualitative data.
- **Hyper research 2.6 (http://www.researchware.com):** This software also analyzes both text and multimedia data, enabling the researcher to code, retrieve, theorize and conduct data analyses.
- Discussion of findings, recommendations, implications, limitations, summary: Word-processing software like Microsoft Office or the open-source software Open Office can be used to create text documents, spreadsheets, tables, graphs and charts as well as PowerPoint presentations for preparing tables and visual displays of the research study findings.
- **Budget:** Computer is very helpful in budgeting. It is an important tool in making analysis of any calculation with short period of time. An important part of any research proposal is an accurate and easy-to-follow budget, especially when the researcher is seeking funding. Various spreadsheet software can help with this, including the spreadsheet available in Open Office (listed above) or Microsoft Excel that comes with MS Office. In addition, budget software such as Quicken can also be useful for this part of the research process.
- **References and bibliography:** Researchers often use style and database software to help them to organize their reference resources and to format their reference and bibliography lists correctly using the common citation styles, such as Vancouver, APA, or Chicago styles. The researcher can easily differentiate between book reviews and journal reviews by the help of a computer. She/he can organize the authors name alphabetically or any other means by the help of a computer.

    Limitations of computer use:
    - The researcher should have the knowledge on computer.
    - Sometime the data can be deleted by improper handling.
    - The internet facilities may not be available for all time and accessible in all areas due to network problem.

Guidelines for Using Computer in Research

There are general guidelines for the use of the internet in research. First, researchers should carefully consider the rationale for incorporating computer technologies in their studies, looking at both the advantages and disadvantages of using a specific computer technology. Consulting with experts will provide insights on the pros and cons of using computer technologies in a specific study. Second, although many studies use computer technologies, potential issues in using the technologies are still being discovered. Thus, researchers should be aware of and sensitive to potential unexpected issues throughout the research process. With the daily advances in computer technologies, researchers frequently encounter unanticipated problems. Indeed, many issues related to security, authenticity, self-reporting, comparison of computer-based instruments to conventional instruments, and contraction with commercial bodies providing computer technologies have been reported. Finally, researchers should be conscious of the limitations of the specific computer technology that they adopt and work to resolve them. For example, current computer technologies may not provide high-resolution images of pictures taken in clinical or home settings, which may be essential for health assessment and monitoring of a specific health condition. Thus, researchers who want to use image transfers need to consider how to supplement and strengthen this strategy using other computer technologies or other design strategies in their health assessment and monitoring process.

SUMMARY

- Whenever an individual undertakes a research project, the commitment includes the responsibility to communicate the completed project to others. A research project cannot be considered complete and there are no values until its results are effectively communicated with its users and consumers.
- There are some common steps for communicating the research. Communication can be done through publication in journals or presentation in any seminars. Before communicating a report for the research must be prepared. There are mainly three types of report. That are; technical report, popular report and oral presentation or verbal report. The final will be written in a concise and objective style and in simple language with avoiding vague expressions which can be send for publication.
- Thesis is also a type of research report which describe details about research. It is especially written in academic purpose. Generally in nursing during completion of BSc nursing, MSc nursing or PhD nursing course the student nurse has to develop a thesis and present to his/her university and college library. Broadly the thesis can be divided into different sections/subsections with appropriate headings for easy understanding of the thesis.
- Nowadays the need for research-based practice is widely accepted. But unfortunately, many current nursing interventions are based on tradition rather than science. Some traditional procedures seem very logical and helpful when considered at face value, but a review of the scientific literature reveals that intervention is not only ineffective, but also potentially harmful.
- A major barrier to research utilization is the absence of published research on specific clinical issues. In addition, published research may have limitations (e.g., sample size or design) that restrict the ability to generalize results to clinical practice settings. Nurses may lack experience reading and critiquing research reports. The most crucial factor in facilitating research utilization is the identification of clinically relevant problems and issues. Other facilitating factors include environments in which individuals are committed to critical thinking and to the research utilization process.
- A research proposal is a document proposing a research project, generally in the sciences or academia, and generally constitutes a request for sponsorship of that research. Proposals are evaluated on the cost and potential impact of the proposed research, and on the soundness

of the proposed plan for carrying it out. It can be written in the educational institutions like nursing colleges specifically for postgraduate degrees for getting approval of universities to conduct a research. There should be a specific format for conducting research.

❖ Advances in computer-based technology have become an important aspect of nursing research. With emphasis on innovation in research by funding agencies, including the National Institutes of Health, nurse researchers are attracted to innovative computer technologies. It is difficult to conceive today a scientific research project without a computer.

QUESTIONS TO TEST YOUR KNOWLEDGE

Q1. What do you mean by communication of research report? Why it is essential? Write the steps for communicating the research report. (3+3+4)

Q2. Explain about the various types of report. Enumerate the guidelines for writing research report. Write the steps in writing report. (5+4+6)

Q3. Write the steps of preparing the manuscript for journal. (15)

Q4. Write short notes on following:
  a. Utilization of research findings
  b. Research proposal
  c. Use of computer in research

Q5. Multiple choice questions:

  I. Why to communicate research results?
   a. To contribute the base of evidence for nursing practice
   b. It allows for other nurses to critique.
   c. It stimulates others to replicate or develop similar studies.
   d. All of the above

  II. When a full written report of the study is required for record keeping or for public dissemination, this is called:
   a. Technical report
   b. Popular report
   c. Verbal report
   d. None of the above

  III. The ultimate outcome of the research process is termed as:
   a. Research results
   b. Research reports
   c. Research publication
   d. Research process
   The Supplementary Information in the research report are

  IV. If the research result have policy implications that report is termed as:
   a. Technical report
   b. Popular report
   c. Verbal report
   d. Written report

  V. Ideally the abstract should consists about how many wards:
   a. 50-100
   b. 150-200
   c. 200-250
   d. 250-300

  VI. In a research report which of the following section consist of fully interpretation and evaluation of results.
   a. Methodology
   b. Introduction
   c. Analysis
   d. Discussion

  VII. Which form of communication of research report can reach highest target population?
   a. Oral presentation in conference
   b. Poster presentation in conference
   c. Journal publication
   d. Thesis/dissertation

VIII. The process of synthesizing, disseminating and using research generated knowledge to make an impact or change in the existing practice in society is termed as:
   a. Research practice
   b. Evidence-based practice
   c. Research efficacy
   d. Research utilization
IX. According to Vancouver style of writing bibliography when et al can be used?
   a. When there is six author or more publishing article
   b. When there is five author or more publishing article
   c. When there is four author or more publishing article
   d. When there is seven author or more publishing article
X. Many quantitative and qualitative journal articles follow a conventional organization called the IMRAD format which is:
   a. Introduction, method, results and discussion
   b. Introduction, method, reviews, analysis and discussion
   c. Introduction, method, recommendations, and discussion
   d. Introduction, method, results and diagnosis

ANSWERS

| I. d | II. a | III. b | IV. b | V. d |
| VI. a | VII. c | VIII. a | IX. a | X. a |

Index

Page numbers followed by *f* refer to figure and *t* refer to table

A

Abstract 56, 78, 381, 413
    statistical 225
Accessible population 54, 199
Accredited Social Health Activist 431, 432
Accuracy, no degree of 215
Acknowledgments 402, 415
Acquired immunodeficiency syndrome 431
Action research 51
    studies 193
Adequate sampling procedures, use of 274
Administrative support 88
    and cooperation, lack of 25
Ambiguous questions 68
American Psychological Association 407
    referencing style 407
Analysis
    approaches in 365
    cleaning data for 280
    preparing data for 48
    solution 9
Analytical research 13
Analyzing data 48
Anemia 428
Anger 270
Anonymity 56
Anxiety 323
Applied research 11, 53
Arithmetic mean 299, 300
    demerits of 301
    merits of 301
Assumptions 54, 107-109, 125, 404
    types of 107, 107*f*
Attitude scales 68
Attribute variables 68, 97
Audience 400
Auditability 390
Authority 5
Authorship, decide on 396
Autobiographical memories 256
Average inter-item correlation 270

B

Bar diagram 291
    types of 291
Bar graph 71
Basic physiology 253
Basic research 10, 54
Beneficence, principles of 148
Bertalanffy general system's theory 133
Bias
    check for 371
    number of 216
Bibliography 121, 405, 430, 438
    list 408, 410
    style of 406
    writing 405, 409
Bimodal distribution, case of 307
Biophysiological methods 252
    advantages 253
    disadvantages 253
    purposes 252
    types 253
Biostatistics 284
    application of 279
Bipolar questions 242
Bivariate study 56, 99
Blind review 77
Brainstorming 84
British nursing index 117
Broad agency announcements 424
Budget 438

C

Cafeteria question 241
Care, timewise sale of 295*t*
Case study 63, 192
    research 51
Central limit theorem 75
Central tendency, measures of 73, 284, 298, 299, 311
Central value, objectives of 298

Certification 402
Charts, use of 398
Checklist 252, 415
Chi-square
    Analysis
        simplest method of 341
        steps of 339
    table 341t
    test 75, 333, 338, 339, 373
Clinical ladder program 422
Clinical nursing
    practice, research in 17
    research 54
Closed-format questions 240
    subtypes of 240
Cluster sampling 208, 212
    advantages 212
    disadvantages 212
    one-stage 212
    two-stage 212
Cohort study 64
Communication factors 420
Community
    bias 218
    residents 221
Comparative
    descriptive design 179
    scales 261
    studies 59
Compilation sheets, summarizing data in 369
Computer
    in quantitative data analysis, use of 333
    in research, guidelines for 438
    technology 439
    use, limitations of 438
Conception, phase of 40
Conceptual framework 57, 124, 136, 137, 404, 436
    development of 138
    ingredients of 139
    purposes of 138
Conceptual model 57, 125
    development of 141
Conceptual research 13
Conclusion 386, 405
Confidence interval 75
Confirmation stage 33
Confounding variable 98
    kinds of 273
Congruity, establishment of 141
Consecutive sampling 217
Construct validity 66
    types of 270
Construction test 255
Content 425
    analysis 63, 193, 365
    deciding about 397
    validity 66
Contingency
    questions 69, 241
    table 72, 289
Contrast data 371
Control group 59
Control over sampling method, lack of 218
Controversial subject 85
Convenience sampling 64, 216
Correlation 59, 323, 331t
    coefficient 59, 326
    value table 326t
Correlational design 179, 180, 180f, 382
Costs 198
Counseling guideline, development of 143
Counterbalanced design 177
Covariance, analysis of 75, 353-355
Cover page 402
Criminal activities 153
Critical appraisal, components of 379
Criticism 192
Critique
    aspects of 378
    emphasizes 376
    skills 378
    types of 379f
Cross-check data 371
Crossover design 174
Cross-sectional
    research design 182
    study 64
    surveys 183
Cumulative frequency 287
    curve 286, 296
    distribution 286, 286t, 287f, 296f
    percentage 288f
        distribution table 287t

D

Data 55, 221, 226
    analysis 279, 335, 385, 388, 405
        methods 437
        plan for 429, 435
        tool for 437
    case of grouped 319
    classification of 281
    coding of 367
    collection 52, 225, 226, 229, 279, 429, 437
        amount of 227
        approaches, dimensions of 224, 224f
        method 221, 225, 229, 381, 383, 384
        plan 223, 228
        procedure 434

six 'W's of 225f
tools of 229
type of 227
compare 371
describing 283
drawing inference of 283
editor window 335
graphical presentation of 291
greater accuracy of 203
groups 279
interpretation of 279, 283, 405
ordering of 367
points 311
precision of 203
preparation 280
presentation of 279
primary 222
representativeness of 371
saturation 52
sheet 265
source of 191, 222, 223t
types of 227
Decision making 344
Delimitation 104
    types of 106
    uses of 105
Delphi technique 69
Demographic variables 69, 99
Dependent T-test 76
Depression 270
Depth interview 235
    characteristics of 235
Descriptive research 12
Descriptive statistics 72, 284, 334
Descriptive studies 59
Descriptive theories 130
Design 418, 439
    considerations 199
    effect 212
Determination, coefficient of 72
Develop well-prepared research team 47
Developing conceptual framework, steps of 140, 140f
Developing data collection plan 223, 225, 396
    steps of 227, 227f
Developmental research design 182
Diabetes mellitus 240
Diagrams 370
    constructing 291
    types of 291
    use of 398
Diarrhea 431
Direct observation 248
Disciplined research, fallibility of 155
Discovery interviews 232
Discussion 386, 405
    section 414

Dispersion, measures of 284, 311
Disproportional stratified sampling 65, 211
Disseminative phase 48
Dissertation 402
    abstracts online 117
    format of 401
    parts of 402
Distribution free statistics 76
Document 423
    schedule 265
Double-barreled questions 69
Draft body 400
Draft preliminary informations 401
Drinking behavior 244

E

Education quality, rating of 241t
Effective interpretations, strategies for 283
Effective observation, steps of 249
Efficiency 203
Electronic book 411
    chapter from 411
Electronic publication 417
Element 65, 162
Emotional attitude 255
Empirical data 54
Empirical generalization 57
Empirical research 13, 14
End matter 405
    annexure 405
    appendix 405
    bibliography 405
    references 405
Ethical barriers 25
Ethical considerations 88, 163, 383
Ethnography 51, 187
Evidence
    evaluate efficacy of 32
    hierarchy of 30
Evidence-based practice 27-29
    and research utilization, concepts of 28
    final steps of 31
    Iowa model of 33, 34
    steps of 30f, 32
    Stetler model of 34
Execution 250
Existential phenomenology 190
Existing theories 83
Experience 5
Experimental research design 168
    characteristics of 168
    classification of 171f
Experimenter effect 59
Explanatory design 181

Explanatory studies 59
Explicate researcher belief 50
Exploratory descriptive design 179
Exploratory studies 59
Explore 3
  phenomena 90
Expression techniques 255
External appraisal 63
External criticism 63
Extraneous variable 60, 98
  source of 227

F

Face validity 67
Face-to-face contact research 229
Factory workers, sociodemographic variables of 289t
Feasibility 163
  evaluate research problem for 91
Field observation log 252
Figures 369
  list of 403
Filler questions 69
Final bibliography, preparation of 401
Final draft, writing 401
Final outline, preparation of 400
Fisher's exact tests 332
Flexible 186
Flowcharts 370
Focus group 64
  discussions 368
  interview 234
Focused ethnography 187, 188
Formal statement, making 333
Framework analysis 365
Freedom, degrees of 75
Free-hand curve 296
Frequency
  distribution 72, 284-286, 294f, 295f, 363
    table 285t, 286t, 289
    types of 284
  form, data in 339
  polygon 72, 294, 295f
Fundamental research and science 27
Funding, lack of 24

G

Galley proofs 78
Gathering relevant information 140
Gaussian curve 358
Gender difference 353
Geometric mean 308
  calculation of 308, 309

Geriatric people 290t
Good literature review 118
Good research
  problem, characteristics of 86, 87f
  question
    characteristics of 238, 238f
    qualities of 89
  report, characteristics of 398
Good sample, characteristics of 202
Good writing, kind of 399
Grand theories 57, 128, 128t
  characteristics of 129
Graphic display 362
Graphic rating scales 262
Graphs
  constructing 291
  limitations of 298
  types of 291
Grounded theory 51, 194, 365
  studies 64
Grouped frequency distribution 285
Guttman scaling 263

H

Handling multiple variables 155
Harmonic mean 309
  calculation of 310
Hawthorne effect 60
Health problems, agewise distribution of 290t
Healthcare
  environment 16
  organization 421
Hepatitis, scattering of 298f
Hermeneutic phenomenology 190
Higher sampling error 212
Histogram 72, 293
Historical research, conducting of 192
Homogeneity 270
Homogeneous units, clusters of 212
Human dignity, principles of respect for 150
Human immunodeficiency virus 431
  prevention of 399
Hyper research 438
Hypertension 240
Hypothesis 55, 58, 101, 109, 333, 376, 404, 436
  alternative 102
  associative 104
  casual 104
  characteristics of 102
  complex 58, 103
  concept 100
  directional 58, 103
  formulate 44, 428
  functions of 102

importance of 101, 101f
nondirectional 103
purposes of 100
testing 344
  procedures 333
types of 102
Hypothyroidism 240

I

Implement plan 205
Implementing research, process of 24
Incidence studies 179
Independent T-test 76
Inferential statistics 72, 283, 331, 385
  concepts related to 332
  tests 385
Information
  detailed 230
  in-depth 230
  kind of 281
  piece of 221
Informed consent 56, 152
  major elements of 152, 152f
Inquiry, cultivate spirit of 29
Institutional factors 24
Instrument 434
  design 384
  developing 227
  selecting 227
Interaction effect 58
Internal consistency 270
  reliability 67
Internal criticism 64
Internal validity 60
Interobserver reliability 67
Interpretation 251
Interquartile range 72
Inter-rater reliability 67, 269
Interval scale 267
Interview 69
  advantages of 237
  benefits of 230
  characteristics of 230
  disadvantages of 237
  guide 260
  limitations of 231
  schedule 69
  types of 231, 231f, 233
Interviewer's bias 232
Intramuscular injection 33
Intuition 5, 84, 190
Investigator's own biases 232

J

Journal 225
  articles
    content of 412
    qualitative 412
    quantitative 412
  impact factor 412
  publication of article in 411
Judgment 136
Judgmental sampling 65, 214
Justice, principles of 151

K

Keywords 414
King's theory 135
Knowledge
  focused triggers 31
  score 286, 287f, 288f, 296f
Kruskal-Wallis tests 332
Kurtosis 363
  types of 364f

L

Laboratory research, minimal possibility of 156
Leptokurtic distributions 363
Likert question 242, 242t
Likert scale 69, 262
Line graph 295, 295f
Linear regression 329
  calculation of 330t
Literature
  critical appraisal of 83
  review 52, 112, 113, 120, 381, 382, 388, 404, 436
    importance of 114
    purposes of 114
    sources of 115
  source of 382
  type of 382
Logical construct, development of 141
Longitudinal research design 182
Longitudinal study 65
Lottery method 209
Low cost 217
Lung cancer 339

M

Magazines 225
Major potential benefits 150

Major potential cost 150
Malaria 431
Malnutrition 290t
　with economic status, association of 339t, 341t
　with socioeconomic status, association of 340t
Manipulation 12, 61, 170
　checking on 227
Mann-Whitney U-tests 332
Manuscript
　preparing 412
　review 416
　submission of 416
Map diagrams 291, 297
Mathematical theory 201
Matrix question 242, 242t
Maturation 61
Mean 72
　deviation 314, 315t, 316t
　standard error of 77
　sum squares 351
Measles 431
Measurement
　and scaling technique, levels of 266
　instrument, consistency of 268
　interval level of 67
Mechanical devices 252
Median in
　continuous series, computation of 303
　discrete series, calculation of 302, 302t
　individual series, calculation of 302
Medline plus 117
Membership, nature of 158
Mental activity 246
Mesokurtic distributions 363
Metaphor
　concept-constructive 139
　conceptual 138
　uses of 138
Methodological studies 61
Methodology 190, 404, 428
　materials 404
Microsoft excel 333
Mid-day meal programme 204
Middle-range theory 57, 129
　characteristics of 129
Mortality 61
Motivation 270
Multigravida mothers 351
Multi-item scales 262
Multiphase sampling 208, 213, 214
Multiple bar diagram 292
　age and sex in 292f
Multiple choice questions 240
Multiple methods 185
Multiple response table 290

Multiple time series design 177
Multistage sampling technique 208, 213, 213f
Multivariate study 56, 99

N

Narrations, data in 369
Narrative analysis 365, 370
National Institutes of Health 435
National Rural Health Mission 431
Natural language description 222
Neonatal deaths 431
Newspapers 225
Nominal scale 266
Noncomparative rating scale 262
Nondirectional research hypothesis 58
Nonequivalent control group design 61
Nonequivalent pretest-post-test control group design 177
Nonexperimental research
　design 178
　classification of 178, 178f
Non-numeric information 364
Nonparametric test 76, 332
Nonparticipant observation 247
　advantages 248
　disadvantages 248
Nonprobability sampling 65, 217, 219
　classification of 214
　use of 214
Nonsymmetrical distribution 73
Normal distribution 73, 356
Normal probability curve 359, 362
　characteristics of 359
　computation of 357
　importance of 361
　uses of 361
Null hypothesis 58, 102
Nurse
　administrators 421
　advances in preparation of 16
　clinicians 422
　educators 420
　factors related to 419
　improve knowledge of 15
　researcher 421
　　ethical responsibilities of 154
Nursing
　administration 395
　　research in 19
　care, rating scale on 261t
　education, research in 18
　practice 376
　　evidence for 395

reinforce identity of 15
research 1, 14, 27, 54, 147, 188
    areas of 16, 16f
    codes of ethics in 147
    computer in 435
    conceptualization of 26
    dilemma in 155
    ethical principles in 148, 148f
    factors 419
    history of 20
    importance of 15
    major milestones of 20, 21
    model for conceptualization of 26
    registry of 117
    scope of 16, 16f
    uses of 23
    utilization of 418
science, conceptualization of 26
theory 126
    concepts of 125
    evolution of 127
    history of 127
Nutrition rehabilitation center 427

O

Observation 245, 246
    guides 252
    method
        advantages of 251
        uses of 249
    planning for 250
    research 70
    schedule 260
    tools 251
Observational method
    characteristics of 246
    classifications of 246
Offline publications 417
Ogive curve 286, 287, 287f, 288f, 296, 296f
One's first punishment memory 256
One's happiest memory 256
One-group pretest-post-test design 61, 175
One-shot case study 61, 174
One-way
    analysis 353
    classification 347
Online publications 417
Open-format questions 239
    advantages 239
    characteristics 239
    disadvantages 240
Oral communication 395
Ordinal scale 267

Organizational factors 419
Organizing data 280, 367
Organizing numeric data, methods of 284
Outcomes research 54
Overdone subject 85
Overt observation 246

P

Pain measurement 257f
Panchayat Raj System 213, 213f
Panel studies 183
Parameter 74
Parametric tests 76, 332
Participant
    observation 247
    selection of 51
Participatory action research 193
Percentage bar diagram 292
Personal bias 215
Personal interview 233
Personally sensitive information 244
Persuasion stage 32
Phenomenological research 189
Phenomenology 51, 189
    assumptions of 190
    importance of 189
    types 190
Phenomenon 125
    nature of 163
Philosophy 125
Pictograms 291, 297, 297f
Picture diagrams 297
Pie diagram 293, 293f
Pilot study 55
    conduction of 47
Pneumonia 431
Popular report 398
Population 55, 197, 198, 200, 206, 209, 218, 434
    concepts of 197
    describing accessible 204
    during selection, eligibility criteria of 198, 198f
    entire 206
    members of 206
    portion of 199
    setting of 433
    standard deviation 319
    value 206
Poster presentation 395
Post-test only control group design 61, 171
Potential bias, analyzing 227
Power analysis 65
Practical tests 271

Practice
    research 27
    science of 27
Practicing nurses, values and qualification of 24
Prediction design 181
Pre-existing data 70
Pre-experimental design 62, 174
Preliminary pages 401
Preproposals 425
Prescriptive theories 130
Pretesting data collection package 228
Pretest-post-test control group design 62, 170
Prevalence studies 179
Probability 355
    curve 360f
    sampling 65, 205, 219
        features of 208
        method 208
        technique 207
        types of 208
Problem
    analysis 8
    solving
        method 6, 7
        process, steps of 8f
Projective techniques 70, 254
    disadvantages of 256
    interviews 236
Proportion bar diagram 292, 293f
Proportional stratified sampling 65, 211
Proposal
    purposes of 424
    type of 424
    writing, golden rules for 425
Prospective research design 180
Public enterprise 395
Pure research 10
Purposive sampling 65, 214
P-value 332
    approach 332

Qualitative method 235
Qualitative research 11, 54, 380
    critique process 387, 387f
    design 167t, 184
        characteristics of 185f
        classification of 187f
    expertise, lack of 156
    methodology 51
    process steps 49
    report 414t
Quality assurance, statistics for 197
Quantitative data 222, 279, 284, 339, 370
    analysis 280, 280f
    steps of 280
Quantitative information, sense of 283
Quantitative research 12, 54, 380
    design 167t
    process
        major phases in 39
        steps of 50f
    report 414, 414t
    studies 101, 385
        critique process for 380, 380f
        types of 383
Quartile
    calculation of 313
    deviation 313
        coefficient of 313
Quasi experimental design 62, 175
Quasi-statistical tables 369, 370
Query letter 78
Question
    construction 243
    types of 238, 239f
Questionnaire 70, 245
    administration, methods of 243
    advantages of 244
    design 235
    disadvantages of 244
Quota sampling 65, 215, 216

Q

Q methodology 70
Q-sort 70, 258
Qualitative data 222, 232, 274, 366, 369
    analysis 364, 366
        problem in 366
        steps of 367
        types of 365
    computer analysis of 372
    display of 370
    establishing validity of 371
    integrating 370

R

Random
    assignment 62
    numbers, table of 66
    sampling technique 201
    table, use of 209
Range, coefficient of 311
Rank order
    questions 241
    scales 261
Rapport building 236
Rating scale, construction of 264

Ratio scale 267
Reading comprehension 270
Recording 251
    devices 251
    sheets 252
References 386, 405, 415, 438
    general rules for 408, 410
    writing 405
Regression 329
    analysis 328
    equation 329
    example 330
    formula 329
    line 329f
Relative cumulative frequency 286, 287
    distribution 287
Reliability, types of 268
Replication study 56
Report
    preparing outline of 397
    title 381
    types of 398
Representative 202
Research 1, 2
    abstracts 56
    articles 395
    based protocol 33
    characteristics of 2
    communication and utilization of 395
    critique 376
        concept of 376
        importance of 377
        principles of 377, 377f
        purposes of 377
    data, types of 222, 222f
    design 55, 162, 221, 376, 383, 437
        and approach 429, 433
        classification of 164
        concepts of 161
        consists of 428
        construction of 44
        elements of 376
        factors affecting selection of 162, 162f
        selection of 45
    dissemination of 397
    ethics committees
        composition of 158
        role of 157
    findings, utilization of 417
    framework 132
    friendly culture 421
    general aims of 3, 3f
    hypothesis 58, 382
    instruments 68, 437
    journal articles, style of 415

    lack of 381
    methodology of 24, 379
    objectives 91, 92, 94
        characteristics of 92, 92f
        importance of 93
        types of 93
    participants 274
        protection of 157
    problem 81, 82, 85, 89, 90f, 381, 436
        formulation of 41
        sources of 82, 82f
    process 39, 279
        step of 380
    project program 422
    proposal 423
        development and presenting 422
        format of 426
        real content of 427
        sample of 430
    purpose of 218, 400
    questions 382, 385
    report 78
        part of 397
        type of 401
        writing 397
    study 101
        type of 229
    title, consists of 426
    tool 68
        principles of construction of 259
        types of 10
    variables 99
Researchers 157
    communicate 398
    competence 89
    convenience 204
    knowledge and experience 164
    obstructiveness 224
    skills of 153
    technical expertise of 89
    thinking 390
Respondents level, determination of 266
Retrospective research design 181
Rogers' theory 32
Rosenthal effect 62
Rotters incomplete sentence blank 255
Rough draft 192
    preparation of 400

S

Sample 384, 429
    allocation techniques, different 211
    characteristics, congruity with 226
    concept of 200

describing main characteristics of 227
error, no possibility of 215
process, selection of 198, 199, 199f
selection of 46
size 286, 384, 418, 439
    appropriate 202
    determine 205
standard deviation 320
T-test 342
Sampling 197, 200, 437
    based on objectives 200
    bias 65, 207, 208
    consecutive 217
    convenient to 203, 216
    distribution 77
    error 65, 206
        reasons of 206
    fractions 211
    frame 66, 204
    importance of 202, 202f
    judgmental 214
    limitations of 203
    principles of 200, 201f
    process 204, 204f
    purposive 214
    technique 201-203, 207, 216, 219, 434
        classification of 207f
    type of 216
    units 199
Scale homogeneity 67
Scaling technique 268
Scatter diagram 74, 291, 297, 297f, 324, 325f
Scientific
    method 6, 9
        characteristics of 10
    papers 395
    research 6, 9, 39
    training, lack of 24
Search relevant literature review 31
Sector diagram 293
Select clinical research problem 31
Semantic scales 263, 264f
Semiquartile range 74
Semistructured format 235
Sentence completion test 254
Sequential sampling 208, 217
Set up hypothesis 344
Sexual attitude 255
Sexual orientation 244
Significance
    level of 76
    one-tailed test of 76
    two-tailed test of 77
Simple bar diagram 291, 292f
Simple hypothesis 58, 103

Simple random sampling 66, 208
    method in 209
    technique 208
Simulation studies 63
Single case study 174
Situation specific theories 129
    characteristics of 130
Skeletal fixation, external 403
Skewed distribution 73
    curve 363f
Skewness 362
Snowball sampling 66, 217
Social attitude 255
Social issues 84
Society 157
Solomon four-group design 63, 172
    numerical presentation of 172t
Spearman rank correlation 332
    coefficient 327
Specific population, locating people of 217
Specify sampling method 204
Split-half reliability 270
Spot map 297
Squares, total sum of 351
Stability reliability 68, 268
Standard deviation 74, 318, 321t, 322t
    distribution of 360f
    solution, calculation of 321t
Standardized tools, lack of 25, 156
Staple scales 263
Static-group comparison design 175
Statistic 74
    application of 283
Statistical hypothesis testing 205
Statistical regularity, law of 201
Statistical software, modified 334
Statistical test
    power of 77, 205
    tabled value for 333
Stratified random sampling 66, 208, 210
    types of 211
Structured interview 231, 234
Structured observation 71, 248
    strengths of 248
Structured Teaching Program 433
Study
    acknowledge limitation of 43
    determine objectives of 41
    location of 429
    need for 428, 431
    objectives of 428
    period 429
    population 429
        selection of 46
    purpose of 163

setting 429
subjects, lack of 25
types of 94
Subject matter, logical analysis of 400
Subsequent class intervals 286
Supplementary information 230
   draft of 400
Survey
   design 183
   studies 63
Symmetrical distributions 74
Synopsis 423
Syntax window 335
Syphilis 240
System reviews, cochrane database of 117
Systematic random sampling 66, 208, 210

T

Table
   analysis 305, 306t
   construction of 287
   list of 402
   of contents 402
   parts of 288
   random
      method, table for 209t
      numbers, use of 209
   types of 289
Tabulation, general principles of 287
Target population 55, 199, 204
Technical language 399
Telephone interview 71, 233
Test
   consistency 268
   hypothesis 227
   retest method 268
Thematic apperception test 256
Theoretical connectedness 391
Theoretical distribution 356
   types of 356
Theoretical framework 58, 124, 132, 133, 137f, 380, 382
   constructing of 133f
Theoretical research 14
Theory 58, 124, 139
   characteristics of 126, 131
   classification of 128f, 130t
   concepts of 125
   purpose of 126
   types of 127, 130
   uses of 131

Thesis 402
   format of 401
   parts of 402
Time 88, 164
   lack of 25
   sampling 71
   series design 63, 177
Title 413, 427
   declarative 413
   interrogative 413
   page 426
   types of 413
Tools 434
   development of 259
   types of 221, 259, 260f
Training data collectors 226
Transcendental phenomenology 190
Traumatic memory 256
Triangulation 64
True experimental design 63, 170
T-test 77, 342
   unpaired 345
Tuberculosis, prevention of 399
Two-way classification 351, 351t

U

Univariate study 56, 99, 179
Universal assumptions 107

V

Vague overall sampling size 218
Validity 60, 68, 270, 385
   concurrent 273
   construct 271
   content 271, 272
   convergent 271
   criterion 271, 272
   diagnostic 271, 275
   divergent 272
   experimental 271, 273
   external 274
   face 271, 272
   internal 273, 274
   predictive 273
   relationship to internal 271, 274
   statistical conclusion 271, 274
   types of 271
Vancouver referencing style 409
Variability, measures of 73

Variables 56
　concept 96
　types of 97, 338
Variance 74, 317
　analysis of 75, 76, 346, 347, 354, 373
　coefficient of 321
Video-assisted teaching module 45
Vignette method 256, 257
Visual aids 399
Visual analogue scale 71, 257, 257f
　advantages of 258
　functions 260
　limitations 258
　rating scale 261
Vulnerable participants 152

W

Warranted assumptions 108
Weaknesses 249
Wilcoxon's matched pairs 332
Word association test 12, 254
Writing reference, style of 406
Writing research report 396
　guidelines for 399
　steps in 400
Writing style 381, 410

Z

Z-score 75